D0593203

BIPOLAR MEDICATIONS
Mechanisms of Action

BIPOLAR MEDICATIONS

Mechanisms of Action

Edited by

Husseini K. Manji, M.D., F.R.C.P.C.
Charles L. Bowden, M.D.
Robert H. Belmaker, M.D.

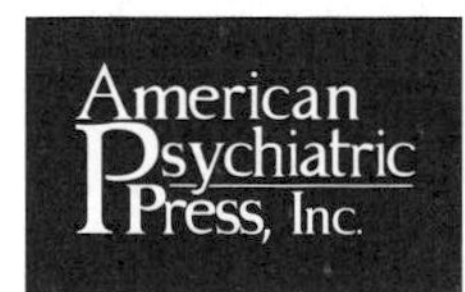

Washington, DC
London, England

Note: The authors have worked to ensure that all information in this book concerning drug dosages, schedules, and routes of administration is accurate as of the time of publication and consistent with standards set by the U.S. Food and Drug Administration and the general medical community. As medical research and practice advance, however, therapeutic standards may change. For this reason and because human and mechanical errors sometimes occur, we recommend that readers follow the advice of a physician who is directly involved in their care or the care of a member of their family.

Manufactured in the United States of America on acid-free paper

03 02 01 4 3 2

First Edition

American Psychiatric Press, Inc.

1400 K Street, N.W., Washington, DC 20005

www.appi.org

Library of Congress Cataloging-in-Publication Data

Bipolar medications: mechanisms of action / edited by Husseini K. Manji, Charles L. Bowden, Robert H. Belmaker. — 1st ed.
p. cm.
Includes bibliographical references and index.
ISBN 0-88048-927-8 (alk. paper)
1. Manic-depressive illness—Chemotherapy. 2. Lithium—Therapeutic use. 3. Depression, Mental—Chemotherapy. 4. Antidepressants. I. Manji, Husseini K., 1959- . II. Bowden, Charles L. III. Belmaker, Robert H.
[DNLM: 1. Bipolar disorder—drug therapy. 2. Antimanic Agents—pharmacology. WM 207 M486 1999]
RC483.5.L5M43 1999
616.89′5061—dc21
DNLM/DLC
for Library of Congress 99-26052
CIP

British Library Cataloguing in Publication Data

A CIP record is available from the British Library.

This book is dedicated to
our families and our patients.

CONTENTS

CONTRIBUTORS

GALILA AGAM, PH.D.
Professor, Stanley Center for Bipolar Research, Psychiatry Research Unit, and Department of Clinical Biochemistry, Faculty of Health Sciences, Ben Gurion University of the Negev, Beersheba, Israel

JOHN R. ATACK, PH.D.
Senior Research Fellow, Merck Sharp and Dohme Research Laboratories, Neuroscience Research Centre, Terlings Park, Harlow, Essex, England

ROBERT H. BELMAKER, M.D.
Hoffer-Vickar Professor of Psychiatry, Beersheba Mental Health Center; Faculty of Health Sciences, Ben Gurion University of the Negev, Beersheba, Israel

AMPARO BENITEZ, D.O.
Child and Adolescent Psychiatrist, Miami, Florida

MATHIAS BERGER, M.D.
Professor and Director, Department of Psychiatry, University of Freiburg, Freiburg, Germany

YULI BERSUDSKY, M.D., PH.D.
Senior Psychiatrist, Beersheba Mental Health Center, Beersheba, Israel

KNUT BIBER, PH.D.
Research Assistant, Department of Medical Physiology, University of Groningen, Groningen, The Netherlands

CHARLES L. BOWDEN, M.D.
Nancy U. Karren Professor and Chairman, Department of Psychiatry, The University of Texas Health Science Center at San Antonio, San Antonio, Texas

JOSEPH R. CALABRESE, M.D.
Professor of Psychiatry, Department of Psychiatry, Case Western Reserve University, Cleveland, Ohio

GUANG CHEN, M.D.
Assistant Professor, Laboratory of Molecular Pathophysiology, Department of Psychiatry and Behavioral Neurosciences, Wayne State University School of Medicine, Detroit, Michigan

JIANG CHEN, M.D., PH.D.
Staff Scientist, Lucent Technologies, Naperville, Illinois

DE-MAW CHUANG, PH.D.
Chief, Section on Molecular Neurobiology, Biological Psychiatry Branch, National Institute of Mental Health, Bethesda, Maryland

MIKE CLARK, PH.D.
Staff Fellow, Biological Psychiatry Branch, National Institute of Mental Health, Bethesda, Maryland

JOHN F. DIXON, B.S.
Assistant Researcher, Department of Pharmacology, University of Wisconsin Medical School, Madison, Wisconsin

PETER GEBICKE, PH.D.
Professor, Department of Psychiatry, University of Freiburg, Freiburg, Germany

GAD M. GILAD, PH.D.
Director, Research and Development, Laboratory of Neuroscience, Research and Development, Assaf Harofeh Medical Center, Zrifin, Israel

VARDA H. GILAD, PH.D.
Research Associate, Laboratory of Neuroscience, Research and Development, Assaf Harofeh Medical Center, Zrifin, Israel

PAUL J. GOODNICK, M.D.
Director, Mood Disorders Program; and Professor of Psychiatry and Behavioral Sciences, University of Miami School of Medicine, Miami, Florida

FREDERICK K. GOODWIN, M.D.
Director, Center on Neurosciences, Medical Progress and Society, Department of Psychiatry, George Washington University, Washington, DC

G. M. GOODWIN, D.PHIL., F.R.C.P.EDIN., F.R.C.PSYCH.
Professor and Honorary Consultant Psychiatrist, Oxford University, Department of Psychiatry, Oxford, England

CAROL A. GRIMES, B.S.
Graduate Student, Department of Psychiatry and Behavioral Neurobiology, University of Alabama at Birmingham, Birmingham, Alabama

LOWELL E. HOKIN, M.D., PH.D.
Professor, Department of Pharmacology, University of Wisconsin Medical School, Madison, Wisconsin

CHRISTOPHER HOUGH, PH.D.
Research Assistant Professor, Uniformed Services University of the Health Sciences, Bethesda, Maryland

JOHN K. HSIAO, M.D.
Chief, Special Projects Program, Schizophrenia Branch, National Institute of Mental Health, Bethesda, Maryland

JENS BITSCH JENSEN, PH.D.
Research Fellow, Department of Pharmacology, The Panum Institute, University of Copenhagen, Copenhagen, Denmark

RICHARD S. JOPE, PH.D.
Professor, Department of Psychiatry and Behavioral Neurobiology, University of Alabama at Birmingham, Birmingham, Alabama

ORA KOFMAN, PH.D.
Senior Lecturer, Department of Behavioral Sciences, Ben Gurion University of the Negev, Beersheba, Israel

ROBERT H. LENOX, M.D.
Karl and Linda Rickels Professor of Psychiatry, Pharmacology and Neuroscience, Department of Psychiatry, University of Pennsylvania, Philadelphia, Pennsylvania

R. A. LESLIE, PH.D.
Director, Neuroscience Research Department, SmithKline Beecham Pharmaceuticals, Neuroscience Research, Harlow, Essex, England

HE LI, PH.D.
Assistant Professor, Uniformed Services University of the Health Sciences, Bethesda, Maryland

PETER P. LI, PH.D.
Associate Professor, Departments of Psychiatry and Pharmacology, Section of Biochemical Psychiatry, Center for Addiction and Mental Health; and University of Toronto, Toronto, Ontario, Canada

XIAOHUA LI, M.D., PH.D.
Chief Resident, Department of Psychiatry and Behavioral Neurobiology, University of Alabama at Birmingham, Birmingham, Alabama

GEORGYI V. LOS, M.D., PH.D.
Associate Scientist, Department of Pharmacology, University of Wisconsin Medical School, Madison, Wisconsin

HUSSEINI K. MANJI, M.D., F.R.C.P.C.
Director, Laboratory of Molecular Pathophysiology, Department of Psychiatry and Behavioral Neurosciences, Wayne State University School of Medicine, Detroit, Michigan

MONICA I. MASANA, PH.D.
Research Assistant Professor, Department of Molecular Pharmacology and Biological Chemistry, Northwestern University, Chicago, Illinois

ROBERT K. MCNAMARA, PH.D.
Assistant Professor of Psychiatry, Department of Psychiatry, University of Pennsylvania, Philadelphia, Pennsylvania

GREGORY J. MOORE, PH.D.
Director, Brain Imaging Program, Department of Psychiatry and Behavioral Neurosciences and Radiology, Wayne State University School of Medicine, Detroit, Michigan

J. M. MOORMAN, PH.D.
Medical Writer, TMG Healthcare Communications Ltd., Abingdon, Oxon, England

ARNE MØRK, PH.D.
Acting Head of Neurobiology Department, The Panum Institute, University of Copenhagen, Copenhagen, Denmark

HIKROKI OZAWA, M.D., PH.D.
Assistant Professor, Department of Neuropsychiatry, Sapporo Medical College, Sapporo, Japan

MARY A. PACHECO, PH.D.
Research Associate, Department of Psychiatry and Behavioral Neurobiology, University of Alabama at Birmingham, Birmingham, Alabama

YARDENA PATISHI, PH.D.
Research Scientist, Beersheba Mental Health Center, Beersheba, Israel

ROBERT M. POST, M.D.
Chief, Biological Psychiatry Branch, National Institute of Mental Health, Bethesda, Maryland

WILLIAM Z. POTTER, M.D., PH.D.
Clinical Research Fellow, Lilly Research Laboratories, Neuroscience Therapeutic Area, Indianapolis, Indiana

MARK M. RASENICK, PH.D.
Professor, Department of Physiology and Biophysics and Department of Psychiatry; Director, Biomedical Neuroscience Training Program; and Member, Committee on Neuroscience, University of Illinois College of Medicine, Chicago, Illinois

HADY SHIMON, M.SC.
Professor, Psychiatry Research Unit, Faculty of Health Sciences, Ben Gurion University of the Negev, Beersheba, Israel

LING SONG, M.D.
Research Associate, Department of Psychiatry and Behavioral Neurobiology, University of Alabama at Birmingham, Birmingham, Alabama

MAURICIO TOHEN, M.D., DR.P.H.
Medical Advisor, Lilly Research Laboratories, Indianapolis, Indiana; and Associate Clinical Professor of Psychiatry, Harvard Medical School, Boston, Massachusetts

GARY D. TOLLEFSON, M.D., PH.D.
President of Neuroscience, Lilly Research Laboratories, Indianapolis, Indiana

M. TINO UNLAP, PH.D.
Research Associate, Department of Psychiatry and Behavioral Neurobiology, University of Alabama at Birmingham, Birmingham, Alabama

DIETRICH VAN CALKER, M.D., PH.D.
Professor, Department of Psychiatry, University of Freiburg, Freiburg, Germany

JÖRG WALDEN, M.D.
Professor, Department of Psychiatry, University of Freiburg, Freiburg, Germany

JERRY J. WARSH, M.D., PH.D.
Professor, Departments of Psychiatry and Pharmacology, Section of Biochemical Psychiatry, Center for Addiction and Mental Health; and Institute of Medical Sciences, University of Toronto, Toronto, Ontario, Canada

DAVID G. WATSON, PH.D.
Associate Scientist, Department of Pharmacodynamics, University of Florida College of Pharmacy, Gainesville, Florida

SUSAN R. B. WEISS, PH.D.
Unit Chief, Unit on Behavioral Biology, Biological Psychiatry Branch, National Institute of Mental Health, Bethesda, Maryland

MARY B. WILLIAMS, PH.D.
Postdoctoral Fellow, Department of Psychiatry and Behavioral Neurobiology, University of Alabama at Birmingham, Birmingham, Alabama

L. TREVOR YOUNG, M.D., PH.D.
Associate Professor, Department of Psychiatry, McMaster University, Hamilton, Ontario, Canada

FOREWORD

Frederick K. Goodwin, M.D.

The introduction of effective psychopharmacological drugs more than four decades ago sparked a revolution that has, over time, reshaped scientific and popular concepts of mental illness. Like all revolutionary periods, the era blazed with activity. Investigators conducted studies of the neurobiological mechanisms that might explain the powerful, specific effects of the new drugs. Manic-depressive illness, now referred to as bipolar disorder, quickly became the clinical mainstay for such research and a model for biological studies on other major mental illness. More homogeneous than nonrecurrent unipolar depression or schizophrenia, bipolar disorder attracted scientific attention for other reasons as well: its genetic diathesis was clear to many clinicians treating the illness, and its cyclic nature gave investigators the opportunity to study the transition phases and to separate the traits intrinsic to the illness from the state changes that accompany being ill.

Not only did lithium launch the psychopharmacology revolution; its effects on both poles of the bipolar subtype also presented an irresistible scientific challenge. However, the nonpatentable lithium ion did not attract pharmaceutical company interest. In addition, the huge second revolution in psychopharmacology of the 1980s and 1990s, with selective serotonin reuptake inhibitors and atypical antipsychotics, seemed to leave bipolar disorder on the sidelines.

That period is now clearly over. Valproic acid, lamotrigine, other new anticonvulsants (and potential antibipolar drugs) still in the pipeline, and possible new inositol monophosphatase inhibitors, glycogen synthase kinase inhibitors, and protein kinase C inhibitors—all these have the potential to revolutionize clinical practice while providing exciting new hypotheses relating to the etiology of bipolar disorder. The present volume reflects the first results of this new wave.

The clinical chapters are state-of-the-art discussions of key issues in the field. Bowden reviews the emergence of valproate as a powerful lithium alternative and/or adjunct, and Calabrese reviews the preliminary but dramatic indications that lamotrigine may offer promise as an even more effective treatment and prophylaxis of the depressive phases of bipolar disorder. Tohen and Tollefson review the growing body of data suggesting that atypical antipsychotics may become important adjunctive agents in the treatment of bipolar disorder. G. M. Goodwin (no relation) presents the single most troubling clinical question about lithium use today: the possibility of withdrawal rebound that could make lithium ineffective or even counterproductive for some patients.

The unique aspect of the volume is its clear future orientation. Atack reviews his work on inositol monophosphatase inhibitors that could mimic lithium action in patients, if the inositol depletion hypothesis is true. The effect of lithium on guanine nucleotide binding proteins (G proteins) is well reviewed by Rasenick and colleagues and Warsh and colleagues, although a G-protein–based therapeutic strategy is not yet in the offing. Manji and colleagues, Jope and colleagues, and Lenox and colleagues review effects of both lithium and valproate on protein kinase C, a research field in which several new inhibitors may soon be in clinical testing as antimanic agents. Agam and Shimon review the antidepressant effects of inositol and how they could relate to lithium's effects as an inositol monophosphatase inhibitor. Gilad and Gilad introduce a relatively new concept of regulation of the polyamine stress response, whereas Hokin and colleagues propose a glutamatergic site of action for both lithium and valproate. Post and colleagues compare lithium, carbamazepine, and valproate and their differential mechanisms, which could form the basis of a rational polypharmacy of bipolar disorder. Kofman and colleagues examine behavioral models in rats, which could be highly important in the screening of new antibipolar compounds; and Leslie and Moorman connect this volume with the molecular biology revolution by reviewing effects of antibipolar compounds on immediate-early genes. Van Calker and colleagues, Mørk and Jensen, and Goodnick and Benitez suggest new directions via adenosine cyclic adenosine monophosphate and calcium channels that make the volume extremely comprehensive.

As coauthor of what has become the standard textbook on bipolar disorder, I especially appreciate this volume because it speaks eloquently to clinicians whose interests and curiosity are beyond the textbook level. Although many of the chapters are patient oriented, they clearly give the reader a real feel for the future and provide solid support for therapeutic optimism.

ACKNOWLEDGMENTS

The editors would like to acknowledge the invaluable contributions of Ms. Donna R. Dolan and Ms. Celia Knobelsdorf, without whom this book would not have been possible. The editors would also like to acknowledge the outstanding editorial assistance of Ms. Elizabeth Gould-Leger and Ms. Alisa Guerzon (American Psychiatric Press, Inc.).

CHAPTER 1

LITHIUM, PHOSPHATIDYLINOSITOL SIGNALING, AND BIPOLAR DISORDER

The Role of Inositol Monophosphatase

John R. Atack, Ph.D.

Despite 50 years having elapsed since the initial report of its efficacy (Cade 1949), lithium remains a mainstay for the treatment of bipolar disorder (Post et al. 1998). However, because of lithium's side-effect profile and narrow therapeutic window, there has been considerable interest in finding a drug that can mimic the therapeutic effects yet is without these liabilities (Atack et al. 1995a; Kofman and Belmaker 1993). The search for such a compound is hampered by the fact that the mechanism of action of lithium remains unknown. Nevertheless, in recent years, attention has focused on the phosphatidylinositol (PI) signal transduction pathway, and more specifically inositol monophosphatase (IMPase), as the therapeutic target for lithium.

In this chapter, the relationship between lithium, bipolar disorder, and PI signaling (Figure 1–1) and the assumptions involved in attributing lithium's therapeutic mechanism of action to modulation of PI signaling (e.g., lack of evidence for either dysfunctional PI signaling in bipolar disorder or the ability of lithium to modulate PI signaling in vivo) are reviewed.

According to this hypothesis, modulation of PI signaling is attributed to the inhibition of IMPase by therapeutically relevant concentrations of lith-

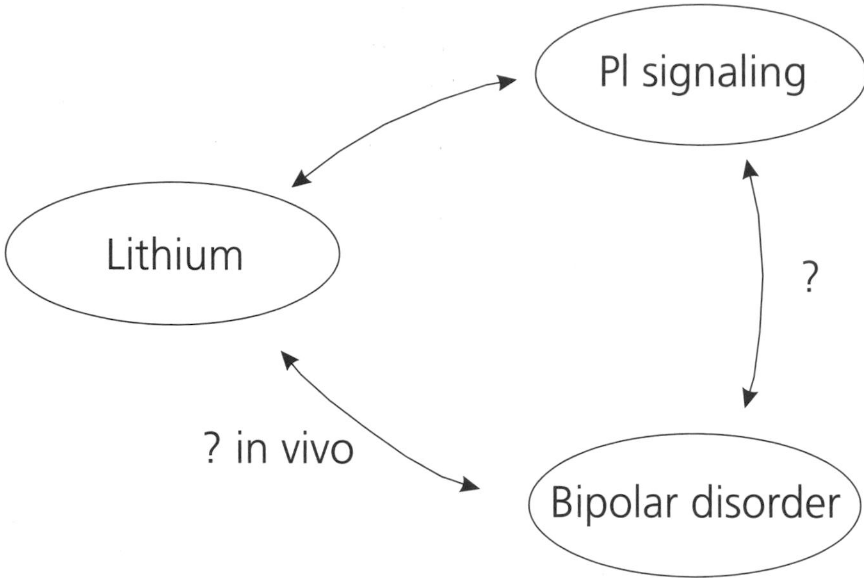

Figure 1–1. The relationship between lithium, phosphatidylinositol (PI) signaling, and bipolar disorder. Although the therapeutic efficacy of lithium in the treatment of bipolar disorder is well established, the evidence that lithium affects PI signaling is restricted to in vitro experiments; it is not known whether therapeutic doses of lithium can attenuate PI signaling in vivo. Furthermore, there is no direct evidence to implicate PI-linked neurotransmitter systems in the pathogenesis of bipolar disorder.

ium. However, lithium possesses a wide range of biochemical and neurochemical effects (Bunney and Garland-Bunney 1987; Wood and Goodwin 1987); therefore, it is difficult to ascribe its effects on PI signaling solely to inhibition of IMPase. In this chapter, the use of substrate-based inhibitors of this enzyme to verify the crucial role of IMPase in PI signaling and the limitations of these compounds (i.e., lack of suitability for in vivo experiments) is described. In addition, the development of novel, non–substrate-based inhibitors is discussed in relation to the structure and mechanism of IMPase.

LITHIUM AND BIPOLAR DISORDER

Lithium was discovered in 1817 by Johann August Arfvedson and accounts for about 0.006% of the earth's crust. It has been used in medicine since the mid-19th century for the treatment of a number of disorders such as gout, bladder stones, and rheumatism. In the late 1940s, lithium was used as a salt substitute in patients with cardiac failure and hypertension, only to be banned by the U.S. Food and Drug Administration (FDA) as a result of reports of lithium-induced fatalities (Johnson 1984). Concurrent with the fall from grace of lithium in the United States, the dramatic effects of lithium in the treatment of mania were described by the Australian physician John Cade, following a remarkable extrapolation from experimental observation to clinical application (Cade 1949).

In the process of investigating the toxicity of urine from patients with mania, depression, and schizophrenia (stored on the top shelf of his kitchen refrigerator; Johnson 1984) in guinea pigs (housed in his back garden; Johnson 1984), Cade observed that urine from subjects with mania was more toxic than that of the other groups. The toxicity turned out to be due to urea, and Cade wondered whether uric acid might be modifying the toxicity of urine in manic patients. In the course of studying the toxicity of uric acid, lithium urate was chosen for injection into guinea pigs, because it was the most soluble of the urates. In controlled experiments, lithium carbonate was injected, and it was noted that "after a latent period of about 2 hours the animals, although fully conscious, became extremely lethargic and unresponsive" (Cade 1978, p. 12) and that "they could be turned on their backs and that, instead of their usual frantic righting reflex behaviour, they merely lay there and gazed placidly back" (Cade 1978, p. 12). These observations in guinea pigs, along with his underlying interest in mania, led Cade to administer lithium citrate to a manic 51-year-old man "who had been in a state of chronic manic excitement for 5 years" (Cade 1949, p. 350). A marked improvement was seen within 5 days, and after 3 months of treatment and observation, the patient was discharged (Cade 1949). The efficacy of lithium in controlling mania was confirmed by others, most notably the controlled, double-blind study of the Danish psychiatrist Mogens Schou (1954), who was to become the major exponent of lithium therapy in Europe.

Concerns about toxicity plagued the use of lithium in the treatment of mania, and for 20 years lithium remained the "Cinderella of psychopharmacology" (Kline 1968, p. 558). However, in 1970 lithium was again approved by the FDA, this time for the treatment of mania. Subsequently, in light of evidence that lithium prevented the recurrence of mania and depressive episodes (Baastrup et al. 1970), in 1974 approval was extended to cover use in the prophylactic treatment of bipolar disorder (Johnson 1984).

Although lithium is remarkably efficacious in the treatment of bipolar disorder, it has, nevertheless, a number of significant limitations. Most notable are the side-effect profile, which can result in an appreciable number of bipolar disorder patients not being able to tolerate lithium therapy, and the relatively narrow range between therapeutic (plasma levels of 0.5–1.0 mEq/L) and toxic (>2 mEq/L) doses of lithium, which necessitates the close monitoring of plasma lithium concentrations. At therapeutic doses of lithium, the side effects often encountered include problems in neurological (hand tremor), gastrointestinal (diarrhea and nausea), endocrine (thyroid function, weight gain), and renal (increased thirst and urine production) function (Janicak and Davis 1987; Weiner 1991). Mild lithium toxicity is characterized by poor concentration and memory, diarrhea, nausea, and tremors, whereas moderate toxicity produces vomiting, sedation, ataxia, excessive thirst, and greatly increased urine production. Severe toxicity results in coma or death at plasma levels >4 mEq/l (Janicak and Davis 1987; Weiner 1991). Furthermore, because the clearance of lithium is associated with the excretion of sodium and water, disruptions in electrolyte homeostasis, such as those produced by a hot day at the beach or gastrointestinal problems, can produce toxic increases in plasma lithium levels (Baraban 1994).

This side-effect profile and toxicity may well be unrelated to the therapeutic mechanism of action of lithium. Consequently, there is the potential to develop compounds that mimic the therapeutic effects of lithium but that are devoid of these undesirable properties (Atack 1995; Kofman and Belmaker 1993). Crucial to the identification of such compounds is an understanding of how lithium exerts its therapeutic effects. However, although lithium is one of the most effective therapies for the treatment of psychiatric disorders (Soares and Gershon 1998), and although 50 years have elapsed since Cade's original description of its therapeutic efficacy (Cade 1949), the mechanism of action of lithium remains unknown—an issue complicated by the diverse range of biochemical and neurochemical effects attributed to lithium (Bunney and Garland-Bunney 1987; Wood and Goodwin 1987).

Any hypothesis of how lithium works should be able to explain the effects of lithium on the presumably distinct neurochemical processes underlying the mania and depression that represent opposite ends of the spectrum of mood (Jope 1999a). Modulation of neurotransmission at the level of the synapse, whether pre- or postsynaptic (e.g., neurotransmitter synthesis release or metabolism, or modulation of the neurotransmitter-receptor interaction) seems unlikely, because it would require that lithium exert distinct actions on the various neurotransmitter systems that mediate mania or depression. Accordingly, attention has focused on the possibility that lithium exerts its therapeutic actions via modulation of postreceptor (i.e., signal transduction) mechanisms that are associated with the neurotransmitter systems responsible for mania and depression (Hudson et al. 1993; Jope 1999b; Jope and Williams 1994; Lenox and Watson 1994; Manji and Lenox 1994, 1998; Manji et al., Chapter 7, in this volume; Lenox et al., Chapter 9, in this volume).

Elucidating the primary postreceptor sites of action of lithium has proved difficult because lithium can produce effects at the level of the transduction of ligand-receptor interactions into intracellular responses either at the membrane (e.g., guanine nucleotide binding protein [G-protein] function and expression) or production of second-messenger molecules (e.g., inositol 1,4,5-trisphosphate [Ins(1,4,5)P_3], diacylglycerol [DAG], cyclic adenosine monophosphate [cAMP]) or further downstream at the level of protein kinase A or C, protein kinase substrates (e.g., myristoylated alanine-rich C kinase substrate [MARCKS], cytoskeletal proteins), or pathways associated with transcription factors and gene expression (e.g., cAMP response element binding protein [CREB], activator protein 1 [AP-1]) (Jope 1999a, 1999b). Most recently, considerable interest has been generated by the observation that lithium inhibits glycogen synthase kinase-3β (GSK-3β) (Klein and Melton 1996; Stambolic et al. 1996). This kinase phosphorylates microtubule-associated proteins such as tau, and therefore its inhibition by lithium results in reduced levels of phosphorylated tau and consequently alterations in the cytoskeleton. In addition, GSK-3_β is inhibitory toward AP-1 such that lithium can activate AP-1 (Jope 1999b).

Of the reported effects of lithium on various aspects of postreceptor signal transduction, the modulation of PI signaling (Figure 1–2) as a consequence of the depletion of intracellular inositol has gained most attention (Baraban et al. 1989; Berridge et al. 1989; Jope and Williams 1994; Snyder 1992). An attractive feature of this inositol depletion hypothesis is that the primary event—inhibition of IMPase by lithium—occurs at therapeutically relevant concentrations of lithium. Furthermore, the fact that lithium has little effect in normal subjects could be explained by the fact that rundown of the PI signaling pathway caused by a depletion of inositol would be expected to take place only under the conditions of excess stimulation presumed to occur in mania or depression (Baraban 1994).

LITHIUM AND PHOSPHATIDYLINOSITOL SIGNALING

The effects of lithium on aspects of PI signaling were originally noted by Allison and colleagues, who observed an accumulation of inositol 1-phosphate [Ins(1)P] and a reduction of inositol in rat brain following an acute (nontherapeutic) dose of lithium (Allison and Blisner 1976; Allison and Stewart 1971; Allison et al. 1976; Sherman 1989). At the time, because the role of inositol phospholipids in cellular signaling was not well characterized, the significance

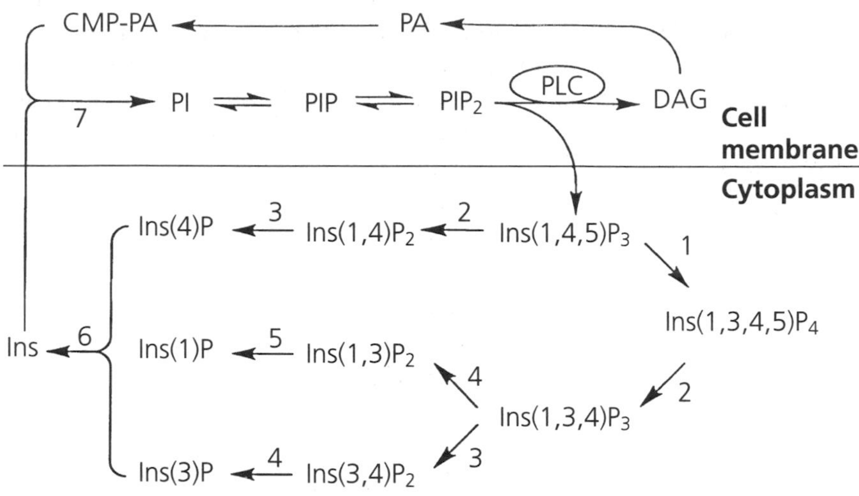

Figure 1–2. Simplified overview of the phosphatidylinositol (PI) signaling pathway, highlighting particularly the metabolism of inositol (Ins) polyphosphates to inositol (for detailed review see Majerus 1992). The agonist-stimulated, phospholipase C (PLC)-mediated hydrolysis of phosphatidylinositol 4,5-bisphosphate (PIP_2) yields the second-messenger molecules diacylglycerol (DAG) and inositol 1,4,5-trisphosphate (Ins(1,4,5)P_3), which activate protein kinase C and mobilize intracellular calcium, respectively. The metabolism of Ins(1,4,5)P_3 proceeds via either of two separate pathways. Hence, Ins(1,4,5)P_3 may be sequentially dephosphorylated to Ins(1,4)P_2 and then inositol 4-phosphate [Ins(4)P]; or, alternatively, it may be phosphorylated to inositol 1,3,4,5-tetrakisphosphate [Ins(1,3,4,5)P_4], which itself is involved in intracellular calcium mobilization. Ins(1,3,4,5)P_4 is then sequentially dephosphorylated to inositol 1,3,4 trisphosphate [Ins(1,3,4)P_3], then inositol 1,3 bisphosphate [Ins(1,3)P_2] or inositol 3,4 bisphosphate [Ins(3,4)P_2], and then inositol 1-phosphate [Ins(1)P] and inositol 3-phosphate [Ins(3)P]. These two separate metabolic pathways for Ins(1,4,5)P_3 converge on a single, common step, which is the dephosphorylation of the inositol monophosphates by inositol monophosphatase to produce inositol, which can then be used for the resynthesis of PI. The proposed lithium-sensitive metabolism of inositol 4,5 bisphosphate [Ins(4,5)P_2] (Jenkinson et al. 1992) is not included, because the exact nature of this pathway remains to be elucidated.

Note. PIP = phosphatidylinositol 4-phosphate; PA = phosphatidic acid; CMP-PA = cytidine monophosphorylphosphatidate. The enzymes involved in the metabolism of the inositol phosphates and the synthesis of PI are 1) inositol 1,4,5-trisphosphate 3-kinase; 2) inositol polyphosphate 5-phosphatase; 3) inositol polyphosphate 1-phosphatase; 4) inositol polyphosphate 4-phosphatase; 5) inositol polyphosphate 3-phosphatase; 6) inositol monophosphatase; 7) PI synthase.

of these observations was uncertain. However, as the importance of the PI signaling pathway became appreciated in the early 1980s, these in vivo effects of lithium, combined with the fact that IMPase is inhibited by therapeutically relevant concentrations of lithium (Hallcher and Sherman 1980; Naccarato et al. 1974), led to the formulation of the inositol depletion hypothesis (Berridge et al. 1982). More specifically, it was proposed that the therapeutic effects of lithium are a consequence of an attenuation of PI signaling caused by a depletion of inositol secondary to an inhibition of IMPase.

IMPase plays a critical role in the recycling of inositol from the inositol phosphates, because it is the final common pathway in their sequential dephosphorylation (Figure 1–2) (Majerus 1992). Moreover, IMPase also controls the de novo synthesis of inositol from glucose 6-phosphate, which proceeds via inositol 3-phosphate [Ins(3)P]. Therefore, in cells in which there are limited uptake mechanisms for extracellular inositol, IMPase regulates the supply of inositol needed to sustain the synthesis of PI and consequently PI-linked signal transduction (Gani et al. 1993).

This hypothesis has been further elaborated with evidence, obtained primarily from cell culture and cortical slice models, showing that lithium not only causes an accumulation of inositol monophosphates [$InsP_1$; i.e., Ins(1)P plus Ins(3)P plus Ins(4)P] but also causes an accumulation of cytidine monophosphorylphosphatidate (CMP-PA)—which in the presence of reduced amounts of its cosubstrate inositol is not used as readily for the synthesis of PI and therefore accumulates (Atack et al. 1995a). Moreover, lithium causes an attenuation of agonist-stimulated $InsP_3$ and $InsP_4$ responses as well as calcium mobilization (Atack et al. 1995a). The depletion of inositol not only makes less inositol available for the synthesis of PI but also attenuates the inositol-induced activation of PI synthase (Batty and Downes 1995).

Initially the specificity of lithium for the brain rather than peripheral PI-linked signaling systems was explained in terms of the blood-brain barrier limiting the supply of inositol from the periphery (Berridge et al. 1989). This would render brain cells particularly dependent on the supply of intracellular inositol (which is regulated by IMPase) and therefore sensitive to the IMPase-inhibitory effects of lithium. However, this theory has been superseded by the suggestion that it is the inositol and lithium transport systems of particular neuronal populations that render them selectively vulnerable to the effects of lithium (Gani et al. 1993). In this regard, it is interesting to note that there are indeed regional differences in the accumulation of inositol in different parts of the brain following intraperitoneal administration (Patishi et al. 1996c) and that chronic lithium produces a selective decrease in hypothalamic inositol levels (Lubrich et al. 1997).

Although the effects of lithium on PI signaling in vitro and in vivo (i.e., accumulation of $InsP_1$ and CMP-PA and attenuation of agonist-stimulated $InsP_3$ and $InsP_4$ and intracellular calcium mobilization responses) are all consistent with the inositol depletion hypothesis and with inhibition of IMPase being the primary action of lithium, there are, nevertheless, several caveats (Jope and Williams 1994). For instance, the possibility that these effects are mediated via other PI-linked mechanisms cannot be ruled out unequivocally, especially since lithium also inhibits other enzymes in the PI signaling pathway, most notably inositol polyphosphate 1-phosphatase (IPP; Inhorn and Majerus 1988; Ragan et al. 1988) and the putative enzyme involved in the metabolism of Ins(4,5)P_2 (Jenkinson et al. 1992).

Furthermore, the various effects of lithium on components of the PI signaling pathway are easily demonstrated in rodent cortical slice and tissue culture models in which inositol can be readily depleted. On the other hand, these effects are not seen in guinea pig, rabbit, or monkey cortical slices (Dixon et al. 1992; Hokin 1993; Lee et al. 1992) or in neuroblastoma cells (Stubbs and Agranoff 1993) in which inositol levels are not as readily depleted.

Additional indirect evidence that lithium produces a depletion of inositol in vivo comes from behavioral studies. Thus, lithium increases the susceptibility of rats and mice to pilocarpine-induced seizures, and these effects can be reversed by *myo*-inositol (Kofman et al. 1993; Tricklebank et al. 1991). Moreover, the inactive stereoisomer of *myo*-inositol, *chiro*-inositol, did not alter the vulnerability of rats to lithium-pilocarpine–induced seizures (Kofman and Belmaker 1993; Kofman et al. 1993; Patishi et al. 1996b). However, an additional reportedly inactive steroisomer, *epi*-inositol, also was found to be active at preventing lithium-pilocarpine seizures (Patishi et al. 1996b; Williams and Jope 1995), suggesting that the effects of *myo*-inositol on reducing the susceptibility to lithium-pilocarpine seizures were unrelated to the reversal of any potential *myo*-inositol depletion in vivo.

To investigate whether *epi*-inositol actually was biochemically inactive with respect to the PI signaling pathway, Richards and Belmaker (1996) used the accumulation of [^{3}H]CMP-PA as a marker of PI cycle turnover in Chinese hamster ovary cells and cortical slices. These results clearly showed that *epi*- and *myo*-inositol were able to prevent the lithium-induced accumulation of [^{3}H]CMP-PA, indicating that both isomers act on the PI pathway. Hence, the effects of *epi*-inositol on the reversal of lithium-pilocarpine–induced seizures were not anomalous; rather, they were consistent with lithium producing an inositol depletion in vivo that could be reversed with either *myo*- or *epi*-inositol (Belmaker et al. 1998).

With respect to the pharmacodynamics of lithium in humans, cerebrospinal fluid (CSF) IMPase activity (Atack et al. 1993b) was measured in psychiatrically healthy subjects before and after therapeutic doses of lithium, and the degree of inhibition of the CSF enzyme was only 9% (Molchan et al. 1994). This number is in contrast to the 80% reduction in erythrocyte IMPase following lithium treatment (Moscovich et al. 1990), but it is consistent with the lower levels of lithium in the CSF compared with plasma (Molchan et al. 1994). This relatively modest inhibition of CSF IMPase might suggest that the attenuating effects of lithium on PI signaling in vivo are not very severe. However, it is unclear to what extent the degree of inhibition of the CSF enzyme reflects inhibition of neuronal IMPase, especially if particular neuronal populations have specific lithium uptake mechanisms (Gani et al. 1993).

These observations highlight a key aspect of the inositol depletion hypothesis as it applies to bipolar disorder: the issue of whether the inhibition of IMPase seen at therapeutic concentrations of lithium is able to produce a depletion of inositol in vivo that is sufficient to compromise PI signaling. In other words, even though lithium may inhibit IMPase and produce a depletion of inositol, it is possible that this process is not enough to slow down the rate of PI synthesis and consequently attenuate the agonist-stimulated production of $InsP_3$. Indeed, in rats and mice, chronic lithium treatment does not decrease $InsP_3$ levels; and under conditions of cholinergic stimulation, $InsP_3$ levels actually increased (Jope et al. 1992; Whitworth et al. 1990). More recently, microdialysis has been used to study the production of $InsP_3$ in vivo (Minisclou et al. 1994). When this technique was applied to the study of the effects of lithium, it was shown that neither basal nor stimulated levels of $InsP_3$ were affected by lithium treatment (Gur et al. 1996).

Although these various data apparently argue against the inositol depletion hypothesis, it is nevertheless possible that lithium exerts its effects on specific neuronal populations. This effect may occur as a result of the inherent PI turnover of these cells (i.e., neurons with a higher PI turnover will be more vulnerable to the inhibitory effects of lithium), or of selective lithium uptake mechanisms, or of susceptibility to inositol depletion (perhaps as a consequence of the lack of an appropriate inositol uptake mechanism; Gani et al. 1993). Consequently, a selective effect of lithium on only certain neuronal populations would be masked by essentially normal PI turnover in the unaffected cells.

It would clearly be advantageous to be able to identify neuronal populations that might be selectively vulnerable to the effects of lithium in vivo. However, although lithium-induced CMP-PA accumulations can be visualized in vitro (Bevilacqua et al. 1994; Hwang et al. 1990), these techniques are not suitable for in vivo use. Moreover, although magnetic resonance imaging techniques can be employed to detect gross changes in inositol or phosphomonoesters (PMEs; see below), they currently lack the anatomical resolution required to identify discrete neuronal populations.

PHOSPHATIDYLINOSITOL SIGNALING IN BIPOLAR DISORDER

A key assumption in the hypothesis that lithium exerts its therapeutic effects in bipolar disorder as a consequence of damping down the PI signaling responses of PI-linked neurotransmitter systems is that these neurotransmitter systems are hyperactive during mania or depression (see Manji et al., Chapter 7; Jope et al., Chapter 8; and Lenox et al., Chapter 9, in this volume). However, there is as yet no *direct* evidence to suggest that abnormal PI signaling is associated with the pathogenesis of this disorder (Atack 1996a). Indirect evidence of altered PI signaling mechanisms in bipolar disorder comes from observations that in peripheral cells (primarily platelets), phosphatidylinositol 4,5-bisphosphate (PIP_2), protein kinase C activity, and agonist-stimulated inositol phosphate accumulation and intracellular Ca^{2+} responses are altered in bipolar disorder (Brown et al. 1993; Dubovsky et al. 1992; Friedman et al. 1993; Kusumi et al. 1991; Mikuni et al. 1991; Soares et al. 1999; van Calker et al. 1993). More recently, IMPase activity has been reported to be lower in transformed lymphoblastoid cell lines from bipolar compared with control subjects (Shamir et al. 1998). However, these data are consistent with, but not proof of, impaired PI signaling in these cells. Moreover, it remains unclear whether these observations in peripheral cells can be reliably extrapolated to predict the status of PI signaling systems within the brain—especially if only some, but not all, PI-linked neurotransmitter systems are dysfunctional (Atack 1996a).

An additional approach has been to examine the genetic variability of lymphocyte IMPase messenger RNA (mRNA) in psychiatrically healthy subjects and subjects with bipolar disorder (Steen et al. 1996), especially because a population variation in IMPase kinetic properties has been reported in transformed lymphocytes (Jarvis et al. 1992). A change of the codon 39 CCA to CCT was detected; but this mutation is silent, because both codons encode for proline. No other genetic variation was observed in either psychiatrically healthy subjects or subjects with bipolar disorder (Steen et al. 1996), suggesting that bipolar disorder is not due to pathological changes in the sequence (and therefore presumably kinetics) of IMPase. Furthermore, the lack of genetic variability in subjects with bipolar disorder who are lithium responders and nonresponders indicates that the lack of lithium responsivity in some patients is *not* due to the presence of a mutated, lithium-insensitive form of the IMPase.

Although these data show that there are no alterations in the coding region of the gene for IMPase, an alteration in the genomic structure of the gene is nevertheless possible, resulting in heterogeneity of bipolar disorder (e.g., distinguishing lithium responders and nonresponders), or the gene itself may be linked to the pathophysiology of bipolar disorder. As a prelude to more detailed analyses of potential polymorphisms, the human gene has been localized to the long arm of chromosome 8 (Sjoholt et al. 1997; Vadnal et al. 1998). However, to date, chromosome 8 has not been highlighted in several linkage studies of bipolar disorder that have implicated loci on chromosomes 4, 6, 13, 15, 18, 21, and X (Baron 1997).

Interestingly, a polymorphism has been identified in the IPP gene (a silent C973A transversion), which differentiated lithium responders and nonresponders in a group of Norwegian bipolar patients but did not differentiate these two populations in a group of Israeli patients (Steen et al. 1998).

Alterations in brain membrane phospholipid metabolism in vivo (Deicken et al. 1995a, 1995b; Kato et al. 1991, 1992, 1993, 1994a, 1994b) have been interpreted as suggesting that PI signaling systems are abnormal in bipolar disorder (Soares and Mallinger 1996). These studies are based mainly on the measurement of the PME peak obtained from phosphorus-31 magnetic resonance imaging. This PME peak contains a contribution from phosphoethanolamine, phosphocholine, and the sugar phosphates, which include $InsP_1$. The initial observation was that PME levels were elevated in the frontal lobe of manic, but not euthymic, lithium-treated subjects with bipolar disorder (Kato et al. 1991). In contrast, subsequent analyses of a larger number of subjects showed that in fact PME levels were unaltered in the manic state but were decreased in the euthymic state (Kato et al. 1992, 1993). These observations have been extended, and PME levels have recently been reported as being decreased in the frontal and temporal lobes of euthymic patients (Deicken et al. 1995a, 1995b).

With respect to PI signaling, the most expedient explanation for these changes in PME levels in bipolar disorder is that they reflect alterations in $InsP_1$ levels. If this were the case, one would expect that lithium treatment, which inhibits IMPase and causes an accumulation of $InsP_1$, would result in an increase in the PME signal. Yet in euthymic bipolar patients, PME levels did not differ before and after initiation of lithium treatment (Kato et al. 1993). Moreover, even if altered PME levels do prove to be a consistent feature of bipolar disorder, and even if the changes in PME levels can be ascribed to changes in $InsP_1$, it does not automatically follow that PI signaling is altered. Thus, changes in the levels of $InsP_1$ do not necessarily mean that the key step in PI signaling—the agonist-stimulated hydrolysis of PIP_2 to produce $InsP_3$ and DAG—is compromised.

Measurements in postmortem brain samples have shown that there is no pathological change in IMPase activity in bipolar subjects (Atack 1996b; Shimon et al. 1997). However, inositol levels are significantly lower in postmortem frontal cortex of bipolar subjects (as well as suicide victims) but normal in occipital cortex and cerebellum (Shimon et al. 1997). However, as with the measurement of other static markers associated with PI signaling, the association between the measurement of IMPase activity or postmortem inositol levels and functional aspects of PI signaling (i.e., agonist-stimulated PI turnover) is uncertain.

To examine the relationship between IMPase and other markers of PI signaling, IMPase activity has been measured in various regions of the rat and human brain (Figure 1–3; Atack 1996b). There do not, however, appear to be any major regional differences in enzyme activity (Patishi et al. 1996a). This relatively homogeneous distribution of enzyme activity, as well as mRNA distribution (Figure 1–4) within the brain, along with the observation that IMPase activity is relatively constant throughout postnatal development (Atack 1996b), is in marked contrast to other components of the PI signaling pathway, which show distinct regional and developmental differences (Balduini et al. 1991; De Smedt et al. 1994; Heacock et al. 1987, 1990; Mailleux et al. 1991, 1993; Mayat et al. 1994; Palmer et al. 1990; Worley et al. 1989).

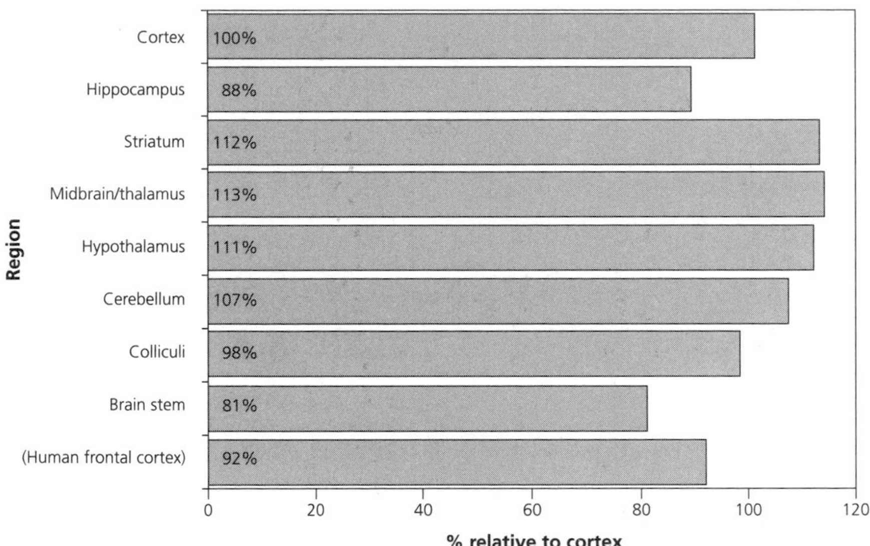

Figure 1–3. Inositol monophosphatase (IMPase) activity in various regions of the rat brain expressed as a percentage of the activity measured in the cortex. For comparative purposes, IMPase activity in a sample of postmortem human frontal cortex is also shown. Absolute activity in the rat cortex was 1.3 nmol/min/mg protein.

This dichotomy between the distribution of IMPase and other PI markers is further emphasized by the situation in Alzheimer's disease: in Alzheimer's disease, a loss of Ins(1,4,5)P_3 receptors occurs (Garlind et al. 1995), yet in post-mortem temporal cortex of subjects, IMPase activity is normal (Figure 1–5). These data, along with the relatively homogeneous distribution and relatively promiscuous substrate specificity (Atack 1996b) of IMPase, suggest that this enzyme may possess functions in the central nervous system unrelated to the ability to hydrolyze $InsP_1$.

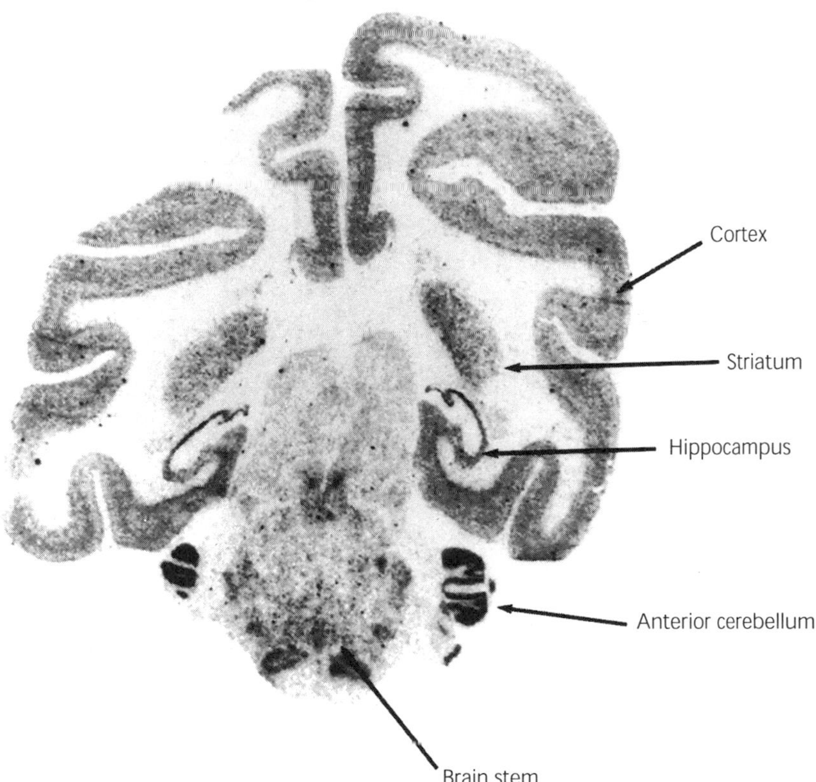

Figure 1–4. In situ hybridization of an antisense oligonucleotide probe directed against amino acids 230–244 of human inositol monophosphatase (IMPase) (the nucleotide sequence of the corresponding sense sequence is shown in Figure 1–8) in squirrel monkey brain. The antisense oligonucleotide showed a relatively homogeneous hybridization pattern to IMPase messenger RNA (mRNA) in different parts of the brain. In contrast, there was essentially no hybridization of sense mRNA (figure not shown).
Source. Data provided by Bob Heavens, Merck Sharp and Dohme Research Laboratories, Neuroscience Research Centre, Harlow, Essex, England.

Moreover, if IMPase is relatively homogeneously expressed despite marked regional differences in the PI turnover of different neuronal populations (as judged, for example, by the distribution of $InsP_3$ receptors), this would result in IMPase being more of a rate-limiting enzyme in neurons with a high PI turnover than in neurons with low PI turnover. This could result in neurons with a high PI turnover being more susceptible to the inhibitory effects of lithium than neurons with low PI turnover.

IMPase INHIBITORS AND THE INOSITOL DEPLETION HYPOTHESIS

One of the caveats of the inositol depletion hypothesis mentioned above is the issue of whether, given the various effects of lithium on various components of

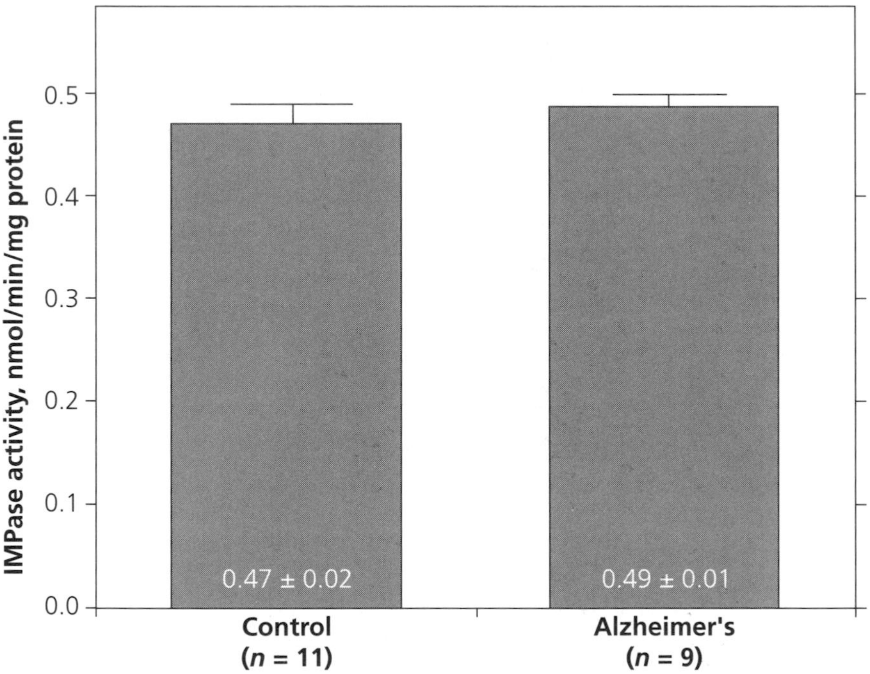

Figure 1–5. Inositol monophosphatase (IMPase) activity (measured at a substrate concentration of 0.1 mM) in homogenates of postmortem temporal cortex from age- and postmortem interval–matched control subjects and subjects with Alzheimer's disease.
Source. Tissue provided by Professor Elaine Perry, MRC Neurochemical Pathology Unit, Newcastle upon Tyne, England.

the PI signaling pathway (and, indeed, other biochemical processes), the effects of lithium on PI signaling can be attributed solely to inhibition of IMPase. This issue has been addressed by using specific inhibitors of IMPase to see whether they can mimic the effects of lithium on the PI cycle, in which case the effects of lithium on PI signaling would be consistent with the primary mechanism of action being inhibition of IMPase.

Various inhibitors of IMPase were synthesized on the basis of the substrate Ins(1)P (Atack and Fletcher 1994), of which the most notable was L-690,330 (Figure 1–6). This compound proved to be a very potent, competitive inhibitor of IMPase, with an IC_{50} of around 300 nM (Atack et al. 1993c). However, because of the highly charged bisphosphonate moiety, this compound did not readily penetrate the cell membrane (Atack et al. 1993c). Nevertheless, and for whatever reason, this compound was able to produce an accumulation of Ins(1)P in vivo, although at very high doses (in the region of 500 mg/kg).

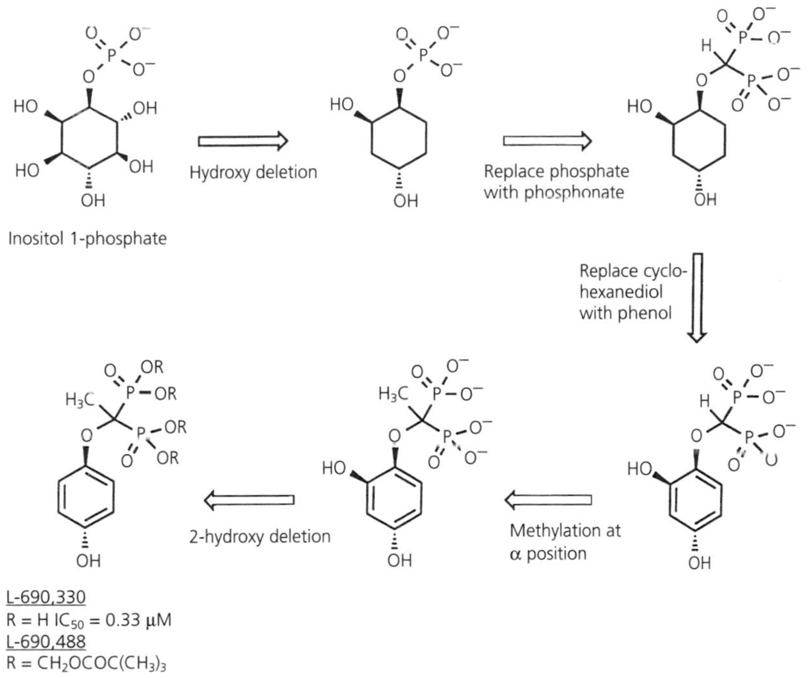

Figure 1–6. Summary of the principal steps in the modification of the substrate inositol 1-phosphate to produce the substrate-based inhibitor L-690,330 and the corresponding tetrapivaloyloxymethyl ester prodrug L-690,488.

The significance of this observation is that it was not known whether a *competitive* inhibitor of IMPase would be able to inhibit the enzyme to an extent sufficient to cause an accumulation of Ins(1)P in vivo (Atack et al. 1993c). Thus, lithium is a *noncompetitive* inhibitor of IMPase and as such exerts a greater effect the faster the enzyme is working (Nahorski et al. 1991). In mechanistic terms, the faster the enzyme is working, the more IMPase is in the E.$Mg_{(1)}$.Pi state (see below), which is the complex that is susceptible to noncompetitive inhibition by lithium. On the other hand, with competitive inhibitors, the substrate can, by definition, compete with the inhibitor for the active site. Consequently, the substrate ($InsP_1$) that accumulates will compete with the inhibitor and tend to alleviate the inhibition. Hence, an accumulation of substrate can overcome the inhibitory effects of a competitive inhibitor. Therefore, the L-690,330–induced accumulation of Ins(1)P in vivo suggests that there is appreciable inhibition of the enzyme in vivo and that the tendency of substrate to accumulate does not overcome the inhibitory effects of the compound.

Because L-690,330 did not readily cross the cell membrane in tissue culture or cortical slice models, the tetrapivaloyloxymethyl ester prodrug of this compound, L-690,488, was synthesized. The rationale for this approach was that by esterification of the bisphosphonate group, the charge of the resulting compound would be greatly reduced, permitting the compound to more readily cross the cell membrane and enter the cell. Once inside the cell, esterases would cleave the esteratic bonds to yield the parent compound L-690, 330, which would then be able to inhibit IMPase. This strategy worked remarkably well in rat cortical slices and Chinese hamster ovary cells transfected with the human muscarinic M_1 receptor (Atack et al. 1994) and human platelets (Figure 1–7). Thus, L-690,488 was much more potent than L-690,330 at causing an accumulation of $InsP_1$, consistent with L-690,488 being much more membrane permeable than L-690,330 (Atack et al. 1994). Moreover, the L-690,488–induced accumulation of $InsP_1$ and CMP-PA and an attenuation of $InsP_3$ and $InsP_4$ responses both mimic the effects of lithium (Atack et al. 1993a).

The fact that a specific inhibitor of IMPase can produce effects on markers of PI signaling, whether it be accumulation of $InsP_1$ and CMP-PA or an attenuation of $InsP_3$ and $InsP_4$ responses, is consistent with the effects of lithium on PI signaling being due primarily to inhibition of IMPase. Unfortunately, however, the lipophilicity of L-690,488 meant that this compound was not suitable for use in vivo. Thus, when L-690,488 was injected into animals, neither it nor the parent compound L-690,330 could be detected in plasma or brain, suggesting that the compound remained at the site of injection.

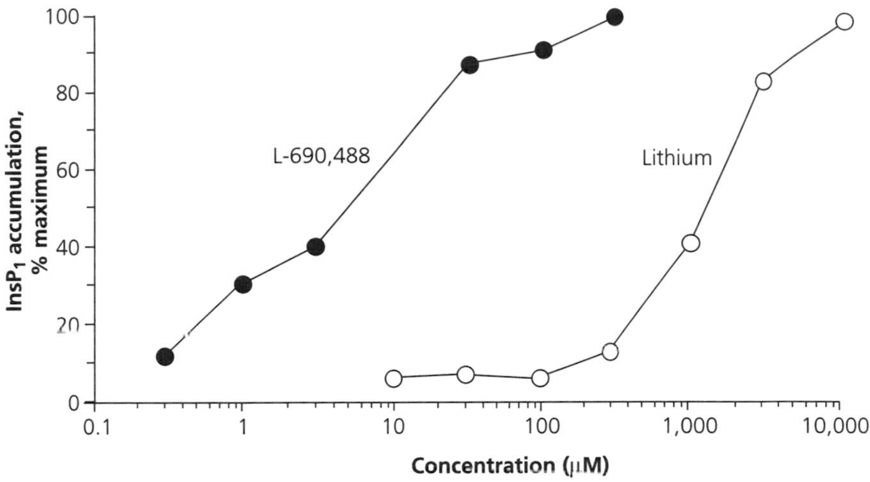

Figure 1–7. Effects of L-690,488 on the thrombin-stimulated accumulation of $InsP_1$ in human platelets showing that L-690,488 is several orders of magnitude more potent than lithium. EC_{50}s in this particular experiment were 4.8 μM for L-690,488 and 1.2 mM for lithium.

IMPase

The search for other, novel inhibitors of IMPase that might be active in vivo was restricted by an absence of detailed information concerning the active site structure, the enzyme substrate hydrolysis, and the lithium inhibition mechanisms. Accordingly, IMPase has been purified, cloned, expressed, and subjected to detailed X-ray crystallographic structural analysis as well as site-directed mutagenesis and enzyme kinetic studies.

Structure

Bovine brain IMPase was purified, cloned, and expressed (Diehl et al. 1990; Gee et al. 1988) and found to be a homodimer with a subunit size of 277 amino acids. The bovine, rat, frog, and human enzymes all share >75% amino acid identity (McAllister et al. 1992; Wreggett 1992), yet IMPase has very little overall identity with other known proteins (Atack et al. 1995b; Parthasarathy et al. 1994). Nevertheless, there are three regions of the enzyme (Figure 1–8, sequences in bold type) that share marked regional homology with the phosphatase enzymes inositol polyphosphate 1-phosphatase (IPP) and fructose

1,6-bisphosphatase (F-1,6-BP; Neuwald et al. 1991). These three regions (amino acids 69–72, 87–100, and 219–233) contain most of the key amino acids involved in substrate and metal binding and enzyme mechanism (see below). Furthermore, corresponding regions occur in a number of other proteins of generally unknown function, suggesting that these proteins may possess phosphatase activity.

Purified IMPase was subjected to X-ray crystallographic studies (Bone et al. 1992, 1994a, 1994b) and found to contain regions of α-helix and β-sheet secondary structure in an αβαβα arrangement (Figure 1–9). Alternating regions of α-helix and β-sheet are also found in IPP and in F-1,6-BP, indicating that this tertiary structure—along with the common occurrence of the three sequences of amino acids shown in bold in Figure 1–8—is responsible for the similar features of these three enzymes: their 1) phosphatase activity, 2) sensitivity to inhibition by lithium, 3) magnesium dependence, and 4) similar two-metal (magnesium)–catalyzed mechanism of action (Atack et al. 1995b).

A striking feature of the structure of IMPase is the hydrophilicity of not only the active site but also the channel leading up to it. This raises the paradoxical situation in which it appears that a hydrophilic, charged compound is required to interact with the primarily polar amino acid residues present in the active site, yet such a compound (like the substrate-based compounds described above) is likely to possess limited permeability through the cell membrane. Because the alternating α-helix and β-sheet secondary structure seems crucial to the function of the enzyme, an alternative approach to developing novel inhibitors might be to identify hydrophobic pockets on the enzyme that are distinct from the active site yet are able to disrupt key structural features of, and thereby inhibit, IMPase.

Mechanism

X-ray crystallographic data of several forms of IMPase (e.g., IMPase alone, IMPase plus either gadolinium [Gd^{3+}], substrate, inhibitor, or manganese; Bone et al. 1992, 1994a, 1994b) were used in conjunction with site-directed mutagenesis (Pollack et al. 1993, 1994) to identify the amino acids involved in substrate and metal (Mg^{2+}) binding and activation of the nucleophile that attacks the substrate. The contributions of these amino acids to the mechanism of IMPase are summarized in Table 1–1.

The initial crystallization of IMPase was performed in the presence of Gd^{3+}, which was used to identify the site at which Mg^{2+}, essential for enzyme activity, binds (Bone et al. 1992). This structure suggested that there was only one metal (Mg^{2+}) binding site per subunit and that this metal possessed nine

1	Met	Ala	Asp	Pro	Trp	Gln	Glu	Cys	Met	Asp	Tyr	Ala	Val	Thr	Leu	Ala	Glu	Gln	Ala	Gly
21	Glu	Val	Val	Cys	Glu	Ala	Ile	Lys	Asn	Glu	Met	Asn	Val	Met	Leu	Lys	Ser	Ser	Pro	Val
41	Asp	Leu	Val	Thr	Ala	Thr	Asp	Gln	Lys	Val	Glu	Lys	Met	Leu	Ile	Ser	Ser	Ile	Lys	Glu
61	Lys	Tyr	Pro	Ser	His	Ser	Phe	Ile	Gly	^{70}Glu	Glu	Ser	Val	Ala	Ala	Gly	Glu	Lys	Ser	Ile
81	Leu	Thr	Asp	Asn	Pro	Thr	Trp	Ile	Ile	^{90}Asp	Pro	^{92}Ile	^{93}Asp	^{94}Gly	^{95}Thr	Thr	Asn	Phe	Val	His
101	Arg	Phe	Pro	Phe	Val	Ala	Val	Ser	Ile	Gly	Phe	Ala	Val	Asn	Lys	Lys	Ile	Glu	Phe	Gly
121	Val	Val	Tyr	Ser	Cys	Val	Glu	Gly	Lys	Met	Tyr	Thr	Ala	Arg	Lys	Gly	Lys	Gly	Ala	Phe
141	Cys	Asn	Gly	Gln	Lys	Leu	Gln	Val	Ser	Gln	Gln	Glu	Asp	Ile	Thr	Lys	Ser	Leu	Leu	Val
161	Thr	Glu	Leu	Gly	Ser	Ser	Arg	Thr	Pro	Glu	Thr	Val	Arg	Met	Val	Leu	Ser	Asn	Met	Glu
181	Lys	Leu	Phe	Cys	Ile	Pro	Val	His	Gly	Ile	Arg	Ser	Val	Gly	Thr	^{196}Ala	Ala	Val	Asn	Met
201	Cys	Leu	Val	Ala	Thr	Gly	Gly	Ala	Asp	Ala	Tyr	Tyr	^{213}Glu	Met	Gly	Ile	His	Cys	Trp	^{220}Asp
221	Val	Ala	Gly	Ala	Gly	Ile	Ile	Val	Thr	Glu	Ala	Gly	Gly	Val	Leu	Met	Asp	Val	Thr	Gly
										5'-GAA	GCT	GGT	GGC	GTG	CTA	ATG	GAT	GTT	ACA	GGT
241	Gly	Pro	Phe	Asp	Leu	Met	Ser	Arg	Arg	Val	Ile	Ala	Ala	Asn	Asn	Arg	Ile	Leu	Ala	Glu
	GGA	CCA	TTT	GAT-3'																
261	Arg	Ile	Ala	Lys	Glu	Ile	Gln	Val	Ile	Pro	Leu	Gln	Arg	Asp	Asp	Glu	Asp			

Figure 1–8. Amino acid sequence of human inositol monophosphatase (IMPase) (McAllister et al. 1992). Three sequences (amino acids 69–72, 87–100, and 219–233) are underlined, and similar motifs occur in a number of other proteins—most notably inositol polyphosphate 1-phosphatase (IPP) and fructose 1,6-bisphosphatase (F-1,6,-BP) (Atack et al. 1995b; Neuwald et al. 1991). These sequences contain most of the key amino acid residues (shown in bold) involved in substrate and metal binding and catalytic mechanism.

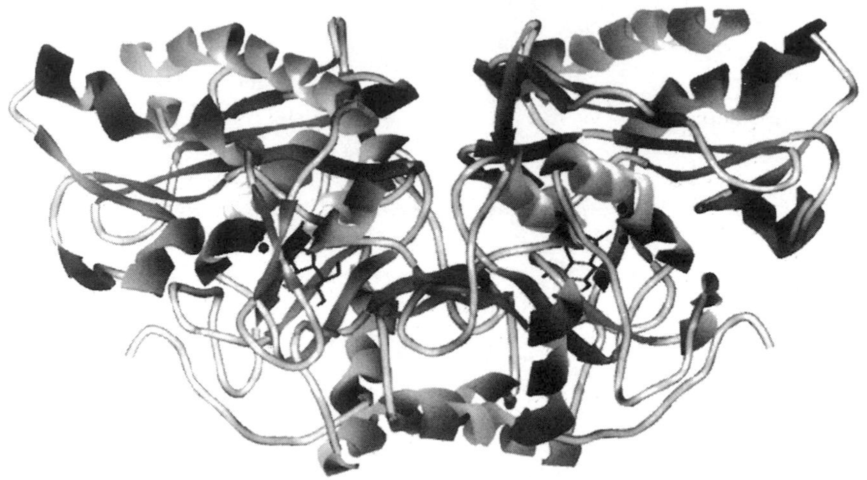

Figure 1–9. Ribbon diagram showing the dimeric structure of human inositol monophosphatase (IMPase); two-metal ions and substrate are also shown in each subunit. α-Helices are shown as thick ribbons, β-sheets as thin ribbons with arrows, and the remainder as a tube.
Source. Courtesy of Dr. Howard Broughton, Merck Sharp and Dohme Research Laboratories, Neuroscience Research Centre, Harlow, Essex, England.

binding interactions. Unfortunately, however, this structure was obtained in the presence of lithium (used for optimum crystal growth conditions), which at the high concentrations used bound at the second metal binding site. Because lithium cannot be observed in the X-ray crystallographic structure, the second metal binding site in this structure was masked. Moreover, since the valence of the trivalent cation Gd^{3+} (3) is different from the physiological divalent cation Mg^{2+} (2), the initial estimate of nine metal-ligand interactions proved to be an overestimate.

Subsequent crystals grown under a number of other different conditions (Bone et al. 1994a, 1994b) confirmed enzymological metal titration curves and molecular modeling studies (Pollack et al. 1994), which suggested that IMPase contains two metal binding sites. Indirect support for the fact that IMPase hydrolyzes substrate via a two-metal mechanism comes from data showing that the IPP and F-1,6-BP, both of which share structural similarities with IMPase, also proceed via a two-metal–catalyzed mechanism (York et al. 1994; Zhang et al. 1993a, 1993b).

The mechanism of hydrolysis of IMPase and the method by which lithium

Table 1–1. Key amino acids involved in substrate and metal binding and enzyme mechanism

Function	Amino acids
Substrate binding	Asp93
	Gly94
	Thr95
	Ala196
	Glu213
	Asp220
Site 1 Mg^{2+}	Glu70
	Asp90
	Ile92
Site 2 Mg^{2+}	Asp90
	Asp93
	Asp220
Nucleophilic water activation	Glu70
	Thr95

inhibits the enzyme are shown in Figure 1–10. In summary, the substrate (InsP) binds to enzyme with Mg^{2+} present in metal binding site 1 (this Mg^{2+} remains bound to the enzyme throughout the catalytic cycle). Following substrate binding, a second Mg^{2+} ion binds and interacts with a trio of aspartate residues (Asp 90, 93, and 220). This Mg^{2+} ion activates the inositol ester oxygen and makes it vulnerable to nucleophilic attack by a water molecule that is activated by Glu70 and Thr95 as well as the site 1 Mg^{2+}. This nucleophilic attack results in hydrolysis of the phosphate bond, leaving the phosphate group complexed with the enzyme and both Mg^{2+} ions. Ordinarily, the second Mg^{2+} rapidly debinds, followed by phosphate to regenerate the enzyme with the site 1 Mg^{2+} bound, ready for the next round of substrate hydrolysis. However, in the presence of lithium, when the second Mg^{2+} debinds from the enzyme/phosphate complex, the second metal binding site becomes occupied by lithium. This process then stops the phosphate group debinding, and the enzyme becomes trapped in this stable, inactive enzyme/phosphate state.

CONCLUSION

Despite the assumptions that remain to be proved (e.g., are PI-linked neurotransmitter systems associated with the pathophysiology of bipolar disorder?

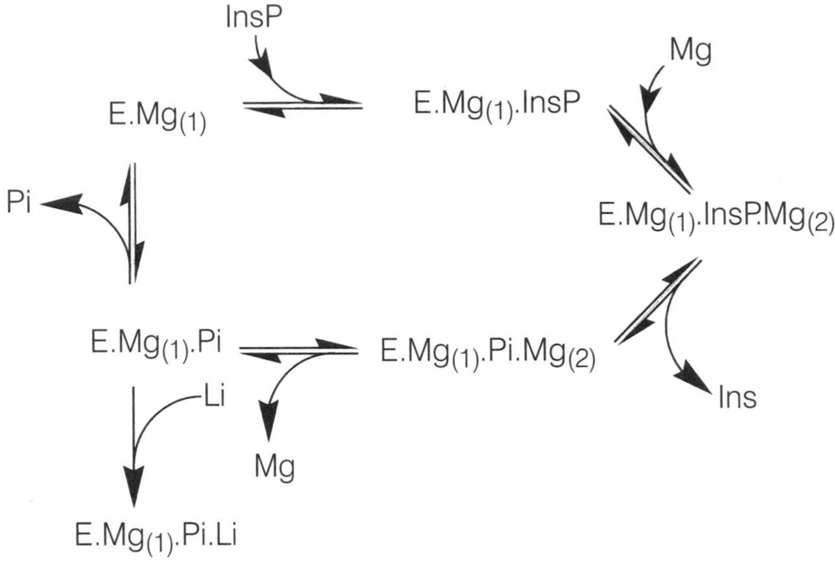

Figure 1–10. Summary of the mechanism of substrate hydrolysis and inhibition by lithium of inositol monophosphatase (IMPase). In brief, magnesium (Mg) remains bound to the enzyme at metal binding site 1 throughout the catalytic cycle. Substrate binds to this $E.Mg_{(1)}$ complex, at which point a second Mg ion occupies metal binding site 2. This process initiates a sequence of events leading to the hydrolysis of the phosphate bond, releasing inositol (Ins). The second Mg then rapidly debinds from the resulting $E.Mg_{(1)}.Pi.Mg_{(2)}$ complex; this process is followed by debinding of inorganic phosphate (Pi) to regenerate the $E.Mg_{(1)}$.
Note. E = enzyme; InsP = inositol 1-phosphate (either inositol 1-, 3-, or 4-phosphate); Li = lithium. $Mg_{(1)}$ and $Mg_{(2)}$ represent magnesium binding at metal binding sites 1 and 2, respectively.

and does inhibition of IMPase by therapeutic doses of lithium deplete intracellular inositol levels to an extent that is sufficient to compromise PI signaling?), the proposal that lithium works via inhibition of IMPase remains arguably the most attractive explanation of how it exerts its effects in the treatment of bipolar disorder. Consistent with this hypothesis, inhibitors of IMPase produce effects on PI signaling that mimic those produced by lithium, the corollary being that the effects of lithium on PI signaling are compatible with inhibition of IMPase being the primary site of action.

Unfortunately, these substrate-based inhibitors of IMPase were not suitable for use in vivo. Therefore, as an alternative approach to the development of inhibitors of IMPase, the structure and mechanism of this enzyme have been elucidated. By understanding the three-dimensional structure of the active site and the mechanism by which the enzyme not only hydrolyzes the substrate but is inhibited by lithium, it may be possible to develop novel inhibitors that may be more amenable to in vivo use than the substrate-based inhibitors. Such compounds could then be useful for the ultimate test of the hypothesis that IMPase is the therapeutic target for lithium by evaluating whether specific inhibitors of this enzyme are effective in the treatment of bipolar disorder.

REFERENCES

Allison JH, Blisner ME: Inhibition of the effect of lithium on brain inositol by atropine and scopolamine. Biochem Biophys Res Commun 68:1332–1338, 1976

Allison JH, Stewart MA: Reduced brain inositol in lithium-treated rats. Nature New Biology 233:267–268, 1971

Allison JH, Blisner ME, Holland WH, et al: Increased brain myo-inositol 1-phosphate in lithium-treated rats. Biochem Biophys Res Commun 71:664–670, 1976

Atack JR: Inositol monophosphatase inhibitors: a novel treatment for bipolar disorder? Biol Psychiatry 37:761–763, 1995

Atack JR: Are platelet and magnetic resonance spectroscopic changes indicative of altered PI signalling in bipolar disorder? Biol Psychiatry 39:462–464, 1996a

Atack JR: Inositol monophosphatase, the putative therapeutic target for lithium. Brain Res Rev 22:183–190, 1996b

Atack JR, Fletcher SR: Inhibitors of inositol monophosphatase. Drugs of the Future 19:857–866, 1994

Atack JR, Prior AM, Griffith D, et al: Characterization of the effects of lithium on phosphatidylinositol (PI) cycle activity in human muscarinic m1 receptor-transfected CHO cells. Br J Pharmacol 110:809–815, 1993a

Atack JR, Rapoport SI, Varley CL: Characterization of inositol monophosphatase in human cerebrospinal fluid. Brain Res 613:305–308, 1993b

Atack JR, Cook SM, Watt AP, et al: In vitro and in vivo inhibition of inositol monophosphatase by the bisphosphonate L-690,330. J Neurochem 60:652–658, 1993c

Atack JR, Prior AM, Fletcher SR, et al: Effects of L-690,488, a prodrug of the bisphosphonate inositol monophosphatase inhibitor L-690,330, on phosphatidylinositol cycle markers. J Pharmacol Exp Ther 270:70–76, 1994

Atack JR, Broughton HB, Pollack SJ: Inositol monophosphatase—a putative target for Li^+ in the treatment of bipolar disorder. Trends Neurosci 18:343–349, 1995a

Atack JR, Broughton HB, Pollack SJ: Structure and mechanism of inositol monophosphatase. FEBS Lett 361:1–7, 1995b

Baastrup P, Poulsen KS, Schou M, et al: Prophylactic lithium: double-blind discontinuation in manic-depressive and recurrent-depressive disorders. Lancet 2:326–330, 1970

Balduini W, Candura S, Costa LG: Regional development of carbachol-, glutamate-, norepinephrine-, and serotonin-stimulated phosphoinositide metabolism in rat brain. Dev Brain Res 62:115–120, 1991

Baraban JM: Toward a crystal-clear view of lithium's site of action. Proc Natl Acad Sci U S A 91:5738–5739, 1994

Baraban JM, Worley PF, Snyder SH: Second messenger systems and psychoactive drug action: focus on the phosphoinositide system and lithium. Am J Psychiatry 146:1251–1260, 1989

Baron M: Genetic linkage and bipolar affective disorder: progress and pitfalls. Mol Psychiatry 2:200–210, 1997

Batty IH, Downes CP: The mechanism of muscarinic receptor-stimulated phosphatidylinositol resynthesis in 1321N1 astrocytoma cells and its inhibition by Li^+. J Neurochem 65:2279–2289, 1995

Belmaker RH, Agam G, van Calker, et al: Behavioral reversal of lithium effects by four inositol isomers correlates perfectly with biochemical effects on the PI cycle: depletion by chronic lithium of brain inositol is specific to hypothalamus, and inositol levels may be abnormal in postmortem brain from bipolar patients. Neuropsychopharmacology 19:220–232, 1998

Berridge MJ, Downes CP, Hanley MR: Lithium amplifies agonist-dependent phosphatidylinositol responses in brain and salivary glands. Biochem J 206:587–595, 1982

Berridge MJ, Downes CP, Hanley MR: Neural and developmental actions of lithium: A unifying hypothesis. Cell 59:411–419, 1989

Bevilacqua JA, Downes CP, Lowenstein PR: Visualization of agonist-stimulated inositol phospholipid turnover in individual neurons of the rat cerebral cortex and hippocampus. Neuroscience 60:945–958, 1994

Bone R, Springer JP, Atack JR: Structure of inositol monophosphatase, the putative target of lithium therapy. Proc Natl Acad Sci U S A 89:10031–10035, 1992

Bone R, Frank L, Springer JP, et al: Structural analysis of inositol monophosphatase complexes with substrates. Biochemistry 33:9460–9467, 1994a

Bone R, Frank L, Springer JP, et al: Structural studies of metal binding by inositol monophosphatase: evidence for two metal ion catalysis. Biochemistry 33:9468–9476, 1994b

Brown AS, Mallinger AG, Renbaum LC: Elevated platelet membrane phosphatidylinositol-4,5-bisphosphate in bipolar mania. Am J Psychiatry 150:1252–1254, 1993

Bunney Jr, WE, Garland-Bunney BL: Mechanisms of action of lithium in affective illness: basic and clinical implications, in Psychopharmacology: The Third Generation of Progress. Edited by Meltzer HY. New York, Raven, 1987, pp 553–565

Cade JFJ: Lithium salts in the treatment of psychotic excitement. Med J Aust 36:349–352, 1949

Cade JFJ: Lithium—past, present and future, in Lithium in Medical Practice. Edited by Johnson FN, Johnson S. Lancaster, United Kingdom, MTP Press, 1978, pp 1–16

De Smedt F, Verjans B, Mailleux P: Cloning and expression of human brain type I inositol 1,4,5-trisphosphate 5-phosphatase: high levels of mRNA in cerebellar Purkinje cells. FEBS Lett 347:67–72, 1994

Deicken RF, Fein G, Weiner MW: Abnormal frontal lobe phosphorus metabolism in bipolar disorder. Am J Psychiatry 152:915–918, 1995a

Deicken RF, Weiner MW, Fein G: Decreased temporal lobe phosphomonoesters in bipolar disorder. J Affect Disord 33:195–199, 1995b

Diehl RE, Whiting P, Potter J, et al: Cloning and expression of bovine brain inositol monophosphatase. J Biol Chem 265:5946–5949, 1990

Dixon JF, Lee CH, Los GV, et al: Lithium enhances accumulation of [^{3}H]inositol radioactivity and mass of second messenger inositol 1,4,5-trisphosphate in monkey cerebral cortex slices. J Neurochem 59:2332–2335, 1992

Dubovsky SL, Murphy J, Thomas M, et al: Abnormal intracellular calcium ion concentration in platelets and lymphocytes of bipolar patients. Am J Psychiatry 149: 118–120, 1992

Friedman E, Hoau Y-W, Levinson D, et al: Altered platelet protein kinase C activity in bipolar affective disorder, manic episode. Biol Psychiatry 33:520–525, 1993

Gani D, Downes CP, Batty I, et al: Lithium and *myo*-inositol homeostasis. Biochim Biophys Acta 1177:253–269, 1993

Garlind A, Cowburn RF, Forsell C, et al: Diminished [^{3}H]inositol(1,4,5)P_3 but not [^{3}H]inositol(1,3,4,5)P_4 binding in Alzheimer's disease brain. Brain Res 681: 160–166, 1995

Gee NS, Ragan CI, Watling KJ, et al: The purification and properties of *myo*-inositol monophosphatase from bovine brain. Biochem J 249:883–889, 1988

Gur E, Lerer B, Newman ME: Acute or chronic lithium does not affect agonist-stimulated inositol trisphosphate formation in rat brain in vivo. NeuroReport 7:393–396, 1996

Hallcher LM, Sherman WR: The effects of lithium ion and other agents on the activity of *myo*-inositol-1-phosphatase from bovine brain. J Biol Chem 255:10896–10901, 1980

Heacock AM, Fisher SK, Agranoff BW: Enhanced coupling of neonatal muscarinic receptors in rat brain to phosphoinositide turnover. J Neurochem 48:1904–1911, 1987

Heacock AM, Seguin EB, Agranoff BW: Developmental and regional studies of the metabolism of inositol 1,4,5-trisphosphate in rat brain. J Neurochem 54:1405–1411, 1990

Hokin LE: Lithium increases accumulation of second messenger inositol 1,4,5-trisphosphate in brain cortex slices in species ranging from mouse to monkey. Adv Enzyme Regul 33:299–312, 1993

Hudson CJ, Young LT, Li PP, et al: CNS signal transduction in the pathophysiology and pharmacotherapy of affective disorders and schizophrenia. Synapse 13:278–293, 1993

Hwang PM, Bredt DS, Snyder SH: Autoradiographic imaging of phosphoinositide turnover in the brain. Science 249:802–804, 1990

Inhorn RC, Majerus PW: Properties of inositol polyphosphate 1-phosphatase. J Biol Chem 263:14559–14565, 1988

Janicak PG, Davis JM: Clinical usage of lithium in mania, in Antimanics, Anticonvulsants and Other Drugs in Psychiatry. Edited by Burrows GD, Norman TR, Davies B. Amsterdam, Elsevier, 1987, pp 21–34

Jarvis MR, Todd RD, Hickok JM, et al: Analysis of myo-inositol monophosphatase in transformed human lymphocytes. Lithium 3:49–54, 1992

Jenkinson S, Challiss RAJ, Nahorski SR: Evidence for lithium-sensitive inositol 4,5-bisphosphate accumulation in muscarinic cholinoceptor-stimulated cerebral-cortex slices. Biochem J 287:437–442, 1992

Johnson FN: The History of Lithium Therapy. London, Macmillan, 1984

Jope RS: A bimodal model of the mechanism of action of lithium. Mol Psychiatry 4:21–25, 1999a

Jope RS: Anti-bipolar therapy: mechanism of action of lithium. Mol Psychiatry 4:117–128, 1999b

Jope RS, Williams MB: Lithium and brain signal transduction systems. Biochem Pharmacol 47:429–441, 1994

Jope RS, Song L, Kolasa K: Inositol trisphosphate, cyclic AMP, and cyclic GMP in rat brain regions after lithium and seizures. Biol Psychiatry 31:505–514, 1992

Kato T, Shioiri T, Takahashi S, et al: Measurement of brain phosphoinositide metabolism in bipolar patients using in vivo ^{31}P-MRS. J Affect Disord 22:185–190, 1991

Kato T, Takahashi S, Shioiri T, et al: Brain phosphorus metabolism in depressive disorders by phosphorus-31 magnetic resonance spectroscopy. J Affect Disord 26:223–230, 1992

Kato T, Takahashi S, Shioiri T, et al: Alterations in brain phosphorus metabolism in bipolar disorder detected by in vivo ^{31}P and ^{7}Li magnetic resonance spectroscopy. J Affect Disord 27:53–60, 1993

Kato T, Shioiri T, Murashita J, et al: Phosphorus-31 magnetic resonance spectroscopy and ventricular enlargement in bipolar disorder. Psychiatry Res 55:41–50, 1994a

Kato T, Takahashi S, Shioiri T, et al: Reduction of brain phosphocreatine in bipolar II disorder detected by phosphorus-31 magnetic resonance spectroscopy. J Affect Disord 31:125–133, 1994b

Klein PS, Melton DA: A molecular mechanism for the effect of lithium on development. Proc Natl Acad Sci U S A 93:8455–8459, 1996

Kline NS: Lithium comes into its own. Am J Psychiatry 125:558–560, 1968

Kofman O, Belmaker RH: Biochemical, behavioral, and clinical studies of the role of inositol in lithium treatment and depression. Biol Psychiatry 34:839–852, 1993

Kofman O, Sherman WR, Katz V, et al: Restoration of brain myo-inositol levels in rats increases latency to lithium-pilocarpine seizures. Psychopharmacology 110:229–234, 1993

Kusumi I, Koyama T, Yamashita I: Serotonin-stimulated Ca^{2+} response is increased in the blood platelets of depressed patients. Biol Psychiatry 30:310–312, 1991

Lee CH, Dixon JF, Reichman M, et al: Li^+ increases accumulation of inositol 1,4,5-trisphosphate and inositol 1,3,4,5-tetrakisphosphate in cholinergically stimulated brain cortex slices in guinea pig, mouse and rat—the increases require inositol supplementation in mouse and rat but not in guinea pig. Biochem J 282:377–385, 1992

Lenox RH, Watson DG: Lithium and the brain: a psychopharmacological strategy to a molecular basis for manic depressive illness. Clin Chem 40:309–314, 1994

Lubrich B, Patishi Y, Kofman O, et al: Lithium-induced inositol depletion in rat brain after chronic treatment is restricted to the hypothalamus. Mol Psychiatry 2:407–412, 1997

Mailleux P, Takazawa K, Erneux C, et al: Inositol 1,4,5-trisphosphate 3-kinase mRNA: High levels in rat hippocampal CA1 pyramidal and dentate gyrus granule cells and in cerebellar Purkinje cells. J Neurochem 56:345–347, 1991

Mailleux P, Takazawa K, Erneux C, et al: Distribution of the neurons containing inositol 1,4,5-trisphosphate 3-kinase and its messenger RNA in the developing rat brain. J Comp Neurol 327:618–629, 1993

Majerus PW: Inositol phosphate biochemistry. Annu Rev Biochem 61:225–250, 1992

Manji HK, Lenox RH: Long-term action of lithium: a role for transcriptional and post-transcriptional factors regulated by protein kinase C. Synapse 16:11–28, 1994

Manji HK, Lenox RH: Lithium: a molecular transducer of mood-stabilization in the treatment of bipolar disorder. Neuropsychopharmacology 19:161–166, 1998

Mayat E, Lebrun F, Sassetti I, et al: Ontogenesis of quisqualate-associated phosphoinositide metabolism in various regions of the rat nervous system. Int J Dev Neurosci 12:1–17, 1994

McAllister G, Whiting P, Hammond EA, et al: cDNA cloning of human and rat brain myo-inositol monophosphatase: expression and characterization of the human recombinant enzyme. Biochem J 284:749–754, 1992

Mikuni M, Kusumi I, Kagaka A, et al: Increased 5-HT-2 receptor function as measured by serotonin-stimulated phosphoinositide hydrolysis in platelets of depressed patients. Prog Neuropsychopharmacol Biol Psychiatry 15:49–61, 1991

Minisclou C, Rouquier L, Benavides J, et al: Muscarinic receptor-mediated increase in extracellular inositol 1,4,5-trisphosphate levels in the rat hippocampus: an in vivo microdialysis study. J Neurochem 62:557–562, 1994

Molchan SE, Atack JR, Sunderland T: Decreased CSF inositol monophosphatase activity after lithium treatment. Psychiatry Res 53:103–105, 1994

Moscovich DG, Belmaker RH, Agam G, et al: Inositol-1-phosphatase in red blood cells of manic-depressive patients before and during treatment with lithium. Biol Psychiatry 27:552–555, 1990

Naccarato WF, Ray RE, Wells WW: Biosynthesis of myo-inositol in rat mammary gland: isolation and properties of the enzymes. Arch Biochem Biophys 164:194–201, 1974

Nahorski SR, Ragan CI, Challiss RAJ: Lithium and the phosphoinositide cycle: an example of uncompetitive inhibition and its pharmacological consequences. Trends Pharmacol Sci 12:297–303, 1991

Neuwald AF, York JD, Majerus PW: Diverse proteins homologous to inositol monophosphatase. FEBS Lett 294:16–18, 1991

Palmer E, Nangel-Taylor K, Krause JD, et al: Changes in excitatory amino acid modulation of phosphoinositide metabolism during development. Brain Res Dev Brain Res 51:132–134, 1990

Parthasarathy L, Vadnal RE, Parthasarathy R, et al: Biochemical and molecular properties of lithium-sensitive myo-inositol monophosphatase. Life Sci 54:1127–1142, 1994

Patishi Y, Belmaker RH, Agam G: Effects of age, sex, steroids, brain region, and genetic strain on brain inositol monophosphatase activity. Biol Psychiatry 40:656–659, 1996a

Patishi Y, Belmaker RH, Bersudsky Y, et al: A comparison of the ability of myo-inositol and epi-inositol to attenuate lithium-pilocarpine seizures in rats. Biol Psychiatry 39:829–832, 1996b

Patishi Y, Lubrich B, Merger M, et al: Differential uptake of myo-inositol in vivo into rat brain areas. Eur Neuropsychopharmacol 6:73–75, 1996c

Pollack SJ, Knowles MR, Atack JR, et al: Probing the role of metal ions in the mechanism of inositol monophosphatase by site-directed mutagenesis. Eur J Biochem 217:281–287, 1993

Pollack SJ, Atack JR, Knowles MR, et al: Mechanism of inositol monophosphatase, the putative target of lithium therapy. Proc Natl Acad Sci U S A 91:5766–5770, 1994

Post RM, Frye MA, Denicoff KD, et al: Beyond lithium in the treatment of bipolar illness. Neuropsychopharmacology 19:206–219, 1998

Ragan CI, Watling KJ, Gee NS, et al: The dephosphorylation of inositol 1,4-bisphosphate to inositol in liver and brain involves two distinct Li^+-sensitive enzymes and proceeds via inositol 4-phosphate. Biochem J 249:143–148, 1988

Richards MH, Belmaker RH: Epi-inositol is biochemically active in reversing lithium effects on cytidine monophosphorylphosphatidate (CMP-PA). J Neural Transm 103:1281–1285, 1996

Schou M, Juel-Nielsen N, Stromgren E, et al: The treatment of manic psychoses by the administration of lithium salts. J Neurol Neurosurg Psychiatry 17:250–260, 1954

Shamir A, Ebstein RP, Nemanov L, et al: Inositol monophosphatase in immortalized lymphoblastoid cell lines indicates susceptibility to bipolar disorder and response to lithium therapy. Mol Psychiatry 3:481–482, 1998

Sherman WR: Inositol homeostasis, lithium and diabetes, in Inositol Lipids in Cell Signalling. Edited by Michell RH, Drummond AH, Downes CP. London, Academic Press, 1989, pp 39–79

Shimon H, Agam G, Belmaker RH, et al: Reduced inositol levels in frontal cortex of post-mortem brain from bipolar patients and suicides. Am J Psychiatry 154:1148–1150, 1997

Sjoholt G, Molven A, Lovlie R, et al: Genomic structure and chromosomal localization of a human myo-inositol monophosphatase gene (IMPA). Genomics 45:113–122, 1997

Snyder SH: Second messengers and affective illness—focus on the phosphoinositide cycle. Pharmacopsychiatry 25:25–28, 1992

Soares JC, Gershon S: The lithium ion: a foundation for psychopharmacological specificity. Neuropsychopharmacology 19:167–182, 1998

Soares JC, Mallinger AG: Abnormal phosphatidylinositol (PI)-signalling in bipolar disorder. Biol Psychiatry 39:461–462, 1996

Soares JC, Mallinger AG, Dippold CS, et al: Platelet membrane phospholipids in euthymic bipolar disorder patients: are they affected by lithium treatment? Biol Psychiatry 45:453–457, 1999

Stambolic V, Ruel L, Woodgett JR: Lithium inhibits glycogen synthase kinase-3 activity and mimics Wingless signalling in intact cells. Curr Biol 6:1664–1668, 1996

Steen VM, Gulbrandsen A-K, Eiken HG, et al: Lack of genetic variation in the coding region of the *myo*-inositol monophosphatase gene in lithium-treated patients with manic depressive illness. Pharmacogenetics 6:113–116, 1996

Steen V, Lovlie R, Osher Y, et al: The polymorphic inositol polyphosphate 1-phosphatase gene as a candidate for the pharmacogenetic prediction of lithium-responsive manic-depressive illness. Pharmacogenetics 8:259–268, 1998

Stubbs EB, Agranoff BW: Lithium enhances muscarinic receptor-stimulated CDP-diacylglycerol formation in inositol-depleted SK-N-SH neuroblastoma cells. J Neurochem 60:1292–1299, 1993

Tricklebank MD, Singh L, Oles RJ: Evidence that a proconvulsant action of lithium is mediated by inhibition of myo-inositol phosphatase in mouse brain. Brain Res 558:145–148, 1991

Vadnal R, Heng HHQ, Parthasarathy L, et al: Human chromosomal localization of a gene for inositol monophosphatase by fluorescence in situ hybridization. NeuroReport 9:683–685, 1998

van Calker D, Förstner U, Bohus M, et al: Increased sensitivity to agonist stimulation of the Ca^{2+} response in neutrophils of manic-depressive patients: effect of lithium therapy. Neuropsychobiology 27:180–183, 1993

Weiner ML: Overview of lithium toxicology, in Lithium in Biology and Medicine. Edited by Schrauzer GN, Klippel K-F. Weinheim, Germany, VCH, 1991, pp 81–99

Whitworth P, Heal DJ, Kendall DA: The effects of acute and chronic lithium treatment on pilocarpine-stimulated phosphoinositide hydrolysis in mouse brain in vivo. Br J Pharmacol 101:39–44, 1990

Williams MB, Jope RS: Modulation by inositol of cholinergic- and serotonergic-induced seizures in lithium treated rats. Brain Res 685:169–178, 1995

Wood AJ, Goodwin GM: A review of the biochemical and neuropharmacological actions of lithium. Psychol Med 17:579–600, 1987

Worley PJ, Baraban JM, Snyder SH: Inositol 1,4,5-trisphosphate receptor binding: autoradiographic localization in rat brain. J Neurosci 9:339–346, 1989

Wreggett KA: Inositol monophosphatase is a highly conserved enzyme having localized structural similarity to both glycerol 3-phosphate dehydrogenase and haemoglobin. Biochem J 286:147–152, 1992

York JD, Chen Z-W, Ponder JW, et al: Crystallization and initial X-ray crystallographic characterization of recombinant bovine inositol polyphosphate 1-phosphatase produced in *Spodoptera frugiperda* cells. J Mol Biol 236:584–589, 1994

Zhang Y, Liang J-Y, Huang S, et al: Crystallographic studies of the catalytic mechanism of the neutral form of fructose-1,6-bisphosphatase. Biochemistry 32:1844–1857, 1993a

Zhang Y, Liang J-L, Lipscomb WN: Structural similarities between fructose-1,6-bisphosphatase and inositol monophosphatase. Biochem Biophys Res Commun 190:1080–1083, 1993b

CHAPTER 2

HUMAN EVIDENCE OF THE ROLE OF INOSITOL IN BIPOLAR DISORDER AND ANTIBIPOLAR TREATMENT

Galila Agam, Ph.D., and Hady Shimon, M.Sc.

Allison and Stewart (1971) first reported that lithium reduces brain levels of inositol. Hallcher and Sherman (1980) showed that this reduction is due to inhibition of the enzyme inositol 1-monophosphatase (IMPase). The K_i of the inhibition is within the therapeutic range (K_i = 0.86 mM; Hallcher and Sherman 1980). Rats treated chronically with lithium show decline in brain inositol levels and buildup of 20- to 40-fold in the substrate, inositol monophosphate (Sherman et al. 1981). Berridge et al. (1989), as they described the widespread role of the phosphatidylinositol (PI) cycle as a second-messenger system, noted the possible psychiatric implications of lithium inhibition of IMPase. Berridge et al. (1982, 1989) suggested that lithium inhibits PI-derived second messengers of activated systems only, without interfering with basal function. This hypothesis was based on the fact that inositol, derived from inositol phosphate breakdown, is essential for the

---

In memory of Professor Avinoam A. Livne, with whom we began inositol monophosphatase research in Beersheba. We wish to thank Dr. Joel Kleinman and Dr. Thomas Hyde for use of material from their postmortem-brain bank. The skillful technical assistance of Dr. Joseph Shapiro and Mrs. Yelena Sobolev in plasma, cerebrospinal fluid, and brain inositol determination is gratefully acknowledged. We thank Professor R. H. Belmaker for critical comments on the manuscript.

resynthesis of PI (Downes et al. 1989). Overactive systems or overstimulated receptors would be dampened by lithium's depletion of the inositol pool available for resynthesis of the parent compound PI, whereas stable systems would be unaffected. This process provides a possible explanation of lithium's paucity of behavioral effects in psychiatrically healthy subjects and its powerful effects in mania and depression.

HUMAN IMPase

The inositol depletion hypothesis was based on animal data concerning the effects of lithium on IMPase. Our group had previously shown species differences in sensitivity of the adenylate cyclase enzyme to lithium inhibition (Belmaker 1981; Ebstein et al. 1976; Newman et al. 1983). We thus questioned whether lithium's effects on IMPase occur in human tissue and in patients after chronic treatment. It also seemed important to ask, if lithium inhibits IMPase, whether the enzyme is present in excessive activity in patients with bipolar disorder who were not treated with lithium. After demonstrating that human erythrocytes possess IMPase with properties (K_m for inositol 1-phosphate (Ins(1)P) and K_i for lithium) similar to those of other tissues in various species (Agam and Livne 1989), we studied the activity of human red blood cell IMPase in bipolar patients untreated with lithium, in psychiatrically healthy control subjects, and in lithium-treated patients with bipolar disorder (Moscovich et al. 1990).

The blood was taken into plastic tubes containing ethylene diaminetetra-acetic acid (EDTA), 1 mg/mL blood. IMPase was measured in fresh red blood cells within 3 hours of venipuncture. After one centrifugation (600 × *g* for 10 min) and aspiration of the plasma and buffy coat, the red blood cells were resuspended in a solution of 150 mM NaCl, 10 mM glucose, and 10 mM Tris-Mops at pH 7.4. Washed red blood cells were obtained by two additional cycles of centrifugation, aspiration, and resuspension in this medium.

IMPase activity was measured in lysates. These were obtained by the addition of 1 volume of a 10-fold concentrated buffer to 9 volumes of packed red blood cells to give a final concentration of 50 mM Tris-HCl, pH 8.0, 0.2 mM KCl, 0.1 mM EDTA, and 0.2% digitonin. Cell lysis was caused by the digitonin.

The reaction mixture for the measurement of IMPase activity contained, in a final volume of 200 μL, 0.7 mM Ins(1)P; 22.5 mM Tris-HCl, pH 7.8; 112.5 mM KCl; 1.35 mM $MgCl_2$, and 90 μL lysate. Incubation was carried out for 1 hour at 37° C, then 10 μL of 6.1 M solution trichloroacetic acid was added to stop the reaction. The mixture was centrifuged for 15 minutes at 20,000 × g at 2° C. Inorganic phosphate in the supernatant was then determined.

To distinguish IMPase activity from nonspecific phosphatases, the inhibition of IMPase activity by Li^+ was used. The phosphatase activity of the red blood cell lysate was measured in the presence and absence of 30 mM Li^+. The IMPase activity was calculated as the difference between these values. Enzyme activity was calculated per red cell (counted in an aliquot before lysis).

Table 2–1 shows the results. Untreated bipolar patients showed activity of IMPase no different from that of control subjects; however, patients treated with lithium at therapeutic concentrations in vivo had almost 80% inhibition of enzyme activity. This finding strengthened the hypothesis that IMPase inhibition could be related to the therapeutic mechanism of lithium in humans.

LITHIUM TREATMENT AND CEREBROSPINAL FLUID INOSITOL LEVELS

One problem with the inositol theory of lithium action is that the dose of lithium injected intraperitoneally necessary for reducing rat brain inositol by 30% is 10 mEq/kg, leading to a peak plasma level of 7.5 mM, far above therapeutic levels (Sherman et al. 1985a, 1985b). Injection of 3 mEq/kg LiCl, leading to

Table 2–1. Inositol monophosphatase activity in lithium-free manic patients, lithium-treated manic patients, and psychiatrically healthy subjects

Group	n	Age ± SD	Inositol monophosphatase activity[a] ± SD
Lithium-free manic patients	10	32 ± 11	5.75 ± 3.2
Lithium-treated manic patients	11	35 ± 11	1.28 ± 1.4[b]
Psychiatrically healthy subjects	9	39 ± 6	6.93 ± 2.7

[a]μmol Pi/10^{10} cells/h.
[b]$F = 14.3$, $P < 0.001$.
Source. Reprinted by permission of Elsevier Science from Moscovich D, Belmaker RH, Agam G, et al.: "Inositol-1-Phosphatase in RBC of Manic-Depressive Patients Before and During Treatment With Lithium." *Biological Psychiatry* 27:552–555, 1990. Copyright 1990 by The Society of Biological Psychiatry.

plasma levels that are therapeutic in humans, reduces rat brain inositol by less than 10%. Perhaps more important, chronic administration of 40 mM LiCl/kg food to rats, leading to therapeutic levels of 0.3–0.6 mM in cortex, lowered brain inositol by a variable percentage not more marked than the effect of a single intraperitoneal dose of 3 mM/kg LiCl. It thus seemed important to study whether lithium treatment in humans reduces cerebrospinal fluid (CSF) inositol levels. If IMPase is the therapeutic site of lithium action, measurement of the hypothesized CSF inositol level reduction could predict response to lithium in patients.

We studied schizophrenic patients willing to participate in a trial of lithium supplementation of ongoing neuroleptic therapy (Agam et al. 1993). None had previously participated in studies of inositol treatment of schizophrenia. All gave written informed consent. The protocol was approved by the hospital Helsinki Committee and the Ministry of Health.

Lithium treatment was given at 1,200 mg/day for 3 days to seven patients. All were males, mean age 42.7 (range 32–55), meeting the DSM-III-R (American Psychiatric Association 1987) criteria for schizophrenia. Lumbar puncture was performed by an experienced neurosurgeon on the morning before starting lithium treatment and on the morning of the fourth day, after a total of 3,600 mg lithium and 12 hours after the last lithium dose. Two additional male patients, ages 42 and 39, were treated with lithium at 1,200 mg/day for 7 days, and lumbar puncture was performed on the morning of the eighth day. Table 2–2 presents the results. Lithium treatment did not reduce CSF inositol levels in the seven patients treated for 3 days or in the two additional patients treated for 7 days.

The lack of effect of lithium treatment on CSF inositol levels appears at first surprising and attributable to methodological reasons, such as the short period of lithium treatment and the relatively low lithium levels achieved in the serum and the CSF. However, in rat studies, an acute large single dose of lithium rapidly reduces brain inositol levels as much as does chronic treatment (Sherman 1991). In the present study, the mean serum lithium level in the patients is 0.5 ±0.2 mM, within the lithium prophylactic therapeutic range, and CSF levels are about one-half to one-third of these levels, as usually expected.

It is possible that lithium did not reduce CSF inositol levels in the present study because CSF inositol derives mainly from the plasma via the choroid plexus (Spector and Lorenzo 1975), and lithium does not lower plasma inositol (Agam et al. 1995), as shown in a study in our laboratory. Moreover, brain inositol levels are about 50 times CSF inositol levels (Spector and Lorenzo 1975). Thus, brain cells must highly concentrate inositol, and lowered brain inositol concentrations might well not be reflected in CSF levels. Another explanation of the above results is that more than one pool of brain inositol ap-

Table 2–2. Human CSF inositol levels before and after lithium treatment

	Inositol (μg/mL)		Lithium (mmol/L)	
Patient no.	Before lithium	After lithium	CSF	Plasma
86	22.5	24.2	0.1	0.4
87	39.2	34.7	0.4	0.7
88	22.7	34.7	0.1	0.3
89	30.5	37.1	0.3	0.7
90	22.7	33.6	0.3	0.6
91	30.0	19.3	0.1	0.6
92	20.7	28.6	0.2	0.7
95	21.1	21.0	0.3	0.5
96	22.2	27.5	0.2	0.4
Mean ± SD	25.7 ± 6.2	27.7 ± 6.3	0.2 ± 0.1	0.5 ± 0.2

Note. CSF = cerebrospinal fluid; SD = standard deviation.
Source. Reprinted from Agam G, Shapiro J, Levine J, et al.: "Short-Term Lithium Treatment Does Not Reduce Human CSF Inositol Levels." *Lithium* 4:267–269, 1993. Used with permission.

pears to exist (Bersudsky et al. 1994; Shayman and Wu 1990) and CSF inositol may equilibrate with the osmolyte-relevant brain pool and not with the neurochemically relevant PI-cycle–related pool, which is more likely to be lowered by lithium inhibition of IMPase.

INOSITOL LEVELS IN POSTMORTEM HUMAN BRAIN

Somewhat paradoxically, in light of the theory that lithium reduces inositol levels, Barkai et al. (1978) reported that inositol is reduced in CSF in both bipolar and unipolar depressed patients. Levine et al. (1993a) gave inositol to 11 unipolar, medication-resistant depressed patients with dramatic results in 7 of the 11. Levine et al. (1995) then performed a controlled double-blind study of 28 depressed patients with 12 g of inositol or placebo for 4 weeks. Inositol treatment reduced Hamilton Rating Scale for Depression scores significantly more than placebo.

Kofman and Belmaker (1990) reported behavioral effects of inositol in rats. Levine et al. (1993b) reported that 12 g daily of inositol orally in humans increased CSF inositol by 70%. Agam et al. (1994) showed that high-dose peripheral inositol in rats could reverse brain effects of lithium on behavior.

These studies support a role for inositol in behavioral disorder. Rahman and Neuman (1993) found that neurophysiological effects of serotonin (5-hydroxytryptamine; 5-HT) on neurons rich in 5-HT_2 receptors could be augmented by inositol, a finding that suggests a connection between serotonergic theories of depression (Ohmori et al. 1992) and the above data on inositol treatment of depression.

We were able to measure inositol levels in postmortem brain specimens from patients with bipolar affective disorder, persons who had committed suicide, and psychiatrically healthy control subjects. Brain specimens in the NIMH brain collection were obtained at autopsy from the Washington, D.C., Medical Examiner's office. Psychiatric diagnosis was determined by independent review of medical records by at least two psychiatrists. After collection from autopsy, the brain tissue was dissected into 1-cm coronal slabs, which were individually frozen in isopentane cooled on dry ice (–40°C). Tissue blocks were stored at –70°C until dissection for this study.

Brain lithium levels were measured by using 100 mg of each sample and homogenization (Downes) in 1 mL of 10% (w/v) perchloric acid. The homogenates were centrifuged at 13,000× g for 30 minutes at room temperature. The entire supernatant was filled up to 5 mL with double-distilled water, and the samples were analyzed by flame-emission spectroscopy (Spectroflame "end on" plasma ICP, with a monochromator for 160–460 nm, and a 5-element polychromator, Spectro, Germany). Sample introduction was manual, through cross-flow nebulizer and glass spray chamber. Lithium was undetectable in all but three bipolar patients with levels of 0.35, 0.48, and 0.23 mmol/kg wet weight.

Human brain free *myo*-inositol levels were analyzed as trimethylsilyl (TMS) derivatives by gas-liquid chromatography, as previously described by Allison et al. (1976), with minor modification. Samples of tissue (approximately 50 mg) were dissected from the various brain areas, weighed, and extracted in 0.5 mL of boiling water containing 400 µg mannitol (as internal standard) for 5 minutes. The denatured tissue was spun down and 250 µL supernatant lyophilized (3-hour Speed Vac SC 110). Silylation of the dried sample was carried out with 200 µL of a mixture of pyridine:bis(TMS) trifluoroacetamide:chlorotrimethylsilan 10:2:1 (v/v/v) for 24 hours at room temperature. Then 2-µL aliquots were chromatographed on a 6-ft column packed with 3% SE-30 on 80/100 mesh gas chrome Q (Supelco), using a Carlo Erba SCU 600 gas chromatograph with a hydrogen flame ionization detector. The oven temperature was isothermal at 220°C, and the carrier gas was nitrogen with a flow of 120 mL/min. The TMS derivatives of mannitol and *myo*-inositol had retention times of 7 and 11 minutes, respectively. Quantitation was performed with the use of TMS derivatives of standard *myo*-inositol and mannitol under the same conditions. Standard curves were run daily, and linearity was verified at the beginning and periodically during the processing of the samples.

Table 2–3 shows the inositol results. Analysis of variance shows a significant difference between the groups for frontal cortex ($F = 3.83$, *df* 2/25, $P = 0.035$), but not for occipital cortex ($F = 1.8$, *df* 2/24, NS) or cerebellum ($F = 0.03$, *df* 2/21, NS). Post hoc *t* test for frontal cortex shows inositol level in frontal cortex of those who committed suicide significantly lower than that of control subjects ($P = 0.01$) and inositol level in frontal cortex of subjects with bipolar disorder significantly less than that of control subjects ($P = 0.01$). There was no significant correlation of age with frontal ($r = -0.06$), occipital ($r = -0.16$), or cerebellar ($r = -0.24$) inositol levels. There was no significant difference in frontal cortex inositol between women (6.7 ± 2.7) and men (7.9 ± 1.9), in occipital cortex inositol between women (7.1 ± 3.1) and men (8.3 ± 2.9), or in cerebellum inositol between women (7.4 ± 2.3) and men (8.4 ± 3.7).

These data suggest that persons with bipolar disorder and persons who committed suicide have a reduction in frontal cortical inositol levels compared with control subjects, with a similar but statistically nonsignificant trend in occipital cortex. Cerebellar inositol shows no difference between the clinical groups. Interestingly, cerebellum also shows no increase in Ins(1)P after lithium treatment (Allison et al. 1976), suggesting that cerebellar inositol may be less involved in neuronal PI-linked signal transduction and more related to osmolyte function. A recent study found that exogenously administered inositol is taken up by cortex, hippocampus, and hypothalamus but not by cerebellum (Patishi et al. 1996).

Inositol levels in the control subjects, about 9 mM, agree well with in vivo results by magnetic resonance spectroscopy (MRS) (Gruetter et al. 1992). Dixon et al. (1992) reported that primate brain inositol levels are 2 times higher than those in the rat. The standard deviation of inositol levels in these postmortem samples is similar in control subjects, in those who committed suicide, and in bipolar patients, suggesting that neither postmortem degradation nor agonal illness in a subgroup of patients is a critical factor in the reduced inositol levels. Moreover, the standard deviation is similar to that in cortex of freshly decapitated rat cortex (Spector and Lorenzo 1975).

Inositol levels do not clearly decline in the first 24 hours postmortem, in human brain covariance analysis (Shimon et al. 1997) or in the rat (Belmaker et al., in press). Inositol is not metabolizable in brain (Sherman 1991). These facts argue against postmortem effects as the cause of the finding of reduced frontal inositol levels. Inositol phosphates that could be metabolized to inositol postmortem are present in very small concentrations compared with

Table 2–3. Inositol levels in postmortem human brain specimens (mmol/kg wet weight)

Brain area and run of samples	Group		
	Bipolar	**Suicide**	**Control**
Frontal			
A	8.18	6.48	11.60
B	7.05	6.35	10.40
C	8.82	5.75	10.50
D	4.90	6.02	7.02
E	4.35	4.37	8.85
F	2.27	5.23	6.55
G	5.90	7.80	4.05
H	5.75	5.40	11.40
I	—	8.45	9.03
J	—	12.10	8.05
Mean ± SD	5.90 ± 2.12	6.74 ± 2.21	8.74 ± 2.39
Occipital			
A	11.20	10.80	7.00
B	7.24	5.55	6.35
C	6.95	5.30	8.15
D	5.55	5.77	9.25
E	—	5.40	12.50
F	1.77	7.65	6.55
G	8.10	9.25	10.8
H	6.05	3.15	16.50
I	—	9.65	9.48
J	—	6.66	4.20
Mean ± SD	6.69 ± 2.84	6.91 ± 2.37	9.08 ± 3.53
Cerebellum			
A	10.55	8.90	5.55
B	5.00	4.35	4.45
C	—	5.55	5.30
D	—	5.57	8.30
E	—	6.91	11.20
F	—	5.55	13.80
G	8.00	15.50	8.35
H	5.35	5.00	7.15
I	—	13.15	8.05
J	—	6.85	4.75
Mean ± SD	7.22 ± 2.58	7.72 ± 3.73	7.69 ± 2.98

Note. Empty cells mean that specimens were unavailable.

inositol (Sherman 1991) and are unlikely to be able to explain the clinical difference.

The pathophysiological implications of low frontal-cortex inositol are not clear. PI synthase may not be saturated at physiological levels of 10 mM inositol (K_m = 4.6 mM) (Ghalayini and Eichberg 1985). Several intracellular pools of inositol may exist (Bersudsky et al. 1994), and the reduction in frontal cortex may be specific to a pool critical for neuronal second-messenger function. Batty and Downes (1994, 1995) reported that inositol may regulate phospholipase C activity in a complex manner unrelated to levels of PI. If inositol levels do regulate PI concentration or phospholipase C activity, which breaks down PI in response to receptor stimulation, then low inositol levels could cause functionally deficient responses to one or more receptors linked to PI, such as 5-HT (Rahman and Neuman 1993).

Inositol functions as an important brain osmolyte (Thurston et al. 1989) and as a second-messenger precursor. Hyponatremia lowers brain inositol, and if those who committed suicide or patients with affective disorders were more likely to be hyponatremic for several days before death than those who were psychiatrically healthy, hyponatremia could artifactually lower brain inositol in the non–neurotransmitter-related pool. However, this effect would not be expected to distinguish between frontal cortex and other areas. Agonal diseases (Hardy et al. 1985) in these patients cannot be ruled out as a cause of the finding. Diabetic ketoacidosis (Kreis and Moss 1992) and Alzheimer's disease (Miller et al. 1993) have been reported to raise brain inositol. Hepatic encephalopathy markedly reduces brain inositol (Haussinger et al. 1994).

COMPARISON WITH MRS MEASUREMENTS OF BRAIN INOSITOL LEVELS

In view of the fact that postmortem brain studies have inherent methodological limitations (Palmer et al. 1988), one should consider that brain inositol can be measured in vivo by magnetic resonance imaging (MRI) (Gruetter et al. 1992). Various groups have used ^{1}H and/or ^{31}P MRS to study possible changes in *myo*-inositol and inositol monophosphate levels in experimental animals and humans. Using ^{1}H MRS, Preece et al. (1992) did not detect changes in *myo*-inositol concentrations following lithium in rats but did find changes in phosphomonoester (PME) by ^{31}P MRS. Kato and colleagues (1991, 1992, 1993) repeatedly reported elevated PME concentrations in patients with bipolar disorder who were in the manic state. Using both ^{1}H and ^{31}P MRS,

Silverstone et al. (1996) conducted a double-blind, placebo-controlled study in human volunteers and found that following chronic lithium administration there were no statistically significant changes either in brain *myo*-inositol concentrations or in concentrations of PME. However, Häussinger et al. (1994) concluded that the ^{1}H-MRS *myo*-inositol signal in the human brain predominantly reflects an osmosensitive inositol pool. Moreover, inositol monophosphates and glycine signals in ^{1}H MRS occur in the same peak as *myo*-inositol (Silverstone et al. 1996). Hence, if *myo*-inositol concentration decreases and Ins(1)P or glycine concentrations increase (Cerdan et al. 1985; Hirvonen 1991; Moats et al. 1993; Sherman et al. 1981), the net effect may be no overall change.

The PME peak includes 1) phosphoethanolamine, which makes the greatest contribution (Gyulai et al. 1984; Preece et al. 1992), 2) phosphocholine, and 3) sugar phosphates, which include the inositol monophosphates (Atack 1996). In view of the fact that, in experimental animals, lithium produces changes in a number of brain phospholipids, including phosphatidylethanolamine and phosphatidylcholine (Joseph et al. 1987; Navidi et al. 1991), the increase in PME levels cannot be attributed solely to inositol monophosphates. Hence, because PME levels appear to be independent of lithium treatment (Deicken et al. 1995a, 1995b; Kato et al. 1993), it may be concluded that altered PME levels in bipolar disorders are not associated with inositol monophosphates. Furthermore, the Ins(1)P brain concentration is 0.05–0.1 mM, whereas the ^{31}P MRS minimum concentration for detection is 0.5–1.0 mM. Thus, a 5- to 10-fold increase is needed to make it detectable. The measurability of changes in Ins(1)P concentrations by ^{31}P MRS in humans remains uncertain (Silverstone et al. 1996). The ^{31}P MRS method relies upon an assumption of equilibrium conditions and intracellular homogeneity—assumptions which may not be valid.

Two seemingly opposing pathophysiological concepts of inositol's relevance to mood disorders have been proposed: 1) Lithium treatment, which causes reduction in brain inositol level (Moore et al. 1998), is effective in affective disorder. 2) Brain inositol levels are reduced in bipolar patients and those who commit suicide; inositol treatment significantly improves depressed patients.

How can we reconcile the two concepts? It may be that lithium does not simply reduce inositol levels but that inositol is involved in a more complex manner in affective disorder and lithium action. Figures 2–1 and 2–2 depict the mechanism of a pendulum as a possible representation of the role of inositol in bipolar disorder. A mechanism of oscillation in signal transduction has already been suggested. Nishizuka (1992) points out that "activation of cell surface receptors often results in the generation of regular oscillation in the intracellular Ca^{2+} concentration" and suggests that "the activities of

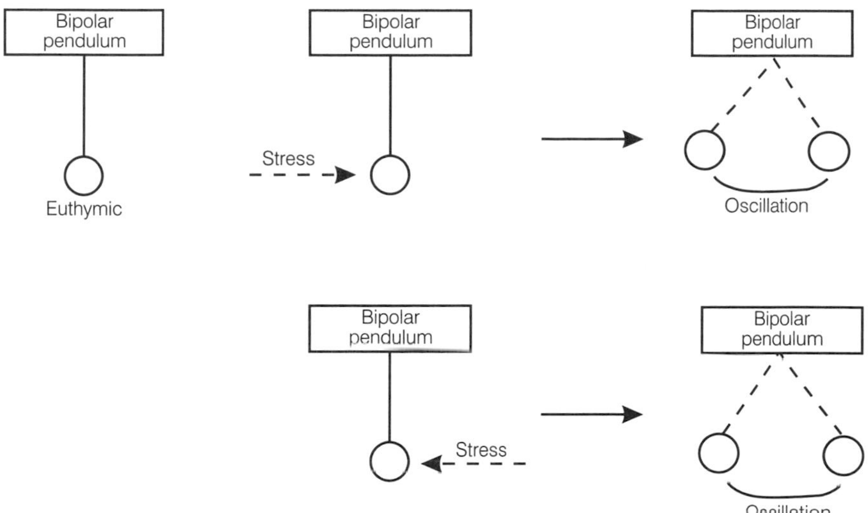

Figure 2–1. Bipolar pendulum: etiology.

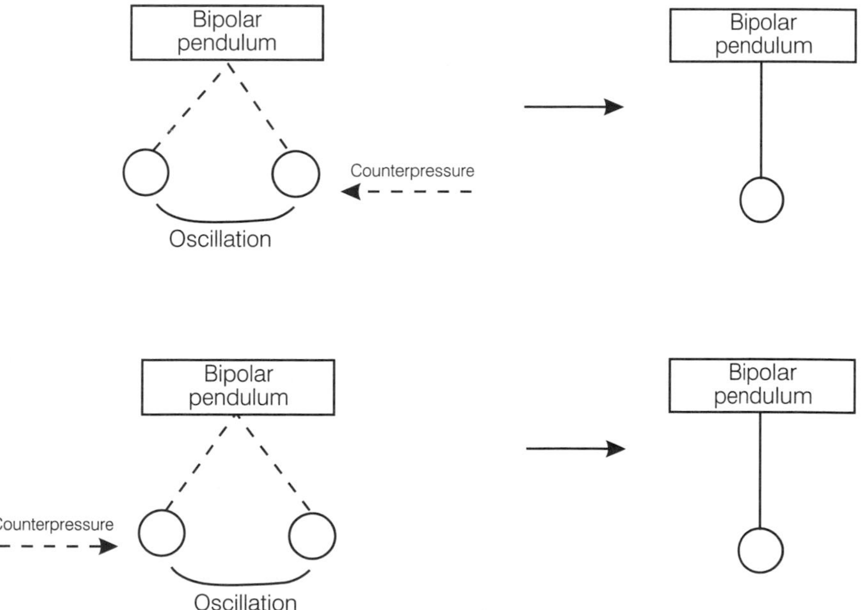

Figure 2–2. Bipolar pendulum: treatment.

phospholipases and PKC and the amounts of diacylglycerol and IP_3 must also be oscillating with a rate or pattern similar to that of Ca^{2+}" (p. 610). It might be that oscillation of inositol concentration also occurs.

Such nonlinear models may be more important in biology than has been traditionally thought.

REFERENCES

Agam G, Livne A: Inositol-1-phosphatase of human erythrocyte is inhibited by therapeutic Li^+ concentrations. Psychiatry Res 27:217–224, 1989

Agam G, Shapiro J, Levine J, et al: Short-term lithium treatment does not reduce human CSF inositol levels. Lithium 4:267–269, 1993

Agam G, Shapiro J, Bersudsky Y, et al: High-dose peripheral inositol raises brain inositol levels and reverses behavioral effects of inositol depletion by lithium. Pharmacol Biochem Behav 49:341–343, 1994

Agam G, Balfour N, Shapiro J, et al: Plasma inositol levels in lithium-treated manic-depressives, schizophrenics and controls. Human Psychopharmacology 10:311–314, 1995

Allison JH, Stewart MA: Reduced brain inositol in lithium-treated rats. Nature: New Biology 233:267–268, 1971

Allison JH, Blisner ME, Holland WM, et al: Increased *myo*-inositol-1-phosphate in lithium-treated rats. Biochem Biophys Res Commun 71:664–670, 1976

American Psychiatric Association: Diagnostic and Statistical Manual of Mental Disorders, 3rd Edition, Revised. Washington, DC, American Psychiatric Association, 1987

Atack JR: Response to a Letter to the Editor: are platelet and magnetic resonance spectroscopic changes indicative of altered PI signalling in bipolar disorder? Biol Psychiatry 39:462–469, 1996

Barkai IA, Dunner DL, Gross HA, et al: Reduced *myo*-inositol levels in cerebrospinal fluid from patients with affective disorder. Biol Psychiatry 13:65–72, 1978

Batty H, Downes CP: The inhibition of phosphoinositide synthesis and muscarinic-receptor-mediated phospholipase C activity by Li^+ as secondary, selective, consequences of inositol depletion in 1321N1 cells. Biochem J 297:529–537, 1994

Batty IH, Downes CP: The mechanism of muscarinic receptor-stimulated phosphatidylinositol re-synthesis in 1321N1 astrocytoma cells and its inhibition by Li^+ ions J Neurochem 65:2279–2289, 1995

Belmaker RH: Receptors, adenylate cyclase, depression and lithium. Biol Psychiatry 16:333–350, 1981

Belmaker RH, Agam G, van Calker D, et al: Behavioral reversal of lithium effects by four inositol isomers correlates perfectly with biochemical effects on the PI cycle; depletion by chronic lithium of brain inositol is specific to hypothalamus; and inositol levels may be abnormal in post-mortem brain for bipolar patients. Neuropsychopharmacology (in press)

Berridge MJ, Downes CP, Hanley MR: Lithium amplifies agonist-dependent phophatidylinositol responses in brain and salivary glands. Biochem J 206:587–595, 1982

Berridge MJ, Downes CP, Hanley MR: Neural and developmental action of lithium: a unifying hypothesis. Cell 59:411–419, 1989

Bersudsky Y, Shapiro J, Agam G, et al: Behavioral evidence for the existence of two pools of cellular inositol. Eur Neuropsychopharmacol 4:463–467, 1994

Cerdan S, Parrilla R, Santoro J, et al: ^{1}H NMR detection of cerebral *myo*-inositol. FEBS Lett 187:167–172, 1985

Deicken RF, Fein G, Weiner MW: Abnormal frontal lobe phosphorus metabolism in bipolar disorder. Am J Psychiatry 152:915–918, 1995a

Deicken RF, Weiner MW, Fein G: Decreased temporal lobe phosphomonoesters in bipolar disorder. J Affect Disord 33:195–199, 1995b

Dixon JF, Los GV, Hokin LE: Lithium enhances accumulation of [^{3}H]inositol radioactivity and mass of second messenger inositol 1,4,5-triphosphate in monkey cerebral cortex slices. J Neurochem 59:2332–2335, 1992

Downes CP, Hawkins PT, Stephens L: Identification of the stimulated reaction in intact cells, its substrate supply and the metabolism of inositol phosphates, in Inositol Lipids in Cell Signalling. Edited by Michell RH, Drummond AH, Downes CP. London, Academic Press, 1989, pp 3–38

Ebstein RP, Belmaker RH, Granhaus L, et al: Lithium inhibition of adrenaline-sensitive adenylate cyclase in humans. Nature 259:411–413, 1976

Ghalayini A, Eichberg J: Purification of phosphatidylinositol synthetase from rat brain by CDP-diacylglycerol affinity chromatography and properties of the purified enzyme. J Neurochem 44:175–182, 1985

Gruetter R, Rothman DJ, Novotny EJ, et al: Localized ^{13}C NMR spectroscopy of *myo*-inositol in human brain in vivo. Magn Reson Med 25:204–210, 1992

Gyulai L, Bolinger L, Leigh JS, et al: Phosphorylethanolamine—the major constituent of the phosphomonoester peak observed by ^{31}P-NMR on developing dog brain. FEBS Lett 178:137–142, 1984

Hallcher LM, Sherman WR: The effect of lithium ion and other agents on the activity of *myo*-inositol-1-phosphatase from bovine brain. J Biol Chem 255:10896–10901, 1980

Hardy JA, Wester P, Winblad B, et al: Patients dying after long terminal phase have acidotic brains; implications for biochemical measurements on autopsy tissue. J Neural Transm 61:253–264, 1985

Häussinger D, Laubenberger J, Dahl V, et al: Proton magnetic resonance spectroscopy studies on human brain *myo*-inositol in hypo-osmolarity and hepatic encephalopathy. Gastroenterology 107:1475–1480, 1994

Hirvonen MR: Cerebral lithium, inositol and inositol monophosphates. Pharmacol Toxicol 69:22–27, 1991

Joseph NE, Renshaw PF, Leigh JS: Systemic lithium administration alters rat cerebral cortex phospholipids. Biol Psychiatry 22:540–544, 1987

Kato T, Shioiri T, Takahashi S, et al: Measurement of brain phosphoinositide metabolism in bipolar patients using in vivo ^{31}P-MRS. J Affect Disord 22:185–190, 1991

Kato T, Takahashi S, Shioiri T, et al: Brain phosphorus metabolism in depressive disorders by phosphorus-31 magnetic resonance spectroscopy. J Affect Disord 26:223–230, 1992

Kato T, Takahashi S, Shioiri T, et al: Alterations in brain phosphorus metabolism in bipolar disorder detected by in vivo ^{31}P and ^{7}Li magnetic resonance spectroscopy. J Affect Disord 27:53–60, 1993

Kofman O, Belmaker RH: Intracerebroventricular *myo*-inositol antagonizes lithium induced suppression of rearing behaviour in rats. Brain Res 534:345–347, 1990

Kreis R, Moss BD: Cerebral metabolic disturbances in patients with subacute and chronic diabetes mellitus: detection with proton MR spectroscopy. Radiology 184:123–130, 1992

Levine J, Gonzalves M, Barbam I, et al: Inositol 6 gm daily may be effective in depression but not in schizophrenia. Human Psychopharmacology 8:49–53, 1993a

Levine J, Rapaport A, Lev L, et al: Inositol treatment raises CSF inositol levels. Brain Res 627:168–170, 1993b

Levine J, Barak Y, Gonsalves M, et al: A double-blind controlled trial of inositol treatment of depression. Am J Psychiatry 152:792–794, 1995

Miller BL, Moats RA, Shonk T, et al: Alzheimer disease: depiction of increased cerebral *myo*-inositol with proton MR spectroscopy. Radiology 187:433–437, 1993

Moats RA, Lien YH, Filippi D, et al: Decrease in cerebral inositols in rats and humans. Biochem J 295:15–18, 1993

Moore GJ, Bebchuk JM, Faulk MW, et al: Longitudinal study of regional brain choline and myo-inositol during lithium therapy in manic depressive illness (abstract). Presented at meeting of American College of Nuclear Physicians, Puerto Rico, 1998

Moscovich D, Belmaker RH, Agam G, et al: Inositol-1-phosphatase in RBC of manic-depressive patients before and during treatment with lithium. Biol Psychiatry 27:552–555, 1990

Navidi M, Yoa FG, Sun GY: Brief chronic effects of lithium administration on rat brain phosphoinositides and phospholipids. J Neurosci Res 28:428–433, 1991

Newman M, Klein E, Birmaher B, et al: Lithium at therapeutic concentrations inhibits human brain noradrenaline-sensitive cyclic AMP accumulation. Brain Res 278:380–381, 1983

Nishizuka Y: Intracellular signaling by hydrolysis of phospholipids and activation of protein kinase C. Science 258:607–614, 1992

Ohmori T, Arora C, Meltzer HY: Serotonergic measures in suicide brain: the concentration of 5-HIAA, HVA and tryptophan in frontal cortex of suicide victims. Biol Psychiatry 32:57–71, 1992

Palmer AM, Lowe SL, Francis PT, et al: Are post-mortem biochemical studies of human brain worth-while? Biochem Soc Trans 16:472–475, 1988

Patishi Y, Lubrich B, Berger M, et al: Differential uptake of *myo*-inositol in vivo into rat brain areas. Eur Neuropsychopharmacol 6:73–75, 1996

Preece NE, Gadian DG, Houseman J, et al: Lithium-induced modulation of cerebral inositol phosphate metabolism in the rat: a multinuclear magnetic resonance study in vivo. Lithium 3:287–297, 1992

Rahman S, Neuman RS: *myo*-Inositol reduces serotonin (5-HT_2) receptor induced homologous and heterologous desensitization. Brain Res 631:349–351, 1993

Shayman JA, Wu D: *myo*-Inositol does not modulate PI turnover in MDCK cells under hyperosmolar conditions. Am J Physiol 258:1282–1287, 1990

Sherman WR: Lithium and the phosphoinositide signalling system, in Lithium and the Cell: Pharmacology and Biochemistry. Edited by Birch NJ. London, Academic Press, 1991, pp 121–157

Sherman WR, Leavitt AL, Honchar MP, et al: Evidence that lithium alters phosphoinositide metabolism: chronic administration elevates primarily D-*myo*-inositol-1-phosphate in cerebral cortex of the rat. J Neurochem 36:1947–1951, 1981

Sherman WR, Honchar MP, Munsell LY: Detection of receptor-linked phosphoinositide metabolism in brain of lithium treated rats, in Inositol and Phosphoinositides: Metabolism and Regulation. Edited by Bleasdale JE, Eichborg J, Hauser C. Clifton, NJ, Humana Press, 1985a, pp 49–65

Sherman WR, Munsell LY, Gish BG, et al: Effects of systemically administered lithium on phosphoinositide metabolism in rat brain, kidney and testis. J Neurochem 44:798–807, 1985b

Shimon H, Agam G, Belmaker RH, et al: Reduced inositol levels in frontal cortex of post-mortem brain from bipolar patients and suicides. Am J Psychiatry 154: 1148–1150, 1997

Silverstone PH, Hanstock CC, Fabian J, et al: Chronic lithium does not alter human *myo*-inositol or phosphomonoester concentrations as measured by ^{1}H and ^{31}P MRS. Biol Psychiatry 40:235–246, 1996

Spector R, Lorenzo AV: Myo-inositol transport in the central nervous system. Am J Physiol 228(5):1510–1518, 1975

Thurston JH, Sherman WR, Hauhart RE, et al: *myo*-Inositol: a newly identified nonnitrogenous osmoregulatory molecule in mammalian brain. Pediatr Res 26:482–485, 1989

CHAPTER 3

THE BRAIN POLYAMINE–STRESS RESPONSE

Development, Recurrence After Repetitive Stressor, and Inhibition by Lithium

Gad M. Gilad, Ph.D., and Varda H. Gilad, Ph.D.

It has been long known that persistent exposure to stressors predisposes vulnerable individuals to affective disorders and exacerbates the symptoms in those who are already affected (Caldecott-Hazard et al. 1991; Gold et al. 1988a, 1988b). As with the general adaptation (stress) syndrome that elicits characteristic behavioral, physiological, and neuroendocrine changes in the affected organism (Selye 1936), so do individual cells respond to life-threatening stressful stimuli by activating, via second-messenger systems, a general intracellular "stress program." The inductive expression of a universal set of stress proteins (Hightower 1991) and increased polyamine (PA) biosynthesis (i.e., the PA response) (Gilad and Gilad 1992) are considered integral components of this stress program.

A rapid but short-lasting transient increase (hours), due to stringent control of the expression of PA-metabolizing enzymes, is the inherent characteristic of the PA response (Tabor and Tabor 1984), and this mode is apparently

This work was supported in part by grants from the German-Israeli Foundation for Scientific Research and Development, the Israel Science Foundation, and the Stanley Foundation.

essential for the positive role of PAs in cellular functions (Gilad and Gilad 1992). In the adult mammalian brain, however, traumatic stress can lead to an incomplete PA response, with persistent accumulation of putrescine (Gilad and Gilad 1992). The fact that the concentrations of the PAs spermidine and spermine in the brain are relatively high, whereas putrescine, the diamine precursor of PAs, is normally low (Seiler and Bolkenius 1985), may suggest that a persistent stress-induced accumulation of putrescine may be harmful (Gilad and Gilad 1992; Paschen et al. 1988). This anomaly in brain PA metabolism may occur during maturation as a result of an altered pattern of gene expression and/or restrictive compartmentalization of the key metabolizing enzymes and their precursors (Gilad and Gilad 1992). Proper regulation of brain PA metabolism, therefore, may be critical for an appropriate response to stressors.

Lithium, the smallest alkali metal cation, is the most efficacious treatment known for bipolar disorder. We demonstrated that, unlike peripheral tissues, the stress-induced PA response in the brain of rats can be prevented by chronic, but not by acute, treatment with lithium (Gilad et al. 1992). This led us to hypothesize that prevention of a maladaptive stress-induced PA response in the brain, may be an important mechanism of lithium's action in the prophylactic treatment of bipolar disorder (Gilad et al. 1992).

The purpose of the series of studies discussed in this chapter was to further characterize the stress-induced PA response and its modulation by lithium in the brain, with the general goal of gaining new knowledge on the biological substrates of bipolar disorder. The experiments had two specific aims.

The first aim was based on the premise that in animals, chronic application of uncontrollable stressors may best approximate stressful life events in humans that exacerbate affective disorders (see Anisman and Zacharko 1990). Accordingly, we sought to characterize the effects of chronic stress application on the PA response in the brain and periphery (liver) and to elucidate how this response is modulated by chronic lithium treatment.

The second aim was based on the fact that an important characteristic of affective disorders is their age dependency, a phenomenon that may be correlated with the regulation and maturation of the hypothalamic-pituitary-adrenocortical (HPA) neuroendocrine system (Goodwin and Jamison 1990). In laboratory rodents, immature individuals undergo a *stress-hyporesponsive period* characterized by a diminished response of the HPA system to stressors (Sapolsky and Meaney 1986). The biochemical mechanisms in the brain that regulate this developmental process and the switch to a stress-responsive system are unclear. It was, therefore, important to characterize the ontogenesis of the brain PA–stress response, and to elucidate any developmental changes that may correspond to the maturation of the HPA stress response.

MATERIALS AND METHODS

Principles of the Study

The experimental design is schematically illustrated in Figure 3–1. All measurements were done 6 hours after the last application of stressor (i.e., 6 hours after dexamethasone or saline injections, and 6 hours after the beginning of restraint stress; Figure 3–1A). For chronic-intermittent-restraint stress experiments, groups of five adult (3-month-old) male rats were used (Figure 3–1B).

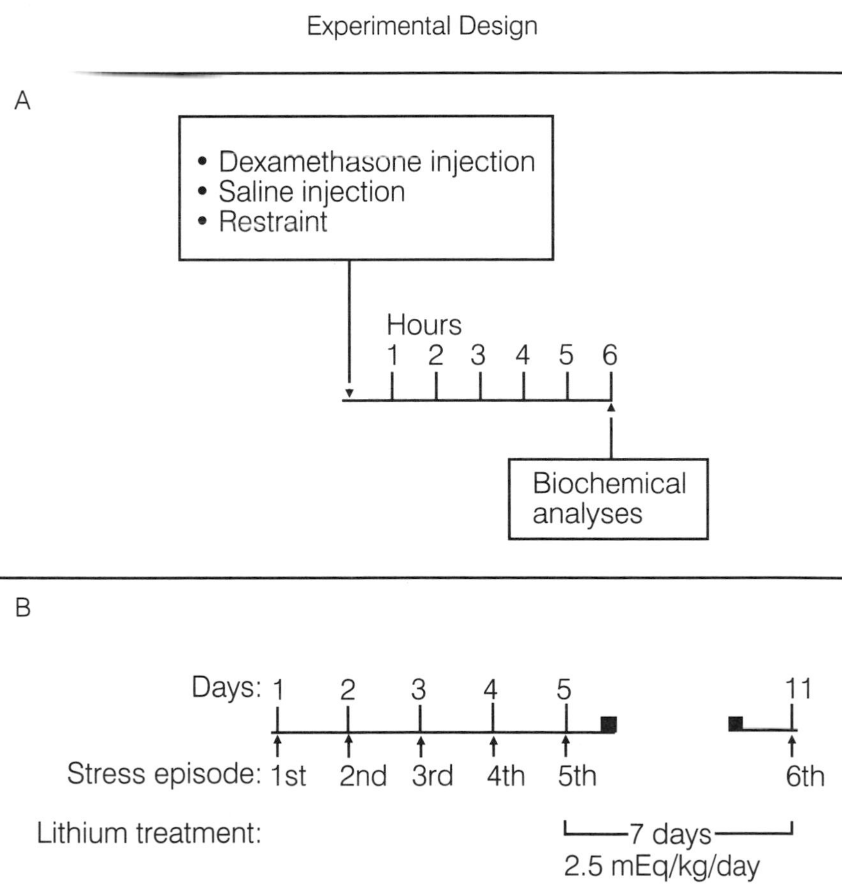

Figure 3–1. The experimental design, illustrating the regimens of (A) acute and (B) chronic stressors, and the time lag for biochemical analyses (A).

They were subjected to one session of restraint stress daily, and one group served for measurements after each stress episode. The last group underwent five daily stress sessions and after a resting period of 7 days was subjected to an additional stress episode. Two additional groups were subjected to an experimental paradigm similar to that for the last group, but during the 7-day resting period between stress sessions, one group received daily injections of 2.5 mEq/kg (106 mg/kg) LiCl, and the other saline (0.9% NaCl). Control animals were left undisturbed in their home cages (unhandled).

Lithium content in the brain, as measured by atomic absorption (Roche Biomedical Laboratories) 6 hours after the last of 7 injections, was 0.7 ±0.2 mM/kg wet weight. This value corresponds to the therapeutic range of plasma levels in human patients maintained on chronic lithium for treatment of bipolar disorder (Goodwin and Jamison 1990; Schou 1957).

In developmental experiments, animals were subjected to a single restraint stress session or to a single dexamethasone injection. Dexamethasone is a synthetic analogue of the stress hormones glucocorticoids and is commonly used to study the stress-induced effects of glucocorticoids. Unhandled animals served as control subjects in the stress experiments, and saline-injected animals served as control subjects in the dexamethasone experiments.

Changes in the two key PA-synthesizing enzymes, ornithine decarboxylase (ODC) and S-adenosylmethionine decarboxylase (SAM-DC) served as markers of the PA-stress response. The enzyme ODC catalyzes the formation of putrescine in the first and rate-limiting step of PA biosynthesis, and SAM-DC catalyzes the formation of the propylamino group needed for the generation of the higher PAs, spermidine and spermine (Tabor and Tabor 1984). The effects of stressors were measured in the hippocampus and striatum—two brain regions known for their response to stressful stimuli (Gilad et al. 1990, 1992)—and in the liver—a peripheral organ long known for its response to stress hormones (Panko and Kenney 1971).

Animals and Treatments

The experiments were done with male Sprague-Dawley rats. They were kept in a temperature-, humidity-, and light-controlled room with a free supply of food and water, in accordance with National Institutes of Health (NIH) guidelines. A dam and her litter of 10 pups were housed in individual cages. Pups were chosen randomly and after treatments were returned to their original home cages for the remainder of the period. Weaning was at age 21 days.

For restraint stress, rats were placed for 2 hours in Plexiglas restrainers adapted to the animal size. Restraint stress was applied daily between 8:30 and 10:30 A.M.

For drug treatments, dexamethasone 21-phosphate (3 mg/kg) was administered by intraperitoneal injection and LiCl (2.5 mmol/kg) by subcutaneous injection.

Tissue Dissection

Six hours after stressor application (Figure 3–1A), the animals were decapitated, and tissues were rapidly dissected on a metal block over ice as reported previously (Gilad et al. 1990), frozen on solid CO_2, and stored at −70°C.

Enzyme Activity Assays

The dissected tissues were homogenized in 5 volumes of ice-cold 50-mM Tris-HCl buffer, pH 7.5, containing 5 mM dithiothreitol, either with or without 40 μM pyridoxal-5′-phosphate for ODC or SAM-DC, respectively.

The activities of ODC and SAM-DC were measured in the tissue homogenates, according to established assays, by the $^{14}CO_2$ evolving method (Gilad and Kopin 1979).

Statistical Analysis

Following analyses of variance (ANOVAs), nonparametric tests (routinely Tukey's post hoc test) were performed; differences were considered significant when $P \leq 0.05$. The data were normalized and group differences expressed as a percentage of control animals.

RESULTS

Effects of Chronic-Intermittent-Restraint Stress in Adults

In the hippocampus, ODC activity increased repeatedly after each daily stress episode to about 150%–175% of control animals (Figure 3–2). In contrast, SAM-DC activity was slightly reduced after the first episode (86% of control

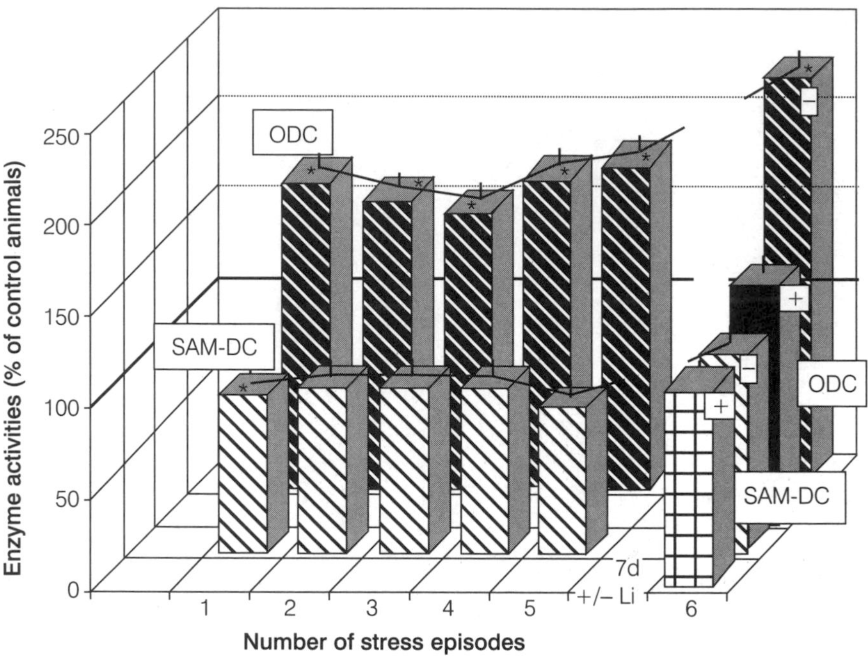

Figure 3–2. Effects of chronic-intermittent-restraint stress on ornithine decarboxylase (ODC) and S-adenosylmethionine decarboxylase (SAM-DC) activities in the hippocampus of adult rats treated with LiCl (+) or with saline (–) during the 7-day interval between the last two stress episodes. Results, mean (±SEM) values of five animals, are expressed as the percentage of unhandled control animals. Control values were 4.1 ± 0.3 pmol/mg protein/h for ODC and 14.7 ± 1.0 nmol/mg protein/h for SAM-DC activity. $^{*}P < 0.01$.

animals), but there were no significant changes thereafter (Figure 3–2).

Although daily restraint stress episodes resulted in a recurring increase of ODC activity in the brain, reaching a similar magnitude again and again, the enzyme activity in the liver was increased only after the first stress episode and remained relatively unchanged thereafter (Figure 3–3).

Effects of a Delayed Stress Episode

After cessation of the repetitive stress session, an additional stress episode 7 days later induced a higher increase in ODC activity (225% of control rats) without a change in SAM-DC activity in the brain (Figure 3–2). After the same experimental paradigm, ODC activity in the liver remained unchanged (Figure 3–3).

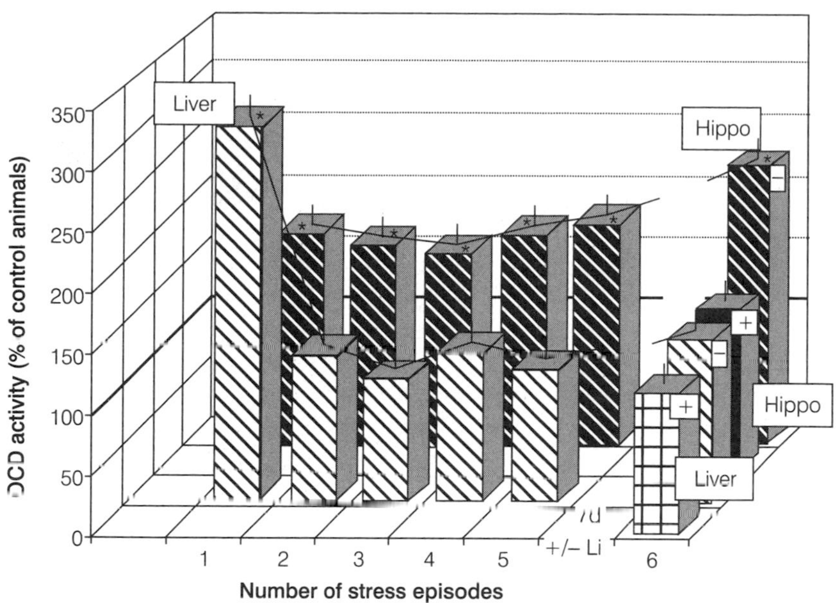

Figure 3–3. Effects of chronic-intermittent-restraint stress on ornithine decarboxylase (ODC) activity in the hippocampus (Hippo) and liver of adult rats treated with LiCl (+) or with saline (–) during the 7-day interval between the last two stress episodes. Results, mean (±SEM) of five animals, are expressed as the percentage of unhandled control subjects. Control values of ODC activity in the hippocampus and liver were 4.1 ± 0.3 and 34.5 ± 3.5 pmol/mg protein/h, respectively. $^{*}P < 0.01$.

Effects of Lithium Treatment

The enhanced ODC increase in the hippocampus after the delayed stress episode was blocked by lithium treatment during the 7-day between-stress interval (Figure 3–3). This lithium treatment had no effect on hippocampal SAM-DC activity (Figure 3–2) or on ODC activity in the liver (Figure 3–3).

Effects of Dexamethasone or Stress During Development

After a single dexamethasone injection, ODC activity in the hippocampus of 10-day-old rats was reduced to 60% of control (Figure 3–4). At age 15 days the activity remained unchanged, and at 30 days it was increased to about 200% of controls (Figure 3–4). In the striatum, however, ODC activity remained at control levels at age 10 days, but it was increased after dexamethasone to about 150% of controls by age 15 days and to about 180% of controls at age 30 days (Figure 3–4).

The activity of SAM-DC in the hippocampus remained unchanged at all ages examined after dexamethasone injection (results not shown).

In contrast, after a single restraint-stress episode, ODC activity in the hippocampus of 10-day-old rats did not change, and it was increased in 60-day-old rats, as expected (Table 3–1). The activity of SAM-DC was not significantly changed after restraint stress at both ages (Table 3–1).

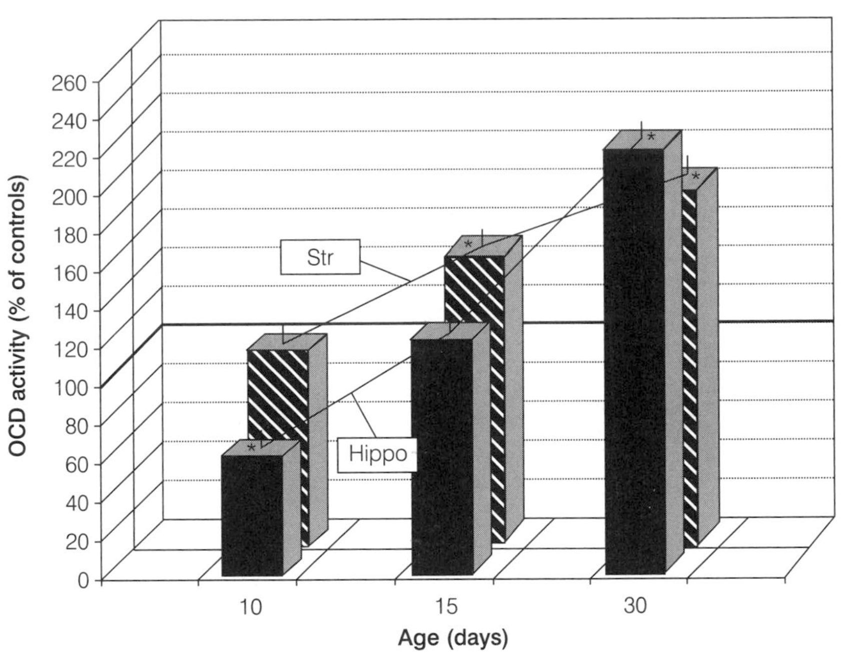

Figure 3–4. Effects of a single dexamethasone injection at different developmental ages on ornithine decarboxylase (ODC) activity in the hippocampus (Hippo) and striatum (Str). Results, mean (±SEM) values of five animals, are expressed as the percentage of saline-injected control rats. Control values of ODC activity (pmol/mg protein/h) in the hippocampus were 14.8 ±2.0, 7.0 ±1.0, and 4.5 ±0.5 at 10, 15, and 30 days, respectively. The values in the striatum were 8.3 ±1.5, 5.0 ±0.7, and 3.2 ±0.3 at 10, 15, and 30 days, respectively. *$P < 0.01$.

Table 3–1. Effect of restraint stress on hippocampal ODC (pmol/mg protein/h) and SAM-DC (nmol/mg protein/h) activities in 10- and 60-day old rats

	ODC			SAM-DC		
Age (days)	**Control**	**Stress**	**% Change**	**Control**	**Stress**	**% Change**
10	15.5 ±2.0	14.5 ±2.0	93.5	3.5 ±0.5	3.1 ±0.5	88.6
60	4.5 ±1.0	8.0 ±1.5	177.8*	15.5 ±1.5	13.2 ±2.0	85.2

Note. ODC = ornithine decarboxylase; SAM-DC = S-adenosylmethionine decarboxylase.
*$P < 0.01$.

DISCUSSION

The PA Response in Chronic Stress and the Effect of Lithium

The results show that daily restraint-stress episodes repetitively induce an increase in brain ODC activity that reaches a similar magnitude again and again. This recurring PA response is unique to the brain, because similar intermittent stress fails to cause a recurrent increase in ODC activity after the first stress episode. Furthermore, after the cessation of the repetitive stress session, an additional stress episode, applied with a delay of 7 days, leads again to increased ODC activity in the brain but not in the liver. The stress-induced increases are unique to ODC, because SAM-DC activity was not altered by stress but rather showed a tendency toward reduction.

Thus, with regard to changes in ODC activity, prior inescapable stressful experience may "condition" both the liver and the brain, but in different manners. In the liver, the experience of a single stress episode leads to a long period of lack of response to subsequent stress applications. In contrast, the hippocampal region of the brain responds repetitively to recurring stress episodes, then expresses an enhanced response when confronted again with the stressor after a time lag.

The influence of prior exposure to a chronic stressor on the response to a subsequent stress application was extensively studied in the peripheral neuroendocrine system (Armario et al. 1988; Cox et al. 1985; Kvetnansky et al. 1979) and in the central noradrenergic system (Nisenbaum et al. 1991; Pol et al. 1992). The neuroendocrine and behavioral response has been termed *adaptation* or *habituation*, and cross-adaptation to different types of stressors may occur (Armario et al. 1988; Weiss et al. 1975). The changes in ODC activity in the liver exemplify such an adaptive response to stress-induced neuroendocrine changes in a peripheral organ, reflected at the molecular biochemical level.

However, behavioral adaptation and cross-adaptation to stressors, especially uncontrollable stressors, may not be of survival advantage, but may be associated with depressive symptoms (Willner 1990). Indeed, such adaptation is not the general rule (Prince and Anisman 1984; Rosellini and Seligman 1977; Willner 1990). It is assumed that specific biochemical mechanisms, which we term the *cellular stress program*, must underlie the ability of the brain to control the behavioral response to chronic stressors. The unique stress-induced PA response in the brain is considered an integral component of this stress program (Gilad and Gilad 1992). Thus, as observed in this chapter, the brain is able to reactivate its PA response to the stressor repeatedly. In this regard, the brain PA response appears to be a unique component of a coordinated cellular stress program, as the expression of another stress protein, *c-fos*, is diminished following repetitive immobilization stress (Umemoto et al. 1994).

It has been long known that persistent exposure to stressors predisposes vulnerable individuals to affective disorders and exacerbates symptoms in those who are already affected (Caldecott-Hazard et al. 1991; Gold et al. 1988a, 1988b). This inability to cope with persistent stressful stimuli may reflect an overactive PA response that, in turn, leads to maladaptive brain response to stressful events. Therefore, the observation that long-term lithium treatment can block the enhanced ODC response after a delayed stress episode is extremely interesting.

How does lithium exert its effect? Lithium does not interfere directly with the activity of PA-metabolizing enzymes (Gilad et al. 1992; Matsui and Pegg 1980; Richards et al. 1990). Therefore, lithium must act on the intact cell and interfere with the generation of intracellular "stress signal(s)" that turn on the PA response—probably at the transcriptional or posttranscriptional levels, although posttranslational changes may also be involved (Obayashi et al. 1992). The putative cellular sites of lithium-PA interactions are illustrated in Figure 3–5. Lithium has been implicated in the regulation of several signal transduction systems (Berridge et al. 1989; Jope and Williams 1994; Lachman and Papolos 1989). In cultured cells challenged with dexamethasone, lithium does not appear to inhibit ODC induction via its known inhibition of phosphatidylinositol turnover (Richards et al. 1990). It has been shown that the inhibitory effect of lithium on phosphatidylinositol turnover in the brain is transient and disappears after chronic treatment (Hirfonen and Savolainen 1991). The effects we observed in the brain occurred only after chronic treatment; this indicates that the inositol lipid-linked signaling pathway may not be involved. This issue is currently under further investigation.

Increased function of guanine nucleotide binding proteins (G proteins) has been implicated in the pathophysiology of bipolar disorder (Avissar et al. 1988; Young et al. 1991). This finding has direct implications for the findings in our studies, because PAs have been found to be stimulatory (Bueb et al. 1992), whereas lithium impairs the function of G proteins. Bearing in mind that PA turnover in the brain is slow (Seiler and Bolkenius 1985), chronic lithium treatment, by preventing the stress-induced PA response, may eventually lead to lowering of the PA concentrations available for stimulating G proteins and may concomitantly enhance its own inhibitory action at this site. The effects of PA-lithium interactions on the functions of G proteins are, therefore, currently under study. It should be noted, however, that other

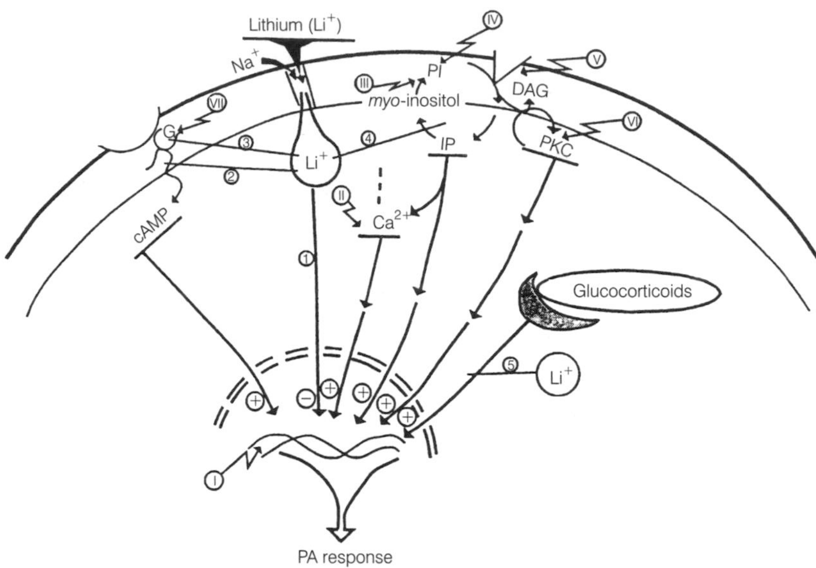

Figure 3–5. Schematic illustration of the putative sites of lithium-polyamine (PA) interactions with second-messenger signaling pathways. It may be envisaged that activation, or induction, of the PA response is a common target of several second-messenger pathways that may be turned on together, or individually, by different stressful stimuli. Increased PA metabolism, in turn, leads to selective modulation of these very second-messenger pathways (indicated by Roman numerals). Several putative modulatory sites are implicated: calcium signaling pathways (II); phosphoinositide signal transduction, where PA inhibition of phosphatidylinositol (PI) formation (III) and hydrolysis (IV) can block the formation of diacylglycerol (DAG) and inositol phosphates (IPs), thus preventing both protein kinase C (PKC) activation and Ca^{2+} mobilization, respectively; direct PKC inhibition (VI); and activation of G proteins (VII), thus modulating cyclic adenosine monophosphate (cAMP) and cyclic guanosine monophosphate (cGMP) formation. In addition, PAs may directly modulate specific membrane receptors (V). Lithium, after entering the cell, mainly via sodium (Na^+) channels, may exert its effects at the several listed key loci (indicated by Arabic numerals) and in this way may directly and indirectly interfere not only with the stress-induced PA response but also with PA action in the neuron. Arabic numerals: 1 = direct genomic effect. 2 = inhibition of guanine-stimulated adenylate cyclase. 3 = attenuation of G proteins. 4 = inhibition of IP phosphatases in the PI cycle. 5 = inhibition of the glucocorticoid-induced PA response.

second-messenger pathways, such as those involving the formation of cyclic adenosine monophosphate (cAMP) (Ebstein et al. 1980; Gilad and Gilad 1992), cyclic guanosine monophosphate (cGMP) (Gilad and Gilad 1992; Schubert et al. 1991), or mechanisms involving regulation of ionic fluxes, such as Na^+,K^+-ATPase (Gilad and Gilad 1992; Kanba et al. 1991), may also be implicated.

Ontogeny of the Stress-Induced PA Response

Unlike mature individuals, immature rats do not show the characteristic stress-induced PA response; rather, a stress-nonresponsive period is evident. The mechanisms that regulate this developmental process and the switch to a stress-responsive system are intriguing. The timing of this period appears to correspond to a similar stress- hyporesponsive period in the development of the HPA system, characterized by a diminished secretion of corticosteroids in response to stressors (Sapolsky and Meaney 1986). These findings may indicate that the developmental regulation of the stress induced activation of the brain PA response is linked to that of the HPA system. In other words, the stress-induced PA response is developmentally regulated, and the switch to the mature pattern corresponds to the cessation of the stress-nonresponsive period in the HPA system.

Interestingly, during this developmental period, corticosteroids are highly cytotoxic to the brain (Bohn 1984; Cotterrell et al. 1972), indicating that immature neurons respond to glucocorticoid challenge in a manner different from that of mature neurons. It is of no surprise, therefore, that dexamethasone treatment causes a reduction in ODC activity in the hippocampus, and the finding is in agreement with previous findings (Anderson and Schanberg 1975). The current finding may indicate that glucocorticoids inhibit the cellular stress (or survival) program by shutting off PA biosynthesis. Similar effects on PA biosynthesis ensue during glucocorticoid-induced apoptosis in the thymus (Brune et al. 1991; Richards 1978) and in embryonic cells (Nguyen-Ba et al. 1994). It appears, therefore, that the developmental nonresponsive period of the HPA system to stressors is highly advantageous for survival; its untimely activation may be suicidal.

The ontogenesis of the dexamethasone-induced alterations in brain PA–synthesizing enzymes is region dependent. The observation that the developmental switch in the PA-stress response occurs earlier in the striatum—a region known to mature early (Bayer 1980)—than in the hippocampus, again indicates the dependence of the response on neuronal maturation. Thus, during development, regional differences in the PA-stress response depend on the stage of neuronal maturation, while in adults regional differences in the intensity of the response are probably regulated by the specificity of neuronal connections.

Of interest is the observation that the period of the developmental switch in the stress-induced PA response occurs between age 15 days and age 30 days, the period of endocrine and sexual maturation in rats. The corresponding period in humans is associated with a high incidence of affective disorders. It is important, therefore, to further elucidate the mechanisms that control this developmental switch and to determine whether and how lithium interferes with these functions.

SUMMARY

The results of the series of studies discussed in this chapter warrant the following conclusions: 1) Repetitive application of stressors results in the recurrence of a PA response in the brain but results in habituation of the response in the liver. 2) The enhanced PA-stress response can be blocked by long-term (days) lithium treatment. 3) The PA-stress response is developmentally regulated, and the switch to the mature pattern corresponds to the cessation of the stress-nonresponsive period in the adrenocortical system. 4) The study implicates an overreactive PA-stress response as a component of the adaptive, or maladaptive, brain response to stressful events and as a novel molecular target for lithium action.

REFERENCES

Anderson TR, Schanberg SM: Effect of thyroxine and cortisol on brain ornithine decarboxylase activity and swimming behavior in developing rat. Biochem Pharmacol 24:495–501, 1975

Anisman H, Zacharko RM: Multiple neurochemical and behavioral consequences of stressors: implications for depression. Pharmacol Ther 46:119–136, 1990

Armario A, Hidalgo J, Giralt M: Evidence that the pituitary-adrenal axis does not cross-adapt to stressors: comparison to other physiological variables. Neuroendocrinology 47:263–267, 1988

Avissar S, Schreiber G, Danon A, et al: Lithium inhibits adrenergic and cholinergic increases in GTP binding in rat cortex. Nature 331:440–442, 1988

Bayer SA: Development of the hippocampal region in the rat, I: neurogenesis examined with ^{3}H-thymidine autoradiography. J Comp Neurol 190:87–114, 1980

Berridge MJ, Downes CP, Hanley MR: Neural and developmental action of lithium: a unifying hypothesis. Cell 59:411–419, 1989

Bohn MC: Glucocorticoid-induced teratologies of the nervous system, in Neurobehavioral Teratology. Edited by Yanai J. Amsterdam, Elsevier, 1984, pp 365–387

Brune B, Hartzell P, Nicotera P, et al: Spermine prevents endonuclease activation and apoptosis in thymocytes. Exp Cell Res 195:323–329, 1991

Bueb J-L, Da Silva A, Mousli M, et al: Natural polyamines stimulate G-proteins. Biochem J 282:545–550, 1992

Caldecott-Hazard S, Guze BH, Kling MA, et al: Clinical and biochemical aspects of depressive disorders, I: introduction, classification, and research techniques. Synapse 8:185–211, 1991

Cotterrell M, Balazs R, Johnson AL: Effects of corticosteroids on the biochemical maturation of rat brain: postnatal cell formation. J Neurochem 19:2151–2167, 1972

Cox RH, Hubbard JW, Lawler JE, et al: Cardiovascular and sympathoadrenal responses to stress in swim-trained rats. J Appl Physiol 58:1207–1214, 1985

Ebstein RP, Hermoni M, Belmaker RH: The effect of lithium on noradrenaline-induced cyclic AMP accumulation in rat brain: inhibition after chronic treatment and absence of supersensitivity. J Pharmacol Exp Ther 213:161–166, 1980

Gilad GM, Gilad VH: Polyamines in neurotrauma: ubiquitous molecules in search of a function. Biochem Pharmacol 44:401–407, 1992

Gilad GM, Kopin IJ: Neurochemical aspects of neuronal ontogenesis in the developing rat cerebellum: changes in neurotransmitter and polyamine synthesizing enzymes. J Neurochem 33:1195–1204, 1979

Gilad GM, Gilad VH, Wyatt RJ, et al: Region-selective and stress-induced increase of glutamate uptake and release in rat forebrain. Brain Res 525:335–338, 1990

Gilad GM, Gilad VH, Wyatt RJ, et al: Chronic lithium treatment prevents the dexamethasone-induced increase of brain polyamine metabolizing enzymes. Life Sci 50:PL149–PL154, 1992

Gold PW, Goodwin FK, Chrousos GP: Clinical and biochemical manifestations of depression: relation to the neurobiology of stress, I. N Engl J Med 319:348–353, 1988a

Gold PW, Goodwin FK, Chrousos GP: Clinical and biochemical manifestations of depression: relation to the neurobiology of stress, II. N Engl J Med 319:413–420, 1988b

Goodwin FK, Jamison KR (eds): Manic-Depressive Illness. New York, Oxford University Press, 1990

Hightower LE: Heat shock, stress proteins, chaperons, and proteotoxicity. Cell 66:191–197, 1991

Hirfonen M-R, Savolainen K: Lithium-induced decrease of brain inositol and increase of brain inositol-1-phosphate is transient. Neurochem Res 16:905–911, 1991

Jope RS, Williams MB: Lithium and brain signal transduction systems. Biochem Pharmacol 47:429–441, 1994

Kanba S, Yagi G, Nakaki T, et al: Potentiation by a sodium channel activator of effects of lithium ion on cyclic AMP, cyclic GMP and inositol phosphates. Neuropharmacology 30:497–500, 1991

Kvetnansky R, McCarty R, Thoa NB, et al: Sympatho-adrenal responses of spontaneously hypertensive rats to immobilization stress. Am J Physiol 246:H457–H462, 1979

Lachman HM, Papolos DF: Abnormal signal transduction: a hypothetical model for bipolar affective disorder. Life Sci 45:1413–1426, 1989

Matsui I, Pegg AE: Effect of thioacetamide, growth hormone or partial hepatectomy on spermidine acetylase activity of rat liver cytosol. Biochim Biophys Acta 633: 87–94, 1980

Nguyen-Ba G, Robert S, Dhalluin S, et al: Modulatory effect of dexamethasone on ornithine decarboxylase activity and gene expression: a possible post-transcriptional regulation by a natural metalloprotease. Cell Biochem Funct 12:121–128, 1994

Nisenbaum LK, Zigmond MJ, Sved AF, et al: Prior exposure to chronic stress results in enhanced synthesis and release of hippocampal norepinephrine in response to a novel stressor. J Neurosci 11:1478–1484, 1991

Obayashi M, Matsui-Yuasa I, Kitano A, et al: Posttranscriptional regulation of spermidine/spermine N^1: acetyltransferase with stress. Biochim Biophys Acta 1131:41–46, 1992

Panko WB, Kenney FT: Hormonal stimulation of hepatic ornithine decarboxylase. Biochem Biophys Res Commun 43:346–350, 1971

Paschen W, Schmidt-Kastner R, Hallmayer J, et al: Polyamines in cerebral ischemia. Neurochem Pathol 9:1–20, 1988

Pol O, Campmany L, Gil M, et al: Behavioral and neurochemical changes in response to acute stressors: influence of previous chronic exposure to immobilization. Pharmacol Biochem Behav 42:407–412, 1992

Prince CR, Anisman H: Acute and chronic stress effects on performance in a forced-swim task. Behav Neural Biol 4:99–119, 1984

Richards JF: Ornithine decarboxylase activity in lymphoid tissues of rats: effects of glucocorticoids. Life Sci 23:1619–1624, 1978

Richards SF, Fox K, Peng T, et al: Inhibition of hormone-stimulated ornithine decarboxylase activity by lithium chloride. Life Sci 47:233–240, 1990

Rosellini RA, Seligman MEP: Failure to escape shock following repeated exposure to inescapable shock. Bulletin of the Psychonomics Society 7:251–253, 1977

Sapolsky RM, Meaney MJ: Maturation of the adrenocortical stress response: neuroendocrine control mechanisms and the stress hyporesponsive periods. Brain Res Brain Res Rev 11:65–76, 1986

Schou M: Biology and pharmacology of the lithium ion. Pharmacol Rev 9:17–58, 1957

Schubert T, Stoll L, Muller WE: Therapeutic concentrations of lithium and carbamazepine inhibit cGMP accumulation in human lymphocytes: a clinical model for a possible common mechanism of action? Psychopharmacology (Berl) 104:45–50, 1991

Seiler N, Bolkenius FN: Polyamine reutilization and turnover in brain. Neurochem Res 10:529–544, 1985

Selye H: A syndrome produced by diverse nocuous agents. Nature 138:32–37, 1936

Tabor CW, Tabor H: Polyamines. Annu Rev Biochem 53:749–790, 1984

Umemoto S, Noguchi K, Kawai Y, et al: Repeated stress reduces the subsequent stress-induced expression of Fos in rat brain. Neurosci Lett 167:101–104, 1994

Weiss JM, Glazer HI, Pohorecky LA, et al: Effects of chronic exposure to stressors on avoidance-escape behavior and on brain norepinephrine. Psychosom Med 37:522–534, 1975

Willner P: Animal models of depression; an overview. Pharmacol Ther 45:425–455, 1990

Young LT, Li PP, Kish SJ, et al: Postmortem cerebral cortex G_s α-subunit levels are elevated in bipolar affective disorder. Brain Res 553:323–326, 1991

CHAPTER 4

ACUTE INHIBITION BUT CHRONIC UPREGULATION AND STABILIZATION OF GLUTAMATE UPTAKE IN SYNAPTOSOMES BY LITHIUM

Lowell E. Hokin, M.D., Ph.D., John F. Dixon, B.S., and Georgyi V. Los, M.D., Ph.D.

The molecular mechanism of action of lithium in the treatment of bipolar disorder is not known. Several theories have been advanced, including brain inositol depletion, amplification of cholinergic neurotransmission, and modulation of several components: guanine nucleotide binding proteins (G proteins), gene expression, protein phosphorylation, and Na^+,K^+ ATPase levels (Jope and Williams 1994). We previously showed that lithium increased accumulation of inositol 1,4,5-trisphosphate [Ins(1,4,5)P_3] in acetylcholine-stimulated cerebral cortex slices of guinea pig, rabbit, and rhesus monkey (Dixon et al. 1992; Lee et al. 1992). In the case of guinea pig and rabbit, inositol 1,3,4,5-tetrakisphosphate [Ins(1,3,4,5)P_4] was also in-

---

The authors wish to thank Terry Hanlon for her assistance in the preparation of this manuscript and Connie Bowes for technical assistance. This work was supported by grants from the University of Wisconsin Medical School Research Committee, the National Institutes of Health (HL 16318), a Young Investigator Award (55588) to G. V. L. from the National Alliance for Research on Schizophrenia and Depression (NARSAD), and an Established Investigatorship Award to L. E. H. from NARSAD.

creased. These effects are in contrast to cholinergically stimulated cerebral cortex slices of rat and mouse, in which lithium decreased accumulation of Ins(1,4,5)P_3 and Ins(1,3,4,5)P_4 (Kennedy et al. 1989; Lee et al. 1992; Whitworth and Kendall 1988). The explanation for the species differences lies in the fact that rat and mouse cerebral cortex slices are less able to accumulate inositol in slices (Allison and Stewart 1971; Lee et al. 1992; Sherman et al. 1986); and in fact if the incubation medium was supplemented with inositol, cerebral cortex slices of these two species also showed lithium-stimulated increases in Ins(1,4,5)P_3 and Ins(1,3,4,5)P_4 (Lee et al. 1992).

In the case of rhesus monkey, neither inositol nor an agonist was required to demonstrate lithium-stimulated accumulation of Ins(1,4,5)P_3 (Dixon et al. 1992). This suggested that an endogenous neurotransmitter was involved in the lithium effect. We have found that beginning at therapeutic concentrations, two antibipolar drugs, lithium and valproate, stimulate the release of glutamate in rhesus monkey or mouse cerebral cortex slices, and that this in turn increases accumulation of Ins(1,4,5)P_3 via activation of the *N*-methyl-D-aspartate (NMDA) receptor. But, unlike lithium, valproate does not cause accumulation of inositol mono- or bisphosphates. Valproate did cause accumulation of Ins(1,4,5)P_3, as predicted from its glutamate-releasing activity. The fact that the two drugs share antibipolar effects and glutamate-releasing and Ins(1,4,5)P_3-accumulating activities—but not stimulation of inositol mono- and bisphosphate accumulation—suggests that inhibition of the respective phosphatases by lithium is not a necessary component for antibipolar action.

RESULTS

Effects of Receptor Antagonists on Lithium-Stimulated Accumulation of Ins(1,4,5)P_3 in Monkey Cerebral Cortex Slices

Figure 4–1 shows the effects of receptor antagonists on lithium-stimulated Ins(1,4,5)P_3 accumulation (Dixon et al. 1994). Atropine, phentolamine, ketanserin, and chlorpheniramine—antagonists at the cholinergic-muscarinic, α_1-adrenergic, 5-HT_2-serotonergic, and H_1-histaminergic receptors, respectively—had no effect on Ins(1,4,5)P_3 accumulation in the presence of lithium. On the other hand, (±)-3-(2-carboxypiperazin-4-yl)-propyl-1-phosphoric acid (CPP), which selectively blocks the ionotropic NMDA receptor in a competitive manner, reduced lithium-stimulated Ins(1,4,5)P_3 accumulation. Dizocilpine [(±)MK-801], ketamine, and 10 mM Mg^{2+}, which block the NMDA ion channel in a noncompetitive manner, also reduced lithium-stimulated Ins(1,4,5)P_3 accumulation. No effect was seen with 10 μM 7-chlorokynurenic acid (7-CKA), which blocks the glycine site on the NMDA receptor (glycine functions cooperatively with glutamate). This is probably because considerable glycine is present in the incubation medium and is not effectively displaced by that concentration of 7-CKA. 6,7-Dinitroquinoxaline-2,3-dione (DNQX), which blocks the α-amino-3-hydroxy-5-methyl-4-isoxazole propionic acid (AMPA) ionotropic receptor, also had no effect on basal or lithium-stimulated Ins(1,4,5)P_3 accumulation. This may be because the permeability of the AMPA channel to Ca^{2+} is much lower than that of the NMDA channel (Mayer and Miller 1990). Note that under the conditions of this experiment, in which slices were incubated with lithium for 1 hour, antagonists at the NMDA receptor/channel complex also reduced Ins(1,4,5)P_3 accumulation in the absence of lithium. Under these conditions, there is considerable accumulation of glutamate in the absence of lithium, which probably accounts for most, if not all, of Ins(1,4,5)P_3 accumulation seen in the absence of lithium (see below). Under different incubation conditions, where the slices were first preincubated in Ca^{2+}-free medium, followed by CPP and finally Ca^{2+} for 20 minutes, with washings in between, CPP selectively abolished the lithium stimulation with no effect on basal Ins(1,4,5)P_3 accumulation (Dixon et al. 1994). Under the latter conditions, there was inhibition of lithium-stimulated Ins(1,4,5)P_3 accumulation with 1 μM (±)MK-801, and this was greater at 10 μM (±)MK-801, without any effect on basal accumulation (Dixon et al. 1994).

Effects of Lithium on Glutamate Release in Monkey Cerebral Cortex Slices

The effects of receptor/channel antagonists described above suggested that the lithium-stimulated accumulation of Ins(1,4,5)P_3 involved glutamatergic neurotransmission at the NMDA receptor. We therefore studied the effects of lithium on glutamate release. Concentrations of lithium ranging from the therapeutic at 1–1.5 mM to the toxic (as high as 25 mM) were studied.

Figure 4–2 shows the effects of increasing concentrations of lithium on accumulation of glutamate in the incubation medium in monkey cerebral cortex slices (Dixon et al. 1994). There was a significant increase in glutamate release at 1.5 mM of lithium, which is the maximum therapeutic concentration. Glutamate release increased progressively with increasing lithium concentrations. Figure 4–3 shows the effect of 10 mM of lithium on the time-dependent

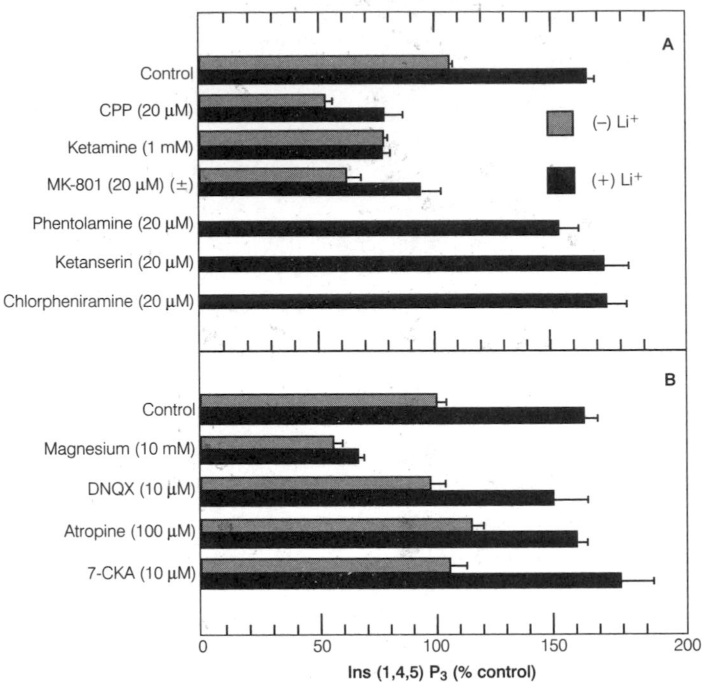

Figure 4–1. Effect of neurotransmitter antagonists on accumulation of inositol 1,4,5-trisphosphate [Ins(1,4,5)P_3] in monkey cerebral cortex slices with and without lithium, as determined by both the [^{3}H]inositol prelabeling technique and the receptor binding mass assay. (A) [^{3}H]Ins(1,4,5)P_3. Cerebral cortex slices, labeled with [^{3}H]inositol, were incubated for 1 hour with ± 25 mM LiCl, as indicated, and with and without various antagonists before perchloric acid quench. The *P* value of the increment due to Li^+ in the control tissue was 0.002. There was no significant increase due to Li^+ in the presence of (±)-3-(2-carboxypiperazin-4-yl)-propyl-1-phosphoric acid (CPP) or ketamine. (B) Ins(1,4,5)P_3 mass. Brain cortex slices were prepared and restored in nominally Ca^{2+}-free Krebs-Henseleit bicarbonate saline (KHBS) and then preincubated for 60 minutes in fresh buffer ± 25 mM LiCl and various antagonists. $CaCl_2$ (2.5 mM, final concentration) was then added and the incubation quenched with perchloric acid after 20 minutes. Ins(1,4,5)P_3 mass was measured by the receptor binding assay, as described by Dixon et al. (1994). Error bars are ±SEM of triplicate tissue incubations. Results are expressed as percentage of the control without lithium. Control = 9.51 ± 0.54 pmol/mg. The *P* values of the increment due to Li^+: control, 0.001; Mg^{2+}, NS; 6,7-dinitroquinoxaline-2,3-dione (DNQX), 0.032; atropine, 0.004; and 7-chlorokynurenic acid (7-CKA), 0.01.

Source. Reprinted from Dixon JF, Los GV, Hokin LE: "Lithium Stimulates Glutamate 'Release' and Inositol 1,4,5-Trisphosphate Accumulation Via Activation of the N-Methyl-D-Aspartate Receptor in Monkey and Mouse Cerebral Cortex Slices." *Proceedings of the National Academy of Sciences USA* 91:8358–8362, 1994. Reproduced by permission of the Proceedings of the National Academy of Sciences USA.

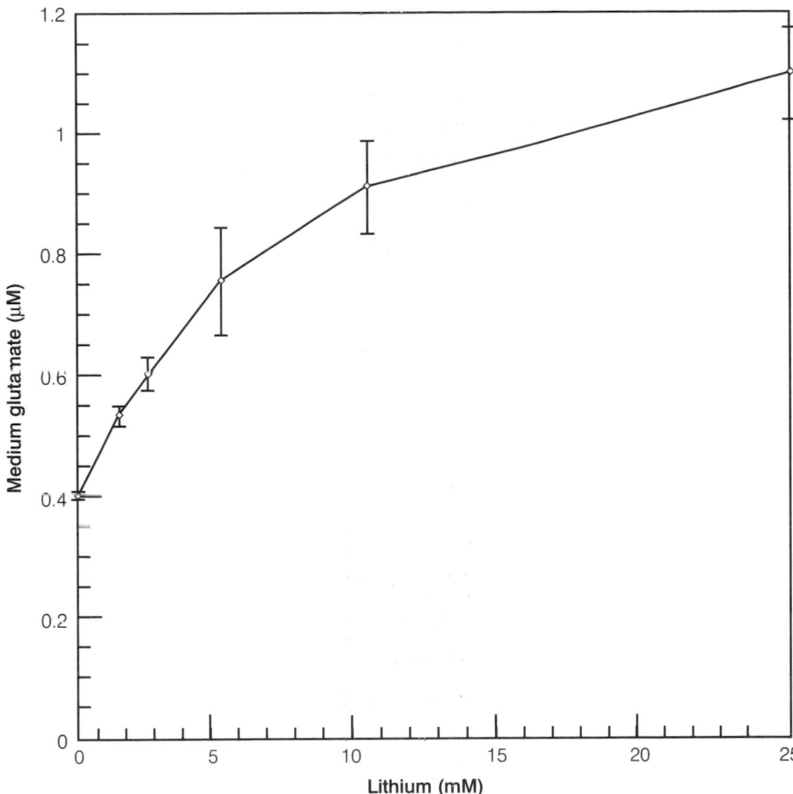

Figure 4–2. Effect of increasing concentrations of lithium (Li) on accumulation of glutamate in the medium during incubation of monkey cerebral cortex slices. Slices were prepared and restored in nominally Ca^{2+}-free Krebs-Henseleit bicarbonate saline (KHBS) in the presence of 10 mM $MgCl_2$. After eight sequential washes in fresh buffer with 1 mM $MgCl_2$, slices were divided into 28 separate aliquots of approximately 100 μL gravity-packed tissue and incubated twice for 30 minutes with complete buffer replacement at the end of each incubation. Medium volume was 3.2 mL throughout. Slices were then incubated with and without various concentrations of Li^+ and with 1.3 mM $CaCl_2$, for 60 minutes before samples of medium were separated from the slices for glutamate analysis. The *P* values of the increment due to Li^+: 0.001 at 1.5, 2.5, and 5 mM LiCl, 0.006 at 10 mM LiCl, and < 0.001 at 25 mM LiCl. Error bars represent ± SEM of four tissue incubations. Tissue averaged 1.16 mg of protein per sample. Medium volume was 3.2 mL.

Source. Reprinted from Dixon JF, Los GV, Hokin LE: "Lithium Stimulates Glutamate 'Release' and Inositol 1,4,5-Trisphosphate Accumulation via Activation of the N-Methyl-D-Aspartate Receptor in Monkey and Mouse Cerebral Cortex Slices." *Proceedings of the National Academy of Sciences USA* 91:8358–8362, 1994. Reproduced by permission of the Proceedings of the National Academy of Sciences USA.

accumulation of glutamate in the incubation medium. After a lag of 10 minutes, lithium progressively increased glutamate release over a 2-hour period. Figure 4–4 shows the effects of 25 m*M* of lithium on the release of glutamate and the accumulation of Ins(1,4,5)P_3. Lithium caused a threefold increase in medium glutamate over control. Ins(1,4,5)P_3 was also increased. In general, the release of glutamate was more responsive to lithium than was the level of Ins(1,4,5)P_3.

Effects of Carbetapentane and CPP on the Release of Glutamate and Ins(1,4,5)P_3 Accumulation in the Presence and Absence of Lithium in Mouse Cerebral Cortex Slices

Lithium also stimulated glutamate release and Ins(1,4,5)P_3 accumulation in mouse cerebral cortex slices (Figure 4–5). To establish that the CPP effects on Ins(1,4,5)P_3 accumulation were specific to the NMDA receptor and not due to any effect on glutamate release, the effect of CPP on glutamate release was studied. CPP markedly inhibited lithium-stimulated Ins(1,4,5)P_3 accumulation, but it had no effect on glutamate release. It is also clear from these results that accumulation of Ins(1,4,5)P_3 is not necessary for lithium stimulation of glutamate release. Carbetapentane, which inhibits depolarization-induced glutamate release (Annels et al. 1991) and which inhibited lithium-stimulated glutamate release in monkey cerebral cortex slices, essentially abolished lithium-stimulated Ins(1,4,5)P_3 accumulation in mouse cerebral cortex slices (Figure 4–6). This further supports the conclusion that lithium-stimulated Ins(1,4,5)P_3 accumulation is due to glutamate release. Carbetapentane also inhibited to some extent basal Ins(1,4,5)P_3 accumulation, suggesting that at least part of the Ins(1,4,5)P_3 seen in the absence of lithium was due to lithium-independent glutamate release.

Effect of Lithium on Ins(1,4,5)P_3 Accumulation in Human Neuroblastoma Cells

Although rhesus monkey shares 94% gene homology with humans, it would be of interest to study the effect of lithium on a human neural model. Obviously, fresh tissue from human brain is not feasible. For human studies we have used human neuroblastoma SH-SY5Y cells (Los et al. 1995), although these cells are cancer cells and differ in many ways from differentiated neurons.

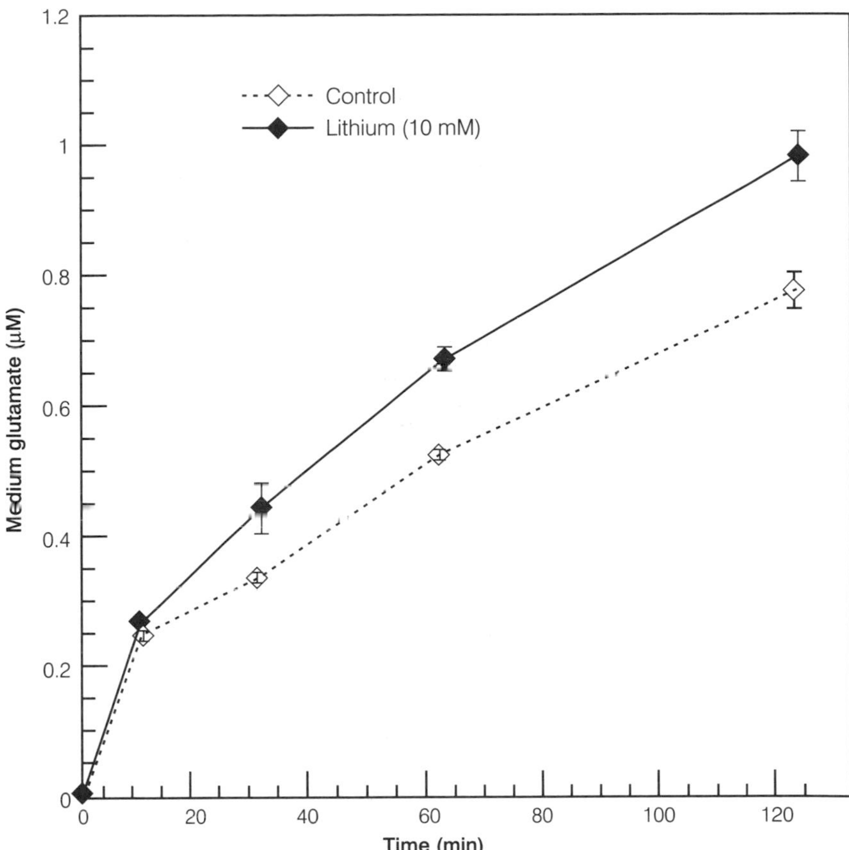

Figure 4–3. Time-dependent accumulation of glutamate in the medium during incubation of monkey cerebral cortex slices ±lithium. Slices were prepared and restored in nominally Ca^{2+}-free Krebs-Henseleit bicarbonate saline (KHBS) with 10 mM $MgCl_2$. The slices were then divided into aliquots and preincubated in 3.2-mL portions of nominally Ca^{2+}-free KHBS with 1 mM $MgCl_2$ for 30 and 60 minutes, with complete buffer replacement after each incubation. The final incubations were initiated by addition of fresh buffer with 1.3 mM $CaCl_2$ and ±10 mM LiCl. The incubations were stopped at the times indicated, the medium removed for glutamate analysis, the tissue homogenized with perchloric acid (3%), and the acid-insoluble protein determined for normalization. Tissue slices averaged 1.14 mg of protein per sample. Error bars show ±SEM of triplicate slice incubations. The *P* values of the increment due to Li^+: 10 minutes, NS; 30 minutes, 0.045; 60 minutes, 0.002; 120 minutes, 0.012.

Source. Reprinted from Dixon JF, Los GV, Hokin LE: "Lithium Stimulates Glutamate 'Release' and Inositol 1,4,5-Trisphosphate Accumulation via Activation of the N-Methyl-D-Aspartate Receptor in Monkey and Mouse Cerebral Cortex Slices." *Proceedings of the National Academy of Sciences USA* 91:8358–8362, 1994. Reproduced by permission of the Proceedings of the National Academy of Sciences USA.

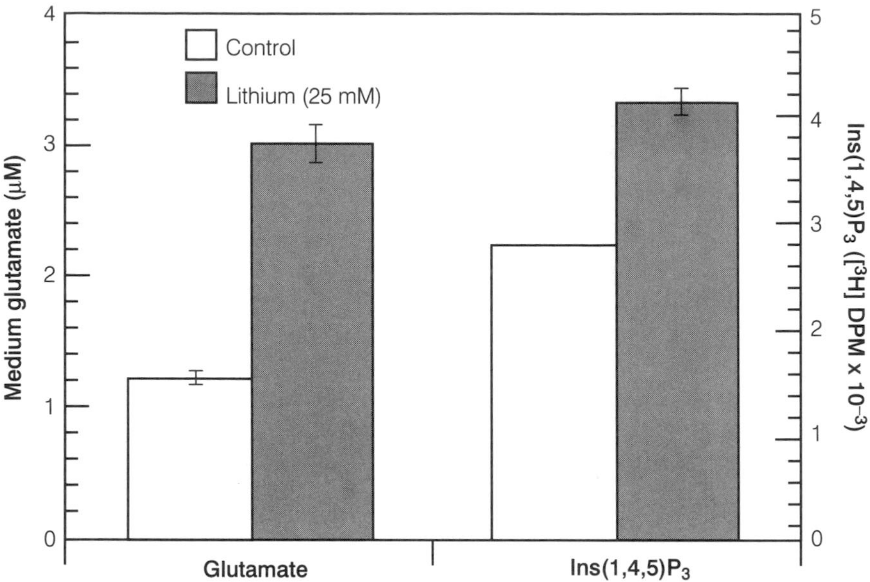

Figure 4–4. Effect of lithium on medium glutamate and [^{3}H]inositol 1,4,5-trisphosphate [Ins(1,4,5)P_3] in monkey cerebral cortex slices. Slices were prepared and prelabeled in nominally Ca^{2+}-free Krebs-Henseleit bicarbonate saline (KHBS) with 10 mM $MgCl_2$, and after eight sequential washes with 1 mM $MgCl_2$, they were separated into aliquots and preincubated for 30 minutes with and without 25 mM LiCl and finally incubated for 20 minutes after addition of $CaCl_2$ (final concentration 1.3 mM). Samples of medium were taken just before quench for glutamate analysis. Error bars are ±SEM of four separate tissue incubations. Tissue averaged 1.58 mg of protein per sample. Medium volume was 3.2 mL. The *P* value of the increment due to Li^+ was 0.001 for both glutamate and Ins(1,4,5)P_3.
Source. Reprinted from Dixon JF, Los GV, Hokin LE: "Lithium Stimulates Glutamate 'Release' and Inositol 1,4,5-Trisphosphate Accumulation via Activation of the N-Methyl-D-Aspartate Receptor in Monkey and Mouse Cerebral Cortex Slices."*Proceedings of the National Academy of Sciences USA* 91:8358–8362, 1994. Reproduced by permission of the Proceedings of the National Academy of Sciences USA.

We found that after 30-minute incubation of SH-SY5Y cells with lithium plus acetylcholine there was a stimulation of Ins(1,4,5)P_3 accumulation by this ion over that of cells incubated with acetylcholine alone (Los et al. 1995). The stimulation by lithium occurred at therapeutic concentrations and increased progressively up to 25 mM of lithium. It appears that in human brain, inositol is not a rate-limiting factor in the presence of lithium. This is consistent with several observations. First, the results of human brain biopsy studies, as well as

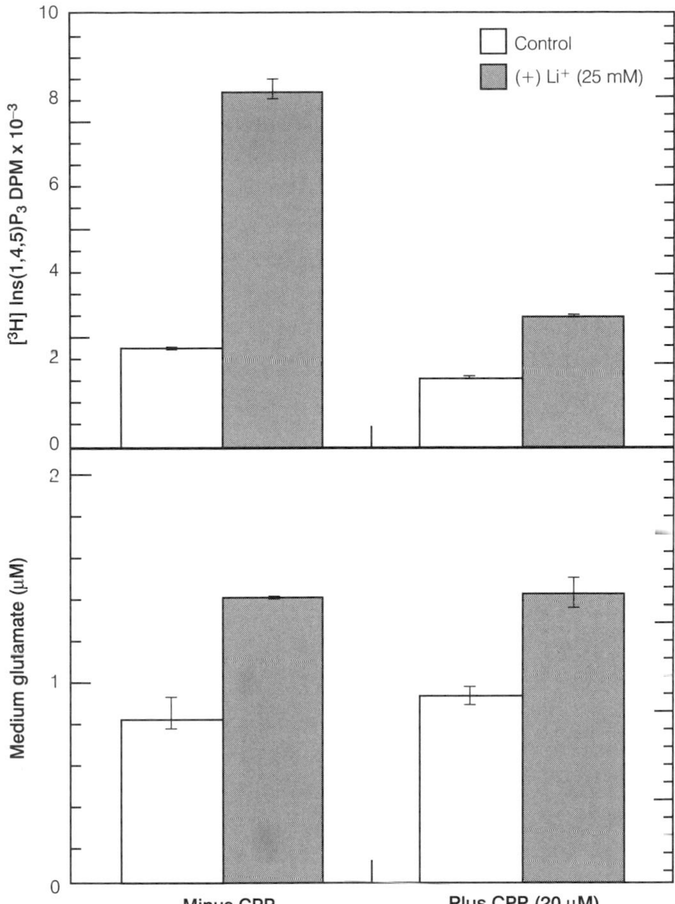

Figure 4–5. Effect of (±)-3-(2-carboxypiperazin-4-yl)-propyl-1- phosphoric acid (CPP) on the lithium-dependent increments in [^{3}H]inositol 1,4,5-trisphosphate [Ins(1,4,5)P_3] and medium glutamate of mouse cerebral cortex slices. Mouse cerebral cortex slices were prepared and prelabeled in nominally Ca^{2+}-free Krebs-Henseleit bicarbonate saline (KHBS), separated into aliquots, preincubated with and without LiCl and CPP for 60 minutes, and then incubated with 1.3 mM $CaCl_2$ for 20 minutes before quench. Samples of incubation medium were taken just before quench for measurement of glutamate. Error bars show ±SEM of four separate tissue incubations. Protein averaged 1.24 mg per sample. CPP significantly reduced Ins(1,4,5)P_3 both with and without Li^+(all *P* values < 0.001). CPP had no significant effect on glutamate in the medium.

Source. Reprinted from Dixon JF, Los GV, Hokin LE: "Lithium Stimulates Glutamate 'Release' and Inositol 1,4,5-Trisphosphate Accumulation via Activation of the N-Methyl-D-Aspartate Receptor in Monkey and Mouse Cerebral Cortex Slices." *Proceedings of the National Academy of Sciences USA* 91:8358–8362, 1994. Reproduced by permission of the Proceedings of the National Academy of Sciences USA.

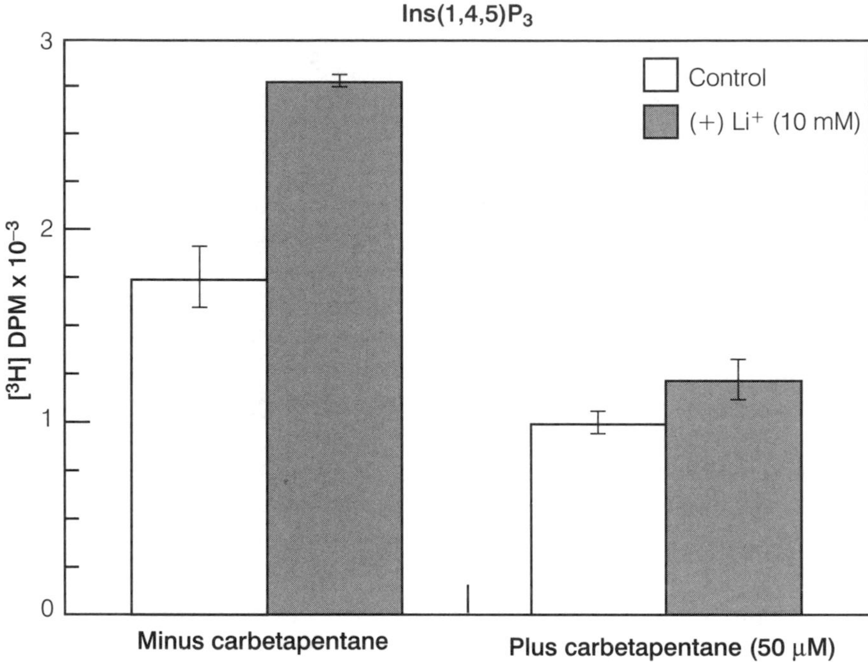

Figure 4–6. Effect of carbetapentane on the lithium-dependent increment in [^{3}H]inositol 1,4,5-trisphosphate [Ins(1,4,5)P_3] in mouse cerebral cortex slices. Mouse cerebral cortex slices were prepared and prelabeled in nominally Ca^{2+}-free Krebs-Henseleit bicarbonate saline (KHBS) and preincubated for 30 minutes ± 10 mM LiCl ± 50 μM carbetapentane. $CaCl_2$ (final concentration 1.3 mM) was then added and the incubation continued for 20 minutes before quench. Error bars show ± SEM of four separate tissue incubations. Tissue averaged 1.29 mg of protein per sample. The *P* value of the decrement due to carbetapentane (–)Li^+ was 0.006 and (+)Li^+ was < 0.001.
Source. Reprinted from Dixon JF, Los GV, Hokin LE: "Lithium Stimulates Glutamate 'Release' and Inositol 1,4,5-Trisphosphate Accumulation via Activation of the N-Methyl-D-Aspartate Receptor in Monkey and Mouse Cerebral Cortex Slices." *Proceedings of the National Academy of Sciences USA* 91:8358–8362, 1994. Reproduced by permission of the Proceedings of the National Academy of Sciences USA.

results of localized proton magnetic resonance spectroscopy in vivo, show that concentration of free *myo*-inositol in gray matter of human brain is 6.2 ± 1.1 mM (Michaelis et al. 1993; Petroff et al. 1989). Second, a K_m value for inositol for phosphatidylinositol (PI) synthase in a crude particulate fraction from rat cerebral cortex is 0.91 ± 0.04 mM (Heacock et al. 1993). The PI synthase from placenta (the only human enzyme described so far) displayed a

K_m of 0.28 mM (Antonsson 1994). The concentration of the brain inositol is thus significantly higher than the K_m for PI synthase. Therefore, in order to affect activity of PI synthase, the level of cellular inositol has to be dramatically reduced. However, chronic or even high acute doses of Li^+produce relatively small decreases in inositol levels in the brain of laboratory animals in vivo (Sherman 1989).

Effects of the Antibipolar Drug Valproate on Glutamate Release and Inositol Phosphate Accumulation in Mouse Cerebral Cortex Slices

It was considered possible that other drugs used in the treatment of bipolar disorder might operate through the same mechanism as lithium—that is, stimulate glutamate release. Valproate, which is an antiepileptic drug, has been found effective in bipolar disorder. Figure 4–7 shows the effect of increasing concentrations of valproate on glutamate release in mouse cerebral cortex slices. Therapeutic concentrations of valproate (approximately 1 mM) released glutamate maximally. But unlike lithium, valproate did not increase accumulation of inositol mono- or bisphosphates, ruling out an inhibitory effect of valproate on their respective phosphatases (Figure 4–8). In fact, Vadnal and Parthasarathy (1995) reported that valproate had no inhibitory effect on inositol monophosphatase enzyme activity.

Valproate did, however, increase Ins(1,4,5)P_3 accumulation, which in all likelihood was due to increased glutamate release—as is the case with lithium (see Table 4–1). The fact that both agents share antibipolar and glutamate-releasing properties but only lithium increases inositol mono- and bisphosphate accumulation suggests that inhibition of their respective phosphatases is not essential for antibipolar action. Rather, glutamate release may be an important component of antibipolar activity.

Lithium Acutely Inhibits Glutamate Uptake by Presynaptic Nerve Endings in Mouse Cerebral Cortex

In the initial studies, it was not clear how lithium increased extracellular glutamate accumulation. Several possibilities existed. Lithium could cause glutamate accumulation by increased release from nerve endings or glial cells. Lithium could inhibit glutamate reuptake in nerve endings or glial cells. To ex-

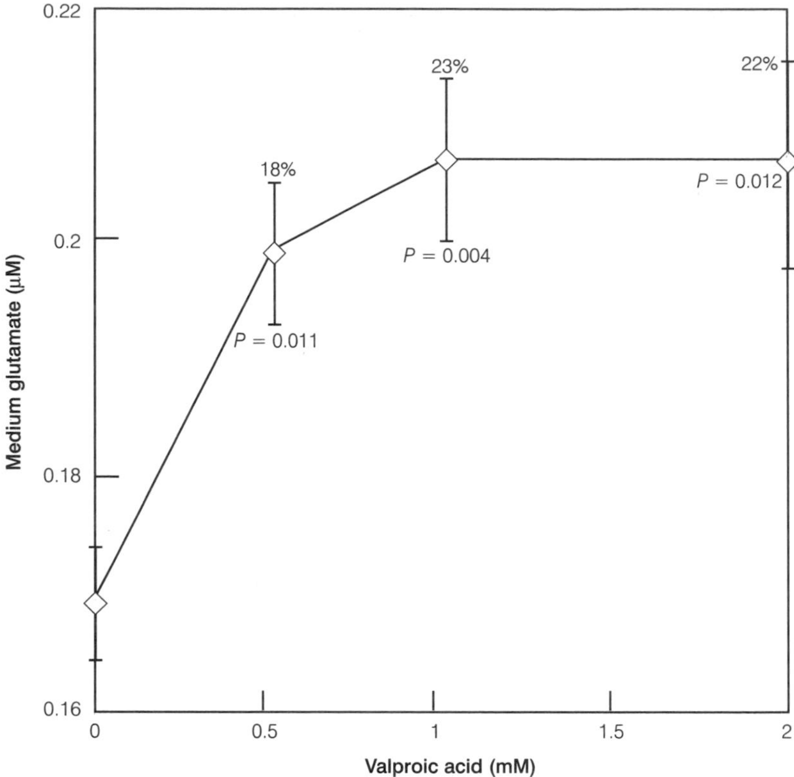

Figure 4–7. Effect of increasing concentrations of valproate on extracellular glutamate in mouse cerebral cortex slices. Mouse cerebral cortex slices were prepared and restored in nominally Ca^{2+}-free Krebs-Henseleit bicarbonate saline (KHBS) with 10 mM $MgCl_2$. Aliquots (average protein = 1.5 mg) were incubated in 3.2 mL nominally Ca^{2+}-free KHBS with 1 mM $MgCl_2$ twice for 30 minutes with complete buffer replacement and then preincubated for 60 minutes with the indicated concentrations of sodium valproate. After addition of Ca^{2+} (1.3 mM, final concentration) the incubation was continued for 20 minutes before removal of aliquots of medium (free of slices) for enzymatic determination of medium glutamate.

amine the second possibility, we studied the effect of lithium on the uptake of [^{3}H]glutamate into cerebrocortical synaptosomes (Dixon and Hokin 1998). At the therapeutic concentration of 1.5 mM, lithium significantly inhibited glutamate uptake. Although this inhibition at 1.5 mM was not great, it should be pointed out that with cerebrocortical slices, when glutamate accumulation was plotted against inhibition of glutamate uptake, accumulation was amplified fivefold over inhibition of uptake (see below). Thus, a 6% inhibition of uptake would be amplified to a 30% increase in accumulation. Inhibition of uptake progressively increased from 6% at 1.5 mM to 35% at 20 mM of lithium. Lith-

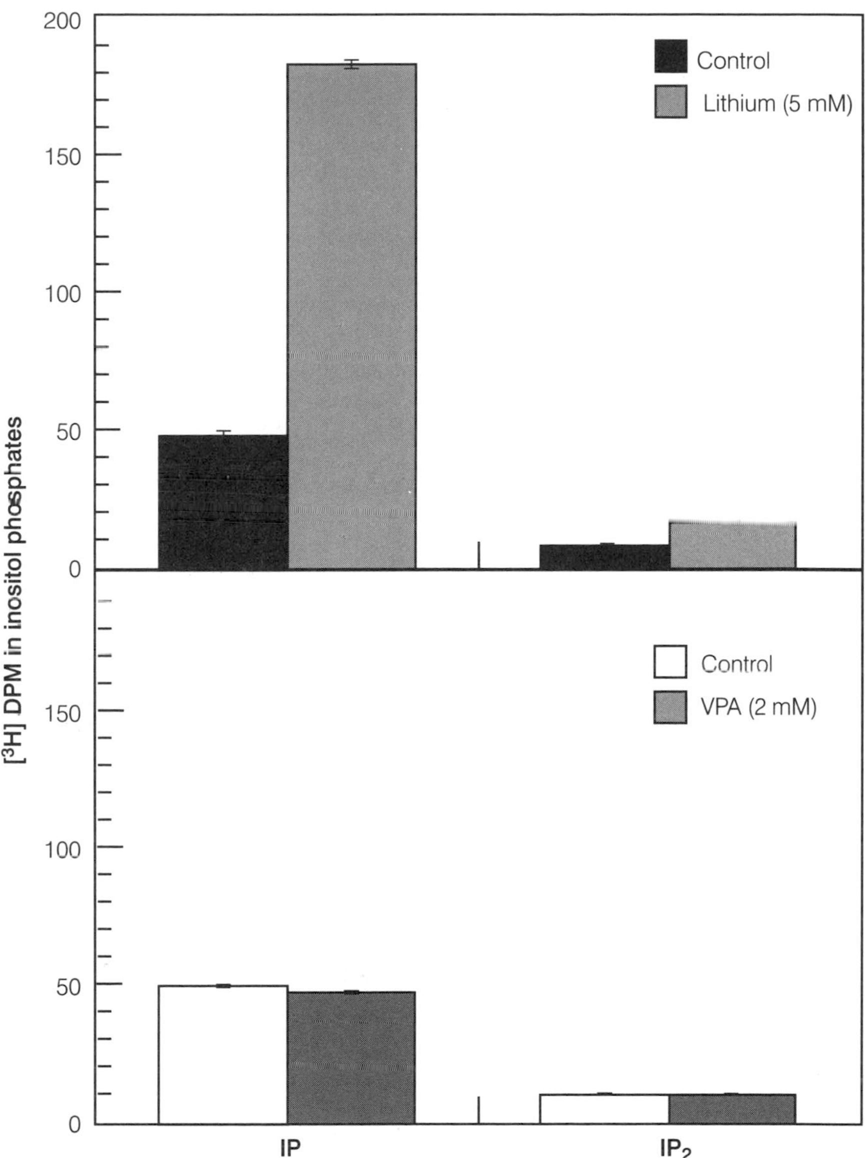

Figure 4–8. Effects of lithium and valproate (VPA) on the accumulation of [^{3}H]inositol monophosphates (IP) and inositol bisphosphates (IP_2) in mouse cerebral cortex slices. Mouse cerebral cortex slices were prelabeled with [^{3}H] *myo*-inositol, prewashed at 37° C with three buffer replacements, preincubated for 60 minutes in nominally Ca^{2+}-free Krebs-Henseleit bicarbonate saline (KHBS) ±LiCl (5 mM) or VPA (2 mM), and then incubated for 20 minutes with 1.3 mM Ca^{2+} before quench and extraction with perchloric acid (3%). Inositol phosphates were separated by high-performance liquid chromatography.

Table 4–1. Effect of valproate on extracellular glutamate and cellular [^{3}H]Ins(1,4,5)P_3 in mouse cerebral cortex slices

	Control[a]	Valproate[a]	% Increase	*P*
Glutamate (nM)	139 ± 5	183 ± 11	31.4	0.008
[^{3}H]Ins(1,4,5)P_3 (DPM)	1,342 ± 62	1,637 ± 28	22	0.003

Note. Mouse cerebral cortex slices were prelabeled and incubated ± sodium valproate (2 mM), as indicated in Figure 4–8. Aliquots of medium (free of slices) were taken for enzymatic determination of medium glutamate, followed immediately by addition of perchloric acid to the tissue. Radioactivity in [^{3}H]Ins(1,4,5)P_3 was measured by liquid scintillation after high-performance liquid chromatography isolation. Abbreviations: DPM = disintegrations per minute. Ins(1,4,5)P_3 = inositol 1,4,5-trisphosphate.
[a]Numbers following ± are standard deviation.

ium had no effect on the K_m for the glutamate transporter but reduced the V_{max}. Thus, lithium inhibited the capacity of the transporter without affecting its affinity for glutamate. This suggested that lithium decreased the number of effective transporter molecules.

Lithium inhibited glutamate uptake in cerebrocortical synaptosomes twice as much as in cerebrocortical slices. We hypothesized that the lesser inhibition of glutamate uptake by lithium in cerebrocortical slices as compared with cerebrocortical synaptosomes might be a result of dampening by other structures in the slice that show no inhibition of uptake. The most likely candidates would be glial cells. In fact, we found no inhibition of uptake in human astrocytes by lithium (G. V. Los, L. E. Hokin, unpublished observations, 1997).

We then studied the effects of L-trans-pyrrolidine-2,4-dicarboxylic acid (PDC) and dihydrokainic acid, two inhibitors of glutamate uptake, on glutamate uptake and accumulation in cerebrocortical slices. The plots of extracellular glutamate accumulation versus inhibition of glutamate uptake for lithium, PDC, and dihydrokainic acid are superimposable. This suggests strongly that inhibition of glutamate uptake by lithium is responsible for the drug's effect on extracellular glutamate accumulation.

Chronic Treatment of Mice With Lithium Upregulates and Stabilizes Glutamate Reuptake by Cerebrocortical Synaptosomes

Lithium is a mood stabilizer; that is, it will normalize mood from the direction of either depression or mania. This requires chronic treatment for 1–2 weeks. The inhibition of synaptosomal uptake of glutamate by lithium occurs immediately. We therefore studied the effects of chronic treatment in mice with a relatively low dose of lithium (0.4% lithium carbonate in mouse chow), achieving a lithium blood level of 0.7–1.0 mM. If we increased the lithium carbonate in the chow to 0.6% to achieve higher blood concentrations, a few fatalities occurred by 2 weeks.

Synaptosomes from the cerebral cortices of mice treated with lithium for 2 weeks showed a small but highly significant ($P < 0.001$) upregulation of glutamate uptake (Figure 4–9). Upregulation would exert an antimanic effect because more excitatory glutamate would be removed from the synaptic cleft. What is perhaps of equal interest is that lithium stabilized glutamate uptake: There was a wide range in glutamate uptake from individual control mice, perhaps representing differing levels of excitability, but uptake in synaptosomes from separate lithium-treated mice was clamped in a narrower range. To express this quantitatively, the variance (σ^2) of uptake in control mice was 0.423, whereas in lithium-treated mice, it was 0.184. This mechanism offers a possible explanation for the fact that clinically, lithium stabilizes mood from the direction of either mania or depression.

DISCUSSION

The results presented here show that our earlier observation of lithium-induced Ins(1,4,5)P_3 accumulation in rhesus monkey cerebral cortex slices in the absence of added agonists is due to lithium-stimulated glutamate release, which elevates Ins(1,4,5)P_3 via activation of the NMDA receptor. Several lines of evidence support this: 1) Most importantly, lithium stimulates glutamate release in monkey and mouse cerebral cortex slices. 2) Antagonists to the NMDA receptor/channel block the elevating effect of lithium on Ins(1,4,5)P_3 accumulation. 3) Carbetapentane, which blocks glutamate release, inhibits both basal and lithium-stimulated Ins(1,4,5)P_3 accumulation. These are criteria that support involvement of a neurotransmitter—in this instance, glutamate.

Although NMDA is not a metabotropic receptor, activation of the NMDA receptor increases Ins(1,4,5)P_3 formation (Mayer and Miller 1990). This would be expected to occur as a result of the increased influx of Ca^{2+}, which activates phospholipase C.

It is of interest that the increase in Ins(1,4,5)P_3 due to lithium is essentially abolished by the highly specific NMDA receptor antagonist, CPP, as well as other NMDA receptor/channel complex antagonists, whereas antagonists to other glutamate receptors had no effect (Figure 4–1 and unpublished observations of J. F. Dixon and L. E. Hokin, January 1994). This is presumably due to

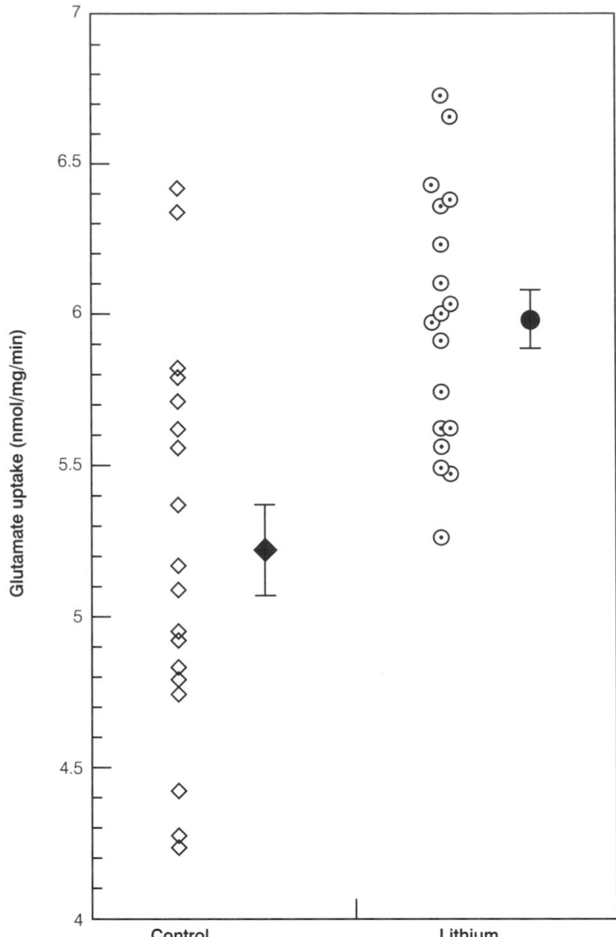

Figure 4–9. Effect of chronic lithium treatment in mice on glutamate uptake by cortical synaptosomes. White male adult mice (average weight 31 g) were fed rodent chow ± 0.4% Li2CO3 for 14 days. Food, water, and saline (0.9% NaCl) were available ad libitum. Water and saline were supplemented with 1% *myo*-inositol. After sacrifice, synaptosomes were prepared from cortical slices from individual mice and the initial rate of uptake of 10 μM L-glutamate determined as described by Dixon and Hokin (1998). Assays were performed in quintuplicate. N = 18 for both conditions. Average control uptake was 5.22 ± 0.15 nmol/mg/min. Average uptake from lithium-treated mice was 5.98 ± 0.1 nmol/mg/min. Lithium differed from control with a significance of $P < 0.001$. The variance (σ^2) for uptake from control mice was 0.423; the variance for uptake from lithium-treated mice was 0.184.
Source. Reprinted from Dixon JF, Hokin LE: "Lithium Acutely Inhibits and Chronically Up-regulates and Stabilizes Glutamate Uptake by Presynaptic Nerve Endings in Mouse Cerebral Cortex." *Proceedings of the National Academy of Sciences USA* 95:8363–8368, 1998. Reproduced by permission of the Proceedings of the National Academy of Sciences USA.

the fact that the EC_{50} for activation of metabotropic receptors by glutamate is one to two orders of magnitude higher than that for the NMDA receptor (Schoepp et al. 1990) and that the concentrations of glutamate achieved at the synapses in cerebral cortex slices in the presence of lithium are insufficient to activate the metabotropic receptors. In addition, the permeability of the AMPA and kainate channels to Ca^{2+} is probably insufficient to cause formation of Ins(1,4,5)P_3.

Earlier studies reported inhibitory effects of lithium on Ins(1,4,5)P_3 accumulation in mouse and rat cerebral cortex slices in the absence of supplementary inositol and in the presence of high concentrations of cholinergic agents (Kennedy et al. 1989; Lee et al. 1992). This is due to inositol depletion in brain cortex slices in these species under these conditions. We have previously discussed the possible reasons for this excessive inositol depletion in rodent brain cortex slices (Dixon et al. 1994): 1) Brain inositol (or its uptake in rodent brain slices) is already limited in mouse and rat as compared to higher species. 2) Lengthy incubation of rat cerebral cortex slices reduces cellular inositol by 80%. 3) High concentrations of cholinergic agents (1 mM carbachol has generally been used) cause a particularly large breakdown of PI, and when lithium is present so as to inhibit inositol monophosphatases and inositol 1-polyphosphatases, large quantities of inositol are trapped in the form of inositol phosphates. 4) Cholinergic agents markedly inhibit inositol uptake into astrocytoma cells (Batty et al. 1993). A similar effect may occur in neuronal cells, or the effect on glial cells may have the secondary effect on neuronal cells of depressing cellular inositol concentrations.

In contrast, as reported here, when mouse cerebral cortex slices were incubated in the absence of added cholinergic agent, lithium increased Ins(1,4,5)P_3 accumulation, even without addition of inositol. Low endogenous levels of glutamate are likely to result in significantly less breakdown of PI than are high levels of cholinergic agents. Thus, minimal amounts of inositol would be trapped in the presence of lithium, and inhibition of Ins(1,4,5)P_3 accumulation would not occur, despite the factors that favor inositol depletion in this species. Also, inhibitory effects of cholinergic agents on inositol uptake would be avoided.

Lithium is excitotoxic at serum levels exceeding 1.5 mM. The excessive release of excitatory glutamate and thus overstimulation of the NMDA receptor at high concentrations of lithium may be a mechanism that contributes to lithium toxicity.

The fact that two antibipolar drugs, lithium and valproate, both stimulate glutamate release and Ins(1,4,5)P_3 accumulation but only lithium causes accumulation of the lower nonmessenger inositol phosphates has implications regarding the mechanism of their antibipolar action. First, the data suggest that increased glutamate release may be important for antibipolar action. Second, the data indicate that inhibition of inositol mono- and bisphosphatase is not essential for antibipolar activity.

Lithium treatment requires 1–2 weeks to exert its antibipolar effect. The chronic effect of lithium on glutamate uptake should mirror the therapeutic effects. We treated mice with lithium for 24 hours and 1 week, in addition to 2 weeks, and measured synaptosomal uptake in the absence of added lithium in the incubation medium (J. F. Dixon and L. E. Hokin, unpublished observations, 1999). Compared with control mice, lithium upregulated synaptosomal uptake of glutamate in treated mice with high statistical significance at 1 and 2 weeks. On the other hand, no upregulation or stabilization of glutamate uptake was seen at 24 hours. Lithium is often referred to as a mood stabilizer because it shifts mood toward normal from the direction of either depression or mania. In addition to upregulating glutamate uptake, lithium stabilized glutamate uptake over the same time span. There was a wide range of glutamate uptake in synaptosomes from individual control mice, but in lithium-treated mice, uptake in synaptosomes from individual mice was clamped in a narrow range In these studies, it is not possible to measure the effect of chronic lithium on extracellular glutamate in vivo. This will require microdialysis or push-pull perfusion in intact animals.

SUMMARY

Beginning at therapeutic concentrations (1–1.5 mM), the antibipolar drug lithium stimulated the release of the major excitatory central neurotransmitter, glutamate, in monkey and mouse cerebral cortex slices in a time- and concentration-dependent manner, and this was associated with increased Ins(1,4,5)P_3 accumulation. CPP, dizocilpine [(±)MK-801], ketamine, and Mg^{2+}—antagonists to the NMDA receptor/channel complex—selectively inhibited lithium-stimulated Ins(1,4,5)P_3 accumulation. Antagonists to cholinergic-muscarinic, α_1-adrenergic, 5-HT_2-serotonergic, and H_1-histaminergic receptors had no effect. Antagonists to non-NMDA glutamate receptors had no effect on lithium-stimulated Ins(1,4,5)P_3 accumulation. Possible reasons for this are discussed. Similar results were obtained in mouse cerebral cortex slices. Carbetapentane, which inhibits glutamate release, inhibited lithium-induced Ins(1,4,5)P_3 accumulation in this model. It is concluded that the primary effect of lithium in the cerebral cortex slice model is stimulation of glutamate release, which, via activation of the NMDA receptor, leads to Ca^{2+} entry. The increased Ins(1,4,5)P_3 accumulation was due to the presumed increased influx of extracellular Ca^{2+}, which activates phospholipase C. These effects may have relevance to the therapeutic action of lithium in the treatment of bipolar disorder as well as its toxic effects, especially at lithium blood levels above 1.5 mM.

As with lithium, therapeutic concentrations of the antibipolar drug valproic acid stimulated glutamate release and Ins(1,4,5)P_3 accumulation but had no effect on accumulation of inositol mono- and bisphosphates in the presence or absence of acetylcholine, showing that valproate does not inhibit inositol mono- or bisphosphatases. Thus, two structurally unrelated antibipolar drugs stimulate glutamate release and Ins(1,4,5)P_3 accumulation, but only lithium causes accumulation of inositol mono- and bisphosphates, suggesting that inhibition of the respective phosphatases is not necessary for antibipolar action.

We report here that the accumulation of extracellular glutamate due to lithium was caused by lithium-induced inhibition of glutamate uptake into cerebrocortical slices or cerebrocortical synaptosomes. Glutamate accumulation was amplified fivefold over inhibition of uptake. When the effects of lithium and the specific glutamate transporter inhibitors, PDC and dihydrokainic acid, were plotted as inhibition of glutamate uptake versus glutamate accumulation, the plots were superimposable. This finding strongly indicates that lithium-induced glutamate accumulation is entirely caused by inhibition of uptake. With cerebrocortical synaptosomes, inhibition of glutamate uptake was twice as great as in slices, suggesting that presynaptic nerve endings are the primary site of inhibition of uptake by lithium. Inhibition of uptake was the result of a progressive lowering of V_{max}, as the lithium concentration was increased, while the K_m remained constant, indicating that lithium inhibited the capacity of the transporter but not its affinity. Chronic lithium treatment in mice, achieving a blood level of 0.7–1.0 mM, which is in the therapeutic range, upregulated synaptosomal uptake of glutamate. This would be expected to exert an antimanic effect because more excitatory glutamate would be removed from the synaptic cleft. Lithium is a mood stabilizer, dampening both the manic and the depressive phases of bipolar disorder. Interestingly, although the uptake of glutamate varied widely in individual control mice, uptake in lithium-treated mice was clamped over a narrow range (variance in control mice, 0.423; in lithium-treated mice, 0.184). This may be responsible for the mood-stabilizing effect of lithium. The therapeutic effect of lithium requires 1–2 weeks of treatment. The upregulation and stabilization of glutamate uptake followed the same time course. No effect was seen at 24 hours, but full upregulation and stabilization were observed at 1 and 2 weeks of treatment.

REFERENCES

Allison JH, Stewart MA: Reduced brain inositol in lithium-treated rats. Nature: New Biology 233:267–268, 1971

Annels SJ, Ellis Y, Davies JA: Non-opioid antitussives inhibit endogenous glutamate release from rabbit hippocampal slices. Brain Res 564:341–343, 1991

Antonsson BE: Purification and characterization of phosphatidylinositol synthase from human placenta. Biochem J 297:517–522, 1994

Batty IH, Michie A, Fennel M, et al: The characteristics, capacity and receptor regulation of inositol uptake in 1321N1 astrocytoma cells. Biochem J 294:49–55, 1993

Dixon JF, Hokin LE: Lithium acutely inhibits and chronically up-regulates and stabilizes glutamate uptake y presynaptic nerve endings in mouse cerebral cortex. Proc Natl Acad Sci U S A 95:8363–8368, 1998

Dixon JF, Lee CH, Los GV, et al: Lithium enhances accumulation of [3H]inositol radioactivity and mass of second messenger inositol 1,4,5-trisphosphate in monkey cerebral cortex. J Neurochem 59:2332–2335, 1992

Dixon JF, Los GV, Hokin LE: Lithium stimulates glutamate "release" and inositol 1,4,5-trisphosphate accumulation via activation of the N-methyl-D-aspartate receptor in monkey and mouse cerebral cortex slices. Proc Natl Acad Sci U S A 91:8358–8362, 1994

Heacock AM, Seguin EB, Agranoff BW: Measurement of receptor-activated phosphoinositide turnover in rat brain: nonequivalence of inositol phosphate and CDP-diacylglycerol formation. J Neurochem 60:1087–1092, 1993

Jope RS, Williams MB: Lithium and brain signal transduction systems. Biochem Pharmacol 47:429–441, 1994

Kennedy ED, Challiss RAJ, Nahorski SR: Lithium reduces the accumulation of inositol polyphosphate second messengers following cholinergic stimulation of cerebral cortex slices. J Neurochem 53:1652–1655, 1989

Lee CH, Dixon JF, Reichman M, et al: Li^+ increases accumulation of inositol 1,4,5-trisphosphate and inositol 1,3,4,5-tetrakisphosphate in cholinergically stimulated brain cortex. Biochem J 282:377–385, 1992

Los GV, Artemenko IP, Hokin LE: Time-dependent effects of lithium on the agonist-stimulated accumulation of second messenger inositol 1,4,5-trisphosphate in SH-SY5Y human neuroblastoma cells. Biochem J 311:225–232,1995

Mayer ML, Miller RJ: Excitatory amino acid receptors, second messengers and regulation of intracellular Ca^{2+} in mammalian neurons. Trends Pharmacol Sci 11:254–260, 1990

Michaelis T, Merboldt K-D, Bruhn H, et al: Absolute concentrations of metabolites in the adult human brain in vivo: quantification of localized proton MR spectra. Radiology 187:219–227, 1993

Petroff OAC, Spencer DD, Alger JR, et al: High-field proton magnetic resonance spectroscopy of human cerebrum obtained during surgery for epilepsy. Neurology 39:1197–1202, 1989

Schoepp D, Bockaert J, Sladeczek F: Pharmacological and functional characteristics of metabotropic excitatory amino acid receptors. Trends Pharmacol Sci 11:508–515, 1990

Sherman WR: Inositol homeostasis, lithium and diabetes, in Inositol Lipids in Cell Signalling. Edited by Michell RH. New York, Academic Press, 1989, pp 39–79

Sherman WR, Gish BG, Honchar MP, et al: Effect of lithium on phosphoinositide metabolism in vivo. Federation Proceedings 46:2639–2646, 1986

Vadnal R, Parthasarathy R: Myo-inositol monophosphatase: diverse effects of lithium, carbamazepine, and valproate. Neuropsychopharmacology 12:277–285, 1995

Whitworth P, Kendall DA: Lithium selectively inhibits muscarinic receptor-stimulated inositol tetrakisphosphate accumulation in mouse cerebral cortex slices. J Neurochem 51:258–265, 1988

CHAPTER 5

EFFECTS OF ANTIDEPRESSANT TREATMENTS ON THE G PROTEIN–ADENYLYL CYCLASE AXIS AS THE POSSIBLE BASIS OF THERAPEUTIC ACTION

Mark M. Rasenick, Ph.D., Jiang Chen, M.D., Ph.D., and Hikroki Ozawa, M.D., Ph.D.

BACKGROUND

Drugs designed to treat depression were first employed on the basis that they facilitate neurotransmission of catecholamines and serotonin. It now appears that an elaborate series of molecular mechanisms underlie the therapeutic effects of the various antidepressant therapies. Despite decades of research, these molecular mechanisms remain a puzzle. This chapter will attempt to provide evidence that facilitated guanine nucleotide binding protein (G-protein)–mediated signal transduction provides at least one piece which can be used to assist in solving it.

Madhavi Talluri is thanked for her superb technical assistance.
Support for this work was provided by the National Institute of Mental Health (MH 39595), the Stanley Foundation, and Abbott Laboratories. M. M. R. is the recipient of a Research Scientist Development Award from the National Institute of Mental Health (MH00699).

G-Protein–Mediated Signal Transduction

Receptors for a variety of biogenic amines, acetylcholine, amino acid neurotransmitters, peptide hormones, and purines are thought to contain seven membrane-spanning domains. These heptaspan receptors couple to G proteins so that the effect of a given agonist can be communicated to the cell interior (Figure 5–1). The multitude of identified and cloned receptors is sufficiently large that any attempt to list them is fruitless, and any such list becomes incomplete as it is written.

G-protein–mediated signaling systems include stimulation (G_s) and inhibition (G_i) of adenylyl cyclase, the gating of K^+(G_i) and Ca^{2+} (G_o) channels, the activation of phosphoinositide phospholipase C (G_q/G_{11}) and Na/H^+ exchange (G_{13}) (Rasenick 1992; Simon et al. 1991). G proteins are heterotrimeric in structure (Table 5–1) and consist of α, β, and γ subunits; α binds guanosine triphosphate (GTP) and possesses intrinsic GTPase. Molecular weights of the α subunits range from 39 to 52 kDa, the βs are about 36 kDa, and the γ subunits range from 8 to 14 kDa. Both the activated α subunit and G β γ subunits appear to regulate effector molecules (Federman et al. 1992; Iyengar 1993; Taussig et al. 1993).

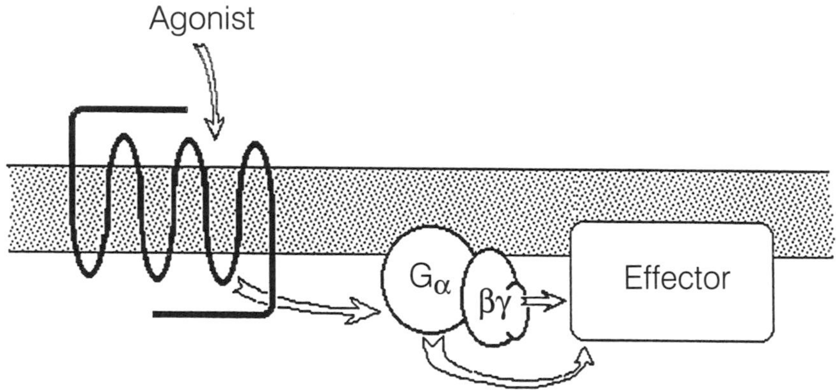

Figure 5–1. Coupling between heptaspan receptors, guanine nucleotide binding protein (G proteins), and effector molecules. The activation of G protein occurs subsequent to agonist occupancy of the receptor, and the activated G protein engages the effector. Depending on the effector, G protein α or βγ subunits are capable of effector regulation. The list of biological processes regulated by G proteins is a partial one. Effectors: Adenylyl cyclase ↑ or ↓; phospholipase (A, C, D); phosphodiesterase; ion flux.
Source. Adapted from Rasenick et al. 1995.

Table 5–1. Biochemical characteristics of heterotrimeric G-protein families

Subfamily	Receptors		Effectors	Second messenger
G_s	β-Adrenoreceptor, dopamine D_1, 5-HT_4	α_s	→ AC	↑ cAMP
			→ Ca^{2+} channels	↑ Ca^{2+} flux
			→ K^+channels	↑ K^+flux
	Odorant	α_{olf}	→ AC	↑ cAMP
G_i	Muscarinic M_2 or M_4 receptor, α_2 adrenoreceptor, dopamine	α_{i1}, α_{i2}, α_{i3}	→ AC	↓ cAMP
			→ PLA_2	↓ Arachidonate release
			→ K^+channels	↑ K^+flux
		α_{oA}, α_{oB}	→ Ca^{2+} channels	↓ Ca^{2+} flux
			→ K^+ channels	↑ K^+ flux
	μ or δ opiate receptors (opiate, 5-HT)?	α_z	→ PLC (via βγ)	↑ IP_3, DAG, CA^{2+}
			→ AC	↓ cAMP
	Rhodopsin	α_t	→ cGMP PDE	↓ cGMP
			→ PLA_2	↓
G_q	Muscarinic, thromboxane A_2, bradykinin, histamine, vasopressin, and 5-HT receptors	α_{15}, α_{16}, α_{14}, α_q, α_{11}	→ PLC-β	↑ IP_3, DAG, Ca^{2+}

(continued)

Table 5–1. Biochemical characteristics of heterotrimeric G-protein families *(continued)*

Subfamily	Receptors		Effectors	Second messenger
G_{12}	Thrombin receptor LPA receptor	$\alpha_{12} \rightarrow NA^+/H^+$ exchanger-1		$\uparrow NA^+/H^+$ exchange
		$\alpha_{13} \rightarrow NA^+/H^+$ exchanger-1 and small G protein and the actin cytoskeleton	Cell proliferation Cell shape changes	
$\beta\gamma$	N/A	$\beta\gamma$	$\rightarrow K^+$ channel	$\uparrow K^+$ flux
			$\rightarrow$ AC-I	$\downarrow$ cAMP
			$\rightarrow$ AC-II and IV	$\uparrow$ cAMP
			$\rightarrow$ Receptor kinases	$\uparrow$ cAMP receptor desensitization
			$\rightarrow$ PLC-β	$\uparrow IP_3$, DAG, Ca^{2+}

Note. The receptor list is not meant to be inclusive. AC = adenylyl cyclase; cAMP = cyclic adenosine monophosphate; cGMP = cyclic guanosine monophosphate; DAG = diacylglycerol; IP_3 = inositol 1,4,5-trisphosphate; PDE = phosphodiesterase; PLA = phospholipase A; PLC = phospholipase C; 5-HT = serotonin.

Although the activation of receptor by agonist and the subsequent activation of G protein by receptor and effector by G protein (whether α or $\beta\gamma$ subunit) has been reviewed extensively, it is often depicted as a linear sequence of events involving agonist binding, G-protein activation and subsequent effector engagement. The actual scenario of events is likely to be far more complex.

G_s and G_i were named for their abilities to stimulate or inhibit (respectively) adenylyl cyclase. Several other functions have also been attributed to these proteins. The sequence similarity among G proteins makes it difficult to assign unique roles to them. Furthermore, many reconstitution studies have demonstrated that the addition of any of several G proteins may elicit an identical effect. Given the multifarious array of G proteins, it is possible that some combination of α, β, and γ subtypes helps to target a given G protein for a specific receptor and effector. Some recent work with antisense probes to different β and γ subunits is consistent with such a hypothesis (Kleuss et al. 1991, 1992, 1993). Furthermore, it is possible that some element of the membrane or cytoskeleton "channels" the appropriate receptor and G protein to the "right" effector. Data from our laboratory lend support to this suggestion (Popova et al. 1997; Roychowdhury and Rasenick 1994; Wang and Rasenick 1991; Wang et al. 1990; Yan et al. 1996).

Adenylyl Cyclase

In this chapter we focus on the effects of antidepressant treatment on G-protein–stimulated adenylyl cyclase. As of this writing, nine forms of the enzyme have been identified by molecular cloning, and each of these forms is found somewhere within the brain (Iyengar 1993). Although all forms of adenylyl cyclase are stimulated by $G_s\alpha$, some (II, IV, VII) are stimulated by $\beta\gamma$ as well. Others (I, III, VIII) are stimulated by calcium/calmodulin, and still others (V, VI) are inhibited by micromolar calcium. Together this allows for a rich regulation of signaling, which may have important ramifications for memory and emotion (Xia et al. 1996).

DEPRESSION AND ANTIDEPRESSANTS

There are three major classes of antidepressant drugs: monoamine oxidase inhibitors, selective serotonin reuptake inhibitors, and typical tricyclic compounds. There are also a variety of atypical antidepressant drugs that defy ready classification. Finally, there is electroconvulsive therapy (ECT). All are clinically effective after chronic treatment (approximately 2–3 weeks). To date, no truly inclusive, unifying hypothesis concerning a mechanism of action for these diverse therapies has been formed.

In the last several decades, research has focused on the effects of the chronic administration of antidepressants on various aspects of neuronal function, and a plethora of studies has demonstrated alterations in the density and/or sensitivity of several neurotransmitter receptor systems (Druker et al. 1989; Okada et al. 1986; Sulser 1984). These results do not explain fully the clinical efficacy of all antidepressants, and the dissociation between receptor numbers and receptor responsiveness has led to the investigation of possible postreceptor sites of actions of these drugs.

Several theories regarding the mechanisms of antidepressant action have been proposed. Neurotransmitter function may be altered indirectly through the regulation of intracellular signaling; and antidepressant agents may be effective, not as a result of effects on a certain neurotransmitter or receptor, but because they modulate converging postsynaptic signals generated in response to multiple endogenous neurotransmitters, including norepinephrine (NE) and serotonin. In this context, the signal-transducing G proteins, which play a major role in the amplification and integration of signals in the central nervous system, are in a unique position to affect the functional balance between neurotransmitter systems.

Theories of antidepressant action might involve several aspects of receptors or G proteins (Figure 5–2):

- The number or affinity of receptors could be altered.
- The coupling between receptor and G protein could be changed.
- The number of G proteins could be changed, or the intrinsic properties of a given G protein (e.g., affinity for GTP or rate of GTP hydrolysis) could be modified.
- The coupling between G proteins and their effectors could be altered, or the effectors themselves could be increased in number or intrinsic activity.

It is also possible that the product of the G protein–adenylyl cyclase axis, cyclic adenosine monophosphate (cAMP) and the myriad proteins phosphorylated by cAMP-dependent protein kinases could be altered by antidepressant treatment (for review, see Hyman and Nestler 1996).

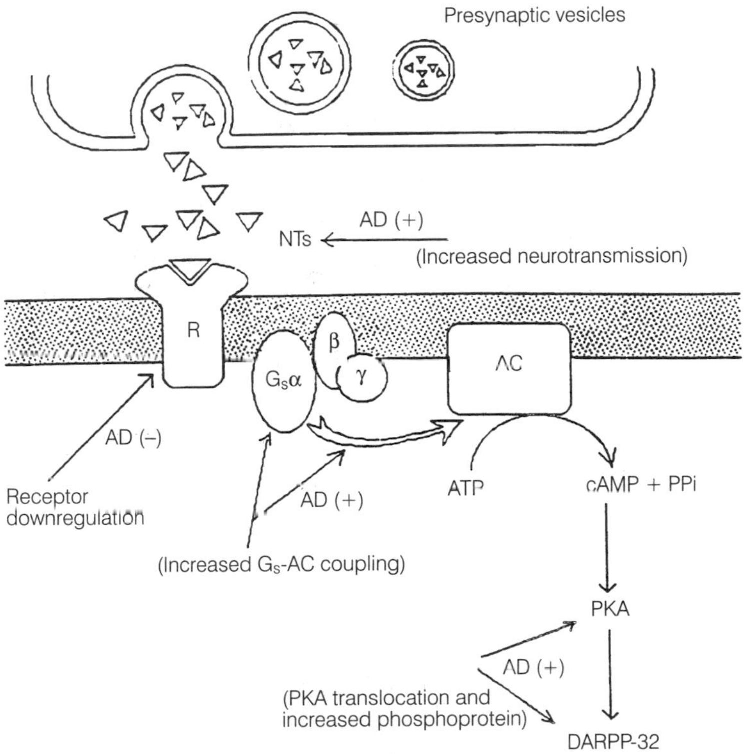

Figure 5–2. Possible targets of antidepressant treatment. The figure depicts processes that might be altered as a result of chronic antidepressant treatment. An affected system need not be the direct target of an antidepressant drug.
Note. AD = antidepressant; NT = neurotransmitter; R = receptor; G_s, $G_s\alpha$ = G proteins that stimulate adenylyl cyclase; β, γ = subtypes of G protein; AC = adenylyl cyclase; ATP = adenosine triphosphate; cAMP = cyclic adenosine monophosphate; PPi = pyrophosphate; PKA = protein kinase A; DARPP-32 = dopamine receptor–associated phosphoprotein.

Antidepressants and β-Receptor Downregulation

The receptor–G protein–adenylyl cyclase system has long been thought to play a role in the therapeutic effects of antidepressant treatment. Vetulani and Sulser (1975) demonstrated that chronic, but not acute, treatment with a variety of antidepressant agents results in a decrease of cAMP production induced by isoproterenol. Reduction of NE-stimulated cAMP levels in different regions of brain have been reported following long-term treatment with a variety of typical and atypical antidepressant agents, as well as with monoamine oxidase inhibitors and ECT. This β-receptor downregulation occurs with a time delay and thus corresponds somewhat with the clinical antidepressant activity.

The mechanism by which antidepressant drugs downregulate β-receptor number and NE-stimulated cAMP production is not known. An initial hypothesis suggested that downregulation of postsynaptic β-adrenergic systems occurs secondary to antidepressant-induced increase in NE within the synaptic cleft. Clearly, many antidepressant compounds (of various types) have this effect. However, in some cultured cells devoid of NE, tricyclic antidepressants have been reported to downregulate β-adrenergic receptors and/or to decrease the cAMP response to isoproterenol (Fishman and Finberg 1987; Hertz and Richardson 1983; Honegger et al. 1986; Manier et al. 1992; Manji et al. 1992). This finding indicates an agonist/receptor–independent mechanism in the regulation of the sensitivity of the β-adrenergic receptor. Studies in our laboratory (University of Illinois College of Medicine, Chicago) have represented a search for a receptor-independent mechanism of antidepressant action. We have chosen the G protein–adenylyl cyclase axis as the site on which to focus our investigation.

Chronic Antidepressant Treatment of Rats and Increase in Coupling Between $G_s\alpha$ and Adenylyl Cyclase

Initial findings concerning G proteins and antidepressant treatment were made more than 15 years ago (Menkes et al. 1983) when it was noted that chronic treatment of rats with amitryptiline or electroconvulsive shock (ECS) increased the ability of a hydrolysis-resistant GTP analog, guanylyl-5′-imidodiphosphate (Gpp(NH)p) to stimulate adenylyl cyclase without modifying the basal activity of that enzyme or the activity in the presence of manganese (which reflected G-protein–independent activation) (Figure 5–3). These effects were absolutely dependent on chronic treatments; treatments of up to 7 days were without effect (Figure 5–4). Further, addition of any of the antidepressant drugs to the adenylyl cyclase assay medium was without effect (Chen and Rasenick 1995a; Ozawa and Rasenick 1989). The notion that increased G_s-mediated activation of adenylyl cyclase resulted from any antidepressant treatment was bolstered by the finding that ECS showed a similar effect (Ozawa and Rasenick 1991) in each parameter examined (Figure 5–5). Thus, it seemed likely that some aspect of G_s function was altered by antidepressant treatment.

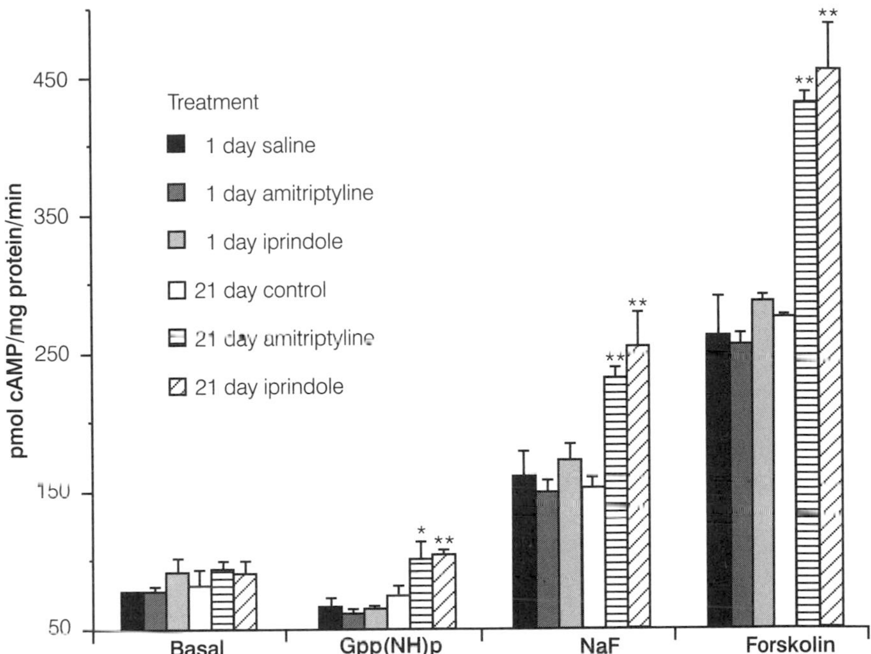

Figure 5–3. Effect of chronic antidepressant treatment in rats on stimulation of adenylyl cyclase. Rats were injected once daily for 21 days with either saline or the indicated compound (10 mg/kg ip). They were sacrificed on the 22nd day. Cerebral cortex membranes were prepared and assayed for adenylyl cyclase as described in Ozawa and Rasenick (1989). Guanylyl-5′-imidodiphosphate (Gpp(NH)p) = 100mM, NaF = 20mM, forskolin (colforsin) = 100mM. Mean values ± SEM of triplicate determinations are shown. Treated groups were compared with corresponding sham groups; $*P < 0.01$, $**P < 0.001$ by two-tailed Scheffé's test after passing the one-way analysis of variance (ANOVA) test. Two other experiments gave similar results. cAMP = cyclic adenosine monophosphate.
Source. Data from Ozawa and Rasenick 1989.

Sensitivity to Gpp(NH)p was not altered by antidepressant treatment: the EC_{50} for Gpp(NH)p was constant in any of the antidepressant treatments (Ozawa and Rasenick 1989, 1991) (Figure 5–5). Furthermore, despite the fact that all tissues would have been exposed to antidepressant drugs, facilitated G-protein activation of adenylyl cyclase was noted only in brain tissue; no effects were seen in liver or renal membranes prepared from antidepressant-treated animals (Menkes et al. 1983; Ozawa and Rasenick 1989).

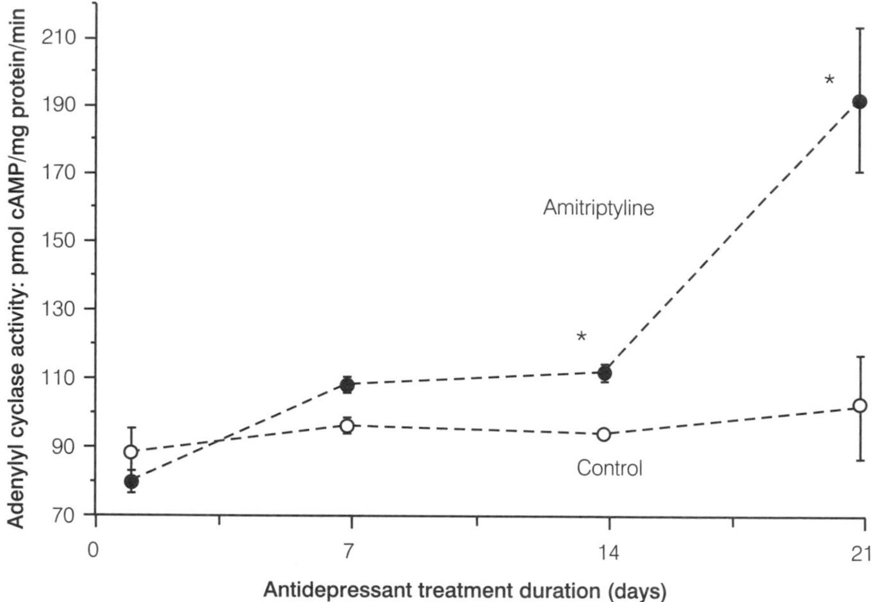

Figure 5–4. Duration of treatment required for antidepressant-induced augmentation of guanylyl-5′-imidodiphosphate (Gpp(NH)p)–activated adenylyl cyclase. Rats were treated with amitriptyline or saline for the indicated period, 21 days. In the treatment (amitriptyline) group, 7 days of treatment means 14 days of saline followed by 7 days of amitryptiline. Membrane preparation and adenylyl cyclase assay were as described in Ozawa and Rasenick (1991). The membranes were assayed in the presence of Gpp(NH)p (100 μM). *$P < 0.01$ compared with control (saline) treatment. *Note.* cAMP = cyclic adenosine monophosphate. *Source.* Adapted from Ozawa and Rasenick 1991.

Antidepressant Treatment and Inhibition of Adenylyl Cyclase

As noted above, adenylyl cyclase can be inhibited through a separate G protein (G_i). In the studies cited in the previous paragraph, it was possible that the increased activation of the enzyme was actually due to diminished inhibition. However, no changes in the activity of G_i were seen, so it was suggested that the antidepressant-induced changes were due to the stimulation of adenylyl cyclase and the G protein thought responsible for that stimulation (G_s). In fact, chemical elimination of G_s eliminated the antidepressant-induced changes in adenylyl cyclase (Ozawa and Rasenick 1989, 1991).

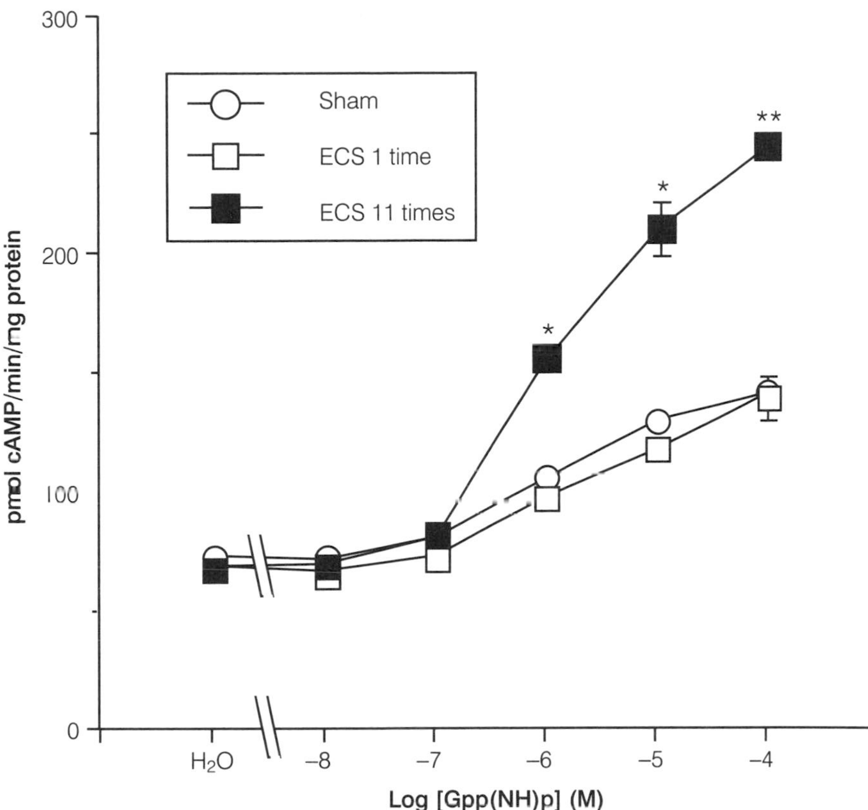

Figure 5–5. Effects of electroconvulsive shock (ECS) on guanylyl-5′-imidodiphosphate [Gpp(NH)p]-stimulated adenylyl cyclase. ECS administration (or sham ECS for control condition) was performed every other day 1 time or 11 times. Rats were sacrificed on the 22nd day, and cerebral cortex membranes were assayed for adenylyl cyclase as described in Chen and Rasenick (1995a). Mean values ± SEM of triplicate determinations are shown. Treated groups compared with corresponding sham groups: $^{*}P < 0.01$, $^{**}P < 0.001$ by two-tailed Scheffé's test after passing the one-way analysis of variance (ANOVA) test. Two other experiments gave similar results. *Note.* cAMP = cyclic adenosine monophosphate. *Source.* Adapted from Chen and Rasenick 1995a.

G-Protein Expression and Antidepressant Treatment

It has been suggested that treatments for affective disorder might alter G-protein content on the synaptic membrane. This possibility was first raised in a study in which GTP binding to brain membranes was performed in rats treated chronically with lithium (Avissar et al. 1988). Changes in isoproterenol-induced GTP binding to membranes were attributed to changes in G-protein content in those membranes. Given the multitude of proteins capable of binding GTP (and the likelihood that the moles of GTP bound far exceeded the molar G-protein content), these results were difficult to interpret. Therefore, several investigators examined G-protein content more directly by using immunoblotting techniques. Small changes in G-protein content were seen by some investigators after certain antidepressant or antimanic treatments (Manji et al. 1995), but no clear consensus has arisen.

Because the potency of Gpp(NH)p for stimulating adenylyl cyclase did not change in response to antidepressant treatment (Figure 5–4), we thought it unlikely that there was an increase in the expression of $G_s\alpha$ protein (or decrease in the expression of $G_i\alpha$). Similarly, the lack of change in manganese-activated adenylyl cyclase rendered it unlikely that antidepressant treatment increased the amount of this enzyme. Immunoblotting studies showed that the amounts of these proteins remained constant, not changing in response to antidepressant treatment (Chen and Rasenick 1995a). It is noteworthy that three series of antidepressant treatments (drugs or ECS) were done for these experiments. For any given G protein, 20%–25% differences between antidepressant and control groups could be seen in a treatment series. In one treatment series, a 25% increase in $G_s\alpha$ was noted for the amitryptiline-treated group, whereas in the next, a 15% decrease was observed. Thus, no reliable and consistent changes in G-protein content could be attributed to antidepressant treatment. Similar results were obtained by Emamghoreishi et al. (1996).

It should be considered that for a given G protein, in many systems the concentration of that protein exceeds by 10-fold that of its cognate receptor. This excess of G protein renders it unlikely that small changes in G protein content would have great physiological significance. It is likely, however, that G proteins have a heterogeneous distribution and are highly compartmentalized in the neuron. Small overall changes could be reflected in large changes in G protein within a given cellular structure. To investigate this possibility, immunocytochemical studies are required.

Antidepressant Treatment and GTP-Binding Properties of G Proteins

It was also possible that changes in the GTP-binding properties of $G_s\alpha$ were altered by chronic antidepressant treatment. This was investigated by exposing synaptic or plasma membranes to the photoaffinity GTP analog, azidoanilido GTP (AAGTP). This compound, which is labeled with ^{32}P in the α phosphate, forms a covalent bond (on ultraviolet irradiation) with the protein to which it is bound. Subsequent to sodium dodecyl sulfate (SDS) polyacrylamide gel electrophoresis, individual G proteins can be identified and AAGTP binding quantified (Rasenick et al. 1994). This was done with membranes prepared from brains of rats subjected to various chronic antidepressant treatments. No changes in intrinsic AAGTP binding were noted. This was consistent with the notion that expression of G proteins was unaltered by antidepressant treatment (Ozawa and Rasenick 1989, 1991). Curiously, interaction among G proteins, as measured by the direct transfer of nucleotide, was facilitated by chronic antidepressant treatment (Ozawa and Rasenick 1991).

Facilitated Interaction Between G_s and Adenylyl Cyclase as Result of Antidepressant Treatment

Increased interaction among G proteins on the synaptic membrane suggested to us that increased activation of G_s might result from increased physical coupling between G_s and adenylyl cyclase. This was investigated by using immunoprecipitation of $G_s\alpha$–adenylyl cyclase complexes with anti-$G_s\alpha$ antibodies. This study also provided independent means to verify that there was no increase in G_s content after antidepressant treatment. The study, done with cerebral cortex membranes from rats treated chronically with amitryptiline or ECS, is illustrated in Figure 5–6. It is noteworthy that, in order to measure significant adenylyl cyclase activity in the immunoprecipitate, G_s must be activated with the hydrolysis-resistant GTP analog Gpp(NH)p. Presumably, this is in order to confer stability on that molecule during the immunoprecipitation process (Halliday et al. 1984). Preactivation with Gpp(NH)p increases the total number of G_s–adenylyl cyclase complexes (independent of antidepressant treatment). At maximum, 50% of the $G_s\alpha$ is immunoprecipitated; this is independent of the association of G_s with adenylyl cyclase. Thus, if there were an increase in the total $G_s\alpha$ after antidepressant treatment, the amount of adenylyl cyclase in the supernatant would increase relative to that in the pellet. It did not, offering independent confirmation that antidepresssant treatment did not increase the amount of $G_s\alpha$. Nonetheless, the total adenylyl cyclase immunoprecipitated by anti-$G_s\alpha$ increased after antidepressant treatment (Figure 5–6), consistent with the idea that antidepressant treatment increases coupling between $G_s\alpha$ and adenylyl cyclase.

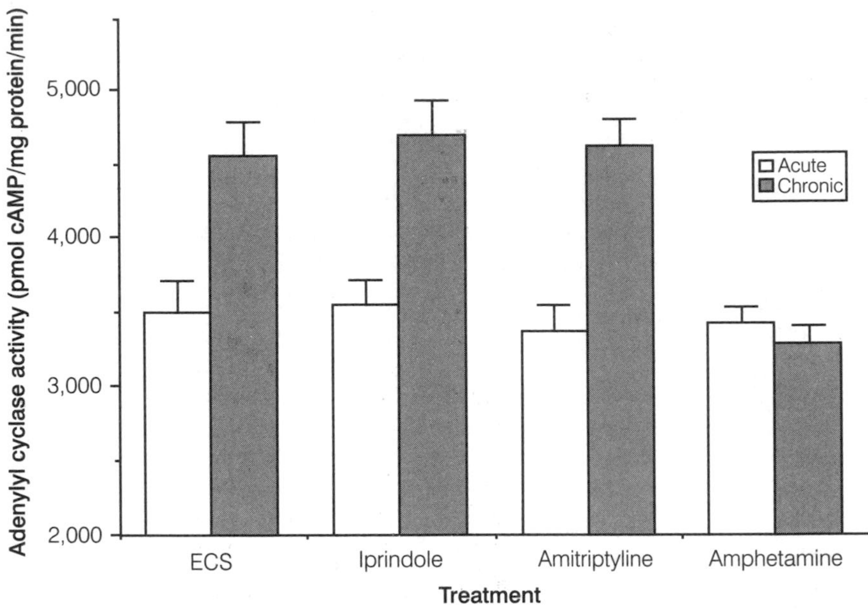

Figure 5–6. Immunoprecipitation of $G_s\alpha$–adenylyl cyclase activity in membrane of rats after chronic antidepressant treatment. Rats were treated with electroconvulsive shock (ECS) (chronic = every other day for 22 days; acute = 1 day) or the indicated drugs (chronic = 21 days; acute = 1 day). Amitriptyline and iprindole were administered at 10 mg/kg intraperitoneally, and 1.5 mg/kg of amphetamine was given intraperitoneally (Chen and Rasenick 1995a). Complexes of $G_s\alpha$–adenylyl cyclase were extracted from cerebral cortex membranes with detergent and immunoprecipitated as described in Chen and Rasenick (1995a). Adenylyl cyclase was assayed in both pellets and supernatants after immunoprecipitation. The total G_s-stimulated adenylyl cyclase was increased ($P < 0.01$) in the chronically treated group, whereas the ratio of adenylyl cyclase immunoprecipitated to that remaining in the supernatant was the same in both groups (about 0.4). This is consistent with the hypothesis that, although chronic antidepressant treatment does not change the amount of G_s, the number of $G_s\alpha$ molecules associated with adenylyl cyclase (coupling between $G_s\alpha$ and adenylyl cyclase) is increased. cAMP = cyclic adenosine monophosphate.

β-Adrenergic Receptors and Antidepressant Action: Use of a Cell Culture System to Resolve the Role of β-Receptor Desensitization and Presynaptic Effects

Treatment of C6 rat glioma cells with a variety of antidepressant drugs has been shown to downregulate the β-adrenergic receptors on those cells

(Fishman and Finberg 1987; Manji et al. 1992). The absence of catecholamine in the culture medium fostered speculation that the effects of the antidepressant compounds were directly on the target neuron, occurring independently of the blockade of neurotransmitter reuptake. This laboratory attempted to determine whether the enhanced coupling between G_s and adenylyl cyclase, similar to that observed in rat brain membranes, could be elicited by incubation of these cells with antidepressant compounds.

Exposure of C6 glioma cells to culture medium containing desipramine (5 μM or 10 μM) for 5 days results in a significant increase in Gpp(NH)p-stimulated adenylyl cyclase activity in cell membranes, which is a pattern similar to that seen in cerebral cortex membrane of rats after chronic (21 days) antidepressant administration (see Figure 5–7). These treatments did not alter the basal activity of adenylyl cyclase. Similar results were observed with two other antidepressant drugs, amitriptyline and iprindole (Table 5–2), suggesting that increased G_s-stimulated adenylyl cyclase activity results after chronic antidepressant exposure in these cells.

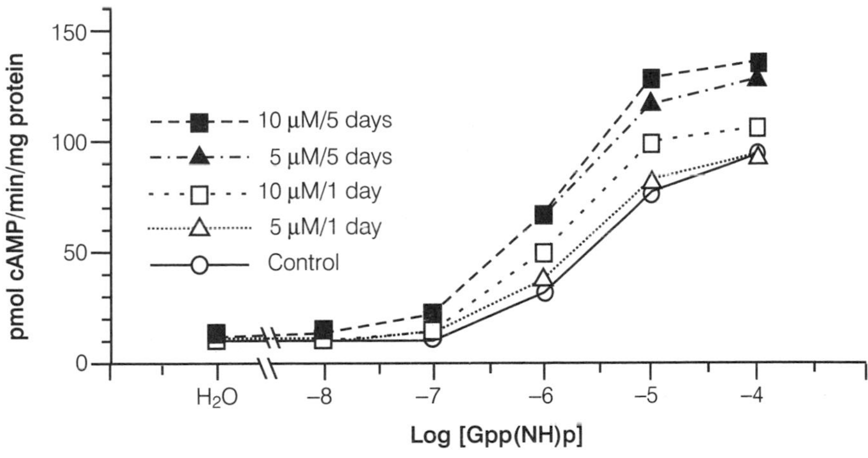

Figure 5–7. Effect of dosage of desipramine and duration of treatment on C6 membrane adenylyl cyclase. Membranes were made from C6 glioma cells exposed to medium containing 5 μM or 10 μM desipramine for 1 day or 5 days. The membranes were assayed as described in Chen and Rasenick (1995b). Values are means ± SEM of individual triplicates. One-way analysis of variance (ANOVA) and two-tailed Scheffé's tests indicated that adenylyl cyclase activity in 5-day treatment groups (for 5 μM) and 1- or 5-day treatment groups (for 10 μM) were significantly higher than that in control groups ($P < 0.05$–0.001). Basal (H_2O) adenylyl cyclase activity was not significantly different among any of the groups. One of two similar experiments is shown. cAMP = cyclic adenosine monophosphate.

Table 5–2. Effect of antidepressants on basal or Gpp(NH)p-stimulated adenylyl cyclase in C6 glioma membranes

Adenylyl cyclase activity	Desipramine (n = 4)	Amitriptyline (n = 4)	Iprindole (n = 3)
Basal (% of control)	96.44 ± 5.92	102.6 ± 2.77	104.8 ± 3.75
Gpp(NH)p (% of control)	171.6 ± 18.22*	171.5 ± 11.76**	153.7 ± 6.77**

Note. C6 glioma cells were exposed to 5 μM of the indicated antidepressant for 5 days. Membranes were prepared and assayed for adenylyl cyclase activity without (basal) or with 1 μM guanylyl-5′-imidodiphosphate [Gpp(NH)p], as described in Chen and Rasenick (1995a). The values shown are means ± SEM of 3–4 independent experiments (see column heads for number of experiments), each performed in triplicate.
*$P < 0.05$. **$P < 0.001$ by Scheffé's test after passing the one-way analysis of variance (ANOVA) test.
Source. Adapted from Chen and Rasenick (1995a).

Effects of Antidepressant Treatment on G-Protein Content in C6 Cells

The primary effect of antidepressant treatment, whether in cells or membranes, was to increase the maximal stimulation of adenylyl cyclase by Gpp(NH)p, forskolin, or sodium fluoride plus aluminum chloride (NaF). Each of these activating agents works best on the adenylyl cyclase–G_s complex. Sensitivity to Gpp(NH)p was little changed by the treatment. Furthermore, immunoblotting revealed that desipramine treatments which increased G_s–adenylyl cyclase coupling in the cells did not change the content of $G_s\alpha$, $G_i\alpha2$, $G_o\alpha$, or $G\beta\gamma$ in the cells (Chen and Rasenick 1995b). This further supports the idea that functional rather than quantitative changes of G proteins contribute to the enhanced activation of adenylyl cyclase after chronic antidepressant treatment. It also strengthens the suggestion that one result of chronic antidepressant treatment is an increase in coupling between G_s and adenylyl cyclase.

Effect of β-Receptor Desensitization on Gpp(NH)p-Stimulated Adenylyl Cyclase

As indicated above, several investigators had noted that antidepressant treatment desensitized β-adrenergic receptors (decreased B_{max}) in C6 cells. These studies suggested that the drugs exerted this effect directly on the "postsynaptic cell." We also noted that the time course of β-receptor desensitization was faster than that required for the increase in G_s activation of adenylyl cyclase (Figure 5–8). A direct uncoupling between β-receptor desensitization was revealed in experiments where C6 cells were incubated with 5 μM isoproterenol for 3 days. This treatment desensitized the β receptors. However, it did not increase Gpp(NH)p-stimulated adenylyl cyclase activity; 5 days' treatment was required for that (Chen and Rasenick 1995b). These results further suggest that enhancement of Gpp(NH)p-stimulated adenylyl cyclase activity by chronic antidepressant treatment is not related to β-receptor desensitization.

Increased "Mobility" of $G_s\alpha$ in the Plasma Membrane Subsequent to Antidepressant Treatment

The increased coupling of $G_s\alpha$ and adenylyl cyclase did not appear to be caused by an intrinsic change in either molecule or receptor-$G_s\alpha$ coupling. Thus, the possibility that some other protein or lipid was changed by chronic antidepres-

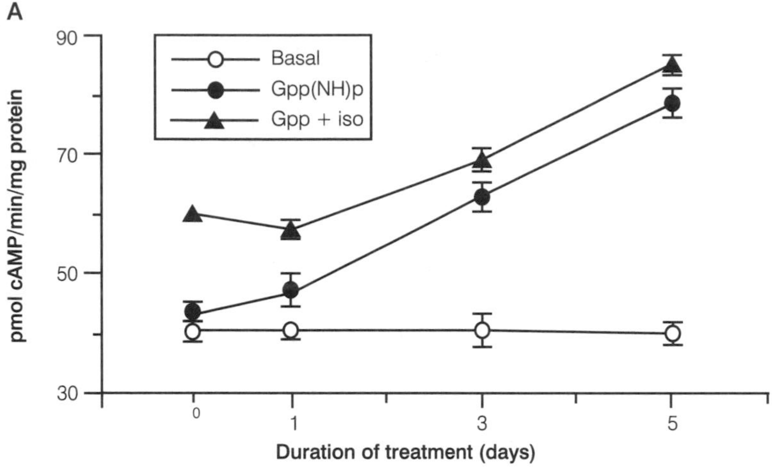

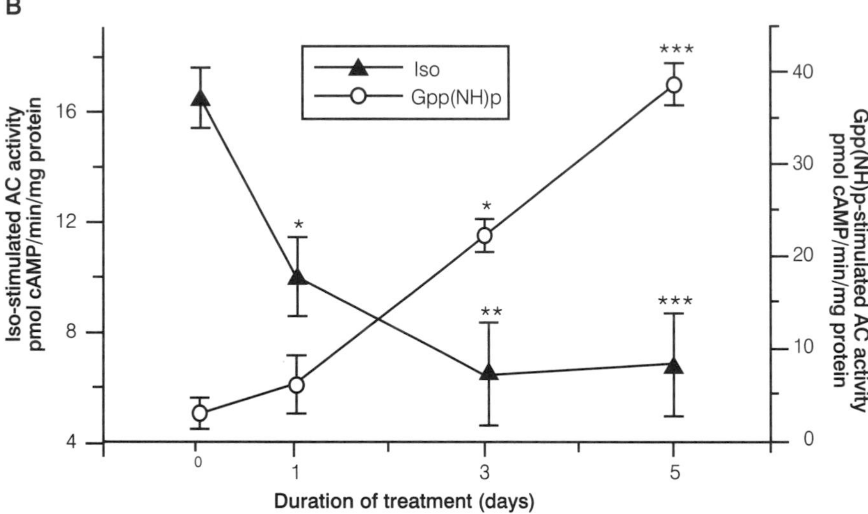

Figure 5–8. Comparison of desipramine-induced β-adrenergic desensitization and guanylyl-5′-imidodiphosphate [Gpp(NH)p]-stimulated adenylyl cyclase (AC) augmentation in C6 glioma cells. C6 glioma cells were exposed to 5 μM for 1 day, 3 days, or 5 days as indicated. Cell membranes were assayed for AC as described in Chen and Rasenick (1995b). In (A), Gpp(NH)p (0.2 μM) or isoproterenol (iso) (1 μM) + Gpp(NH)p-stimulated AC activities were plotted. In order to see the net effect of each reagent, the fractions of Gpp(NH)p-stimulated AC activity (over basal activity) and iso-stimulated activity (over Gpp(NH)p-stimulated activity) were calculated (B) and compared with corresponding controls. Note that β-receptor desensitization occurs before increased Gpp(NH)p-stimulated AC. *$P < 0.05$; **$P < 0.02$; ***$P < 0.01$ by one-way analysis of variance (ANOVA) and Scheffé's tests. *Note.* cAMP = cyclic adenosine monophosphate.

sant treatment was investigated. The hypothesis was that chronic treatment with antidepressants would interact with some membrane target and would allow $G_s\alpha$ to effect a more facile interaction with adenylyl cyclase. This theory was initially investigated by determining the extraction of $G_s\alpha$ from the plasma membrane of C6 cells by two detergents. The detergents, Triton X-100 and Triton X-114, delineate a moderately hydrophobic and a more hydrophobic membrane fraction. $G_s\alpha$ is normally ensconced to a larger extent in the Triton X-114 fraction than in the Triton X-100 fraction. Chronic antidepressant (amitriptyline, desipramine, iprindole, or fluoxetine) treatment increased the amount of $G_s\alpha$ that was extracted by Triton X-100. Only $G_s\alpha$ was altered. The detergent extraction properties of the other G proteins were not altered by antidepressant treatment (Toki et al. 1999).

The Search for an "Antidepressant Receptor"

The evidence presented in this chapter suggests that chronic antidepressant treatment, either in rats or in C6 glioma cells, modifies adenylyl cyclase by some intervention between $G_s\alpha$ and the enzyme. Because in the case of C6 cells no "presynaptic" site is involved (and no neurotransmitter is in the media), it seems likely that antidepressants exert a direct effect on the target cells. This does not mean that G_s or adenylyl cyclase represents a molecular target for drugs designed to combat affective disorder. Given the chemically diverse nature of therapeutic agents, it is likely that the initial "receptor" is not a single entity, but rather several molecular targets forwarding information to a system that ultimately modifies the interaction between G_s and adenylyl cyclase. Given the delay between onset of drug exposure and antidepressant action (whether measured clinically or in terms of increased G_s–adenylyl cyclase coupling), it is unlikely that antidepressants act simply by regulating the expression of a gene. Rather, we have hypothesized that some structural rearrangement accompanies long-term antidepressant treatment. Work from our laboratory has established that elements of the cytoskeleton regulate G-protein function (Popova et al. 1997; Wang et al. 1990; Yan et al. 1996). G proteins also appear to modify the cytoskeleton (Roychowdhury et al. 1999). Perhaps some element of the cytoskeleton modifies its association with G proteins as a result of treatment with antidepressant drugs or ECS. Perhaps cytoskeketal or membrane properties, or the articulations between membrane and cytoskeleton, occur after chronic antidepressant treatments. Investigations into these possibilities are under way.

REFERENCES

Avissar S, Schreiber G, Danon A, et al: Lithium inhibits adrenergic and cholinergic increases in GTP binding in rat cortex. Nature 331:440–442, 1988

Banerjee SP, Kung LS, Riggi SJ, et al: Development of β-adrenergic receptor subsensitivity by antidepressants. Nature 268:455–456, 1977

Chen J, Rasenick MM: Chronic antidepressant treatment facilitates G protein activation without altering G protein content. J Pharmacol Exp Ther 275:509–517, 1995a

Chen J, Rasenick MM: Chronic treatment of C6 glioma cells with antidepressant increases functional coupling between a G protein (Gs) and adenylyl cyclase. J Neurochem 64:724–732, 1995b

Druker BJ, Mamon HJ, Roberts TM: Oncogenes, growth factors, and signal transduction. N Engl J Med 321:1383–1391, 1989

Emamghoreishi M, Warsh J, Sibong D, et al: Lack of effect of chronic antidepressant treatment on G_s and G_i alpha subunit protein and mRNA levels in the rat cerebral cortex. Neuropsychopharmacology 15:281–287, 1996

Federman AD, Conklin BR, Schrader KA, et al: Hormonal stimulation of adenylyl cyclase through Gi-protein βγ subunits. Nature 356:159–161, 1992

Fishman PH, Finberg JPM: Effect of the tricyclic antidepressant, desipramine on β adrenergic receptors in cultured rat C6 glioma cells. J Neurochem 49:282–289, 1987

Halliday K, Stein P, Chernoff N, et al: Limited trypsin proteolysis of photoreceptor GTP-binding protein: light- and GTP-induced conformational changes. J Biol Chem 259:516–525, 1984

Hertz L, Richardson J: Acute and chronic effects of antidepressant drugs on beta-adrenergic function in astrocytes in primary cultures: an indication of glial involvement in affective disorders? J Neurosci Res 9:173–182, 1983

Honegger UE, Disler B, Wiesmann UN: Chronic exposure of human cells in culture to the tricyclic antidepressant desipramine reduces the number of beta-adrenoceptors. Biochem Pharmacol 35:1899–1902, 1986

Hyman SE, Nestler EJ: Initiation and adaptation: a paradigm for understanding psychotropic drug action. Am J Psychiatry 153:151–162, 1996

Iyengar R: Molecular and functional diversity of mammalian Gs-stimulated adenylyl classes. FASEB J 7:768–775, 1993

Kleuss C, Hescheler J, Ewel C, et al: Assignment of G-protein subtypes to specific receptors inducing inhibition of calcium currents. Nature 353:43–48, 1991

Kleuss C, Scherubl H, Hescheler J, et al: Different β-subunits determine G-protein interaction with transmembrane receptors. Nature 358:424–426, 1992

Kleuss C, Scherubl H, Hescheler J, et al: Selectivity in signal transduction determined by gamma subunits of heterotrimeric G proteins. Science 259:832–834, 1993

Manier DH, Bieck PR, Duhl DM, et al: The β-adrenoceptor-coupled adenylate cyclase system in rat C6 glioma cells. Neuropsychopharmacology 7:105–112, 1992

Manji HK, Chen G, Bitran JA, et al: Idazoxan down-regulates β-adrenoreceptors on C6 glioma cells in vitro. Eur J Pharmacol 227:275–282, 1992

Manji HK, Potter WZ, Lenox RH: Signal transduction pathways: molecular targets for lithium's actions. Arch Gen Psychiatry 52:531–543, 1995

Menkes DB, Rasenick MM, Wheeler MA, et al: Guanosine triphosphate activation of brain adenylate cyclase: enhancement by long-term antidepressant. Science 219:65–67, 1983

Okada F, Tokumitsu Y, Ui M: Desensitization of β-adrenergic receptor-coupled adenylate cyclase in cerebral cortex after in vivo treatment of rats with desipramine. J Neurochem 47:454–459, 1986

Ozawa H, Rasenick MM: Coupling of the stimulatory GTP-binding protein Gs to rat synaptic membrane adenylate cyclase is enhanced subsequent to chronic antidepressant treatment. Mol Pharmacol 36:803–808, 1989

Ozawa H, Rasenick MM: Chronic electroconvulsive treatment augments coupling of the GTP-binding protein Gs to the catalytic moiety of adenylyl cyclase in a manner similar to that seen with chronic antidepressant drugs. J Neurochem 30:330–338, 1991

Popova JS, Garrison JC, Rhee SG, et al: Tubulin, Gq and phosphatidylinositol 4,5-bisphosphate interact to regulate phospholipase C β1 signaling. J Biol Chem 272:6760–6705, 1997

Rasenick MM: G's (poem). Trends Biochem Sci 17:71, 1992

Rasenick MM, Talluri M, Dunn WJ III: Photoaffinity guanosine $5'$ triphosphate analogs as a tool for the study of GTP-binding proteins. Methods Enzymol 237:100–110, 1994

Rasenick MM, Caron MG, Dolphin AC, et al: Receptor-G protein-effector coupling: coding and regulation of the signal transduction process, in Pharmacological Sciences: Perspectives for Research and Therapy in the Late 1990s. Edited by Cuello AC, Collier B. Basel, Birkhauser, 1995, pp 91–103

Roychowdhury S, Rasenick MM: Tubulin-G protein association stabilizes GTP binding and activates GTPase: cytoskeletal participation in neuronal signal transduction. Biochemistry 33:9800–9805, 1994

Roychowdhury S, Panda D, Wilson L, et al: G protein α subunits activate tublin GTPase and modulate microtubule polymerization dynamics. J Biol Chem 274:13485–13490, 1999

Simon M, Strathman M, Gautam N: Diversity of G proteins in signal transduction. Science 252:802–808, 1991

Sulser F: Antidepressant treatments and regulation of norepinephrine-receptor-coupled adenylate cyclase systems in brain. Adv Biochem Psychopharmacol 39:249–261, 1984

Taussig R, Iniguez-Lluhi J, Gilman A: Inhibition of adenylyl cyclase by $G_i\alpha$. Science 261:218–221, 1993

Toki S, Donati RJ, Rasenick MM: Treatment of C6 glioma cells and rats with antidepressant drugs increases the detergent extraction of $G_s\alpha$ from plasma membrane. J Neurochem 73:1114–1120, 1999

Vetulani J, Sulser F: Action of various antidepressant treatments reduces reactivity of noradrenergic cyclic AMP-generating system in limbic forebrain. Nature 257:495–497, 1975

Wang N, Rasenick MM: Tubulin-G protein interactions involve microtubule polymerization domains. Biochemistry 30:10957–10965, 1991

Wang N, Yan K, Rasenick MM: Tubulin binds specifically to the signal-transducing proteins, Gsαand Giα1. J Biol Chem 265:1239–1242, 1990

Xia Z, Choi E, Storm DR, et al: Do the calmodulin-stimulated adenylyl cyclases play a role in neuroplasticity? Behav Brain Sci 18:429–440, 1996

Yan K, Greene E, Belga F, et al: Synaptic membrane G proteins are complexed with tubulin *in situ*. J Neurochem 66:1489–1495, 1996

CHAPTER 6

EFFECTS OF LITHIUM AND OTHER MOOD-STABILIZING AGENTS ON THE CYCLIC ADENOSINE MONOPHOSPHATE SIGNALING SYSTEM IN THE BRAIN

Arne Mørk, Ph.D., and Jens Bitsch Jensen, Ph.D.

Since the introduction of lithium in the treatment of manic illness by Cade (1949), numerous reports have documented the therapeutic value of lithium in manic-depressive illness (bipolar disorder). Thus, lithium is effective in the acute treatment of mania, in prophylaxis of recurrent mania and depression, and in prophylaxis of unipolar depression. Furthermore, lithium augments the effect of antidepressants in the treatment of therapy-resistant depression (Austin et al. 1991). In most industrialized countries, 1 person out of every 1,000 in the population is undergoing lithium treatment (Schou 1991).

Although the neurochemical basis for the mood-stabilizing actions of lithium is still unknown, studies in the 1990s have indicated that lithium affects neuronal signal transduction beyond receptors. Several experiments on brain slices and homogenates have demonstrated that lithium affects the levels of second messengers generated by adenylate cyclases and phospholipase C (Avissar and Schreiber 1992; Batty and Downes 1994; Jope and Williams 1994; Mørk et al. 1990; Newman 1991). However, the molecular mechanisms by which lithium affects the synthesis of cyclic adenosine monophosphate (cAMP) and the hydrolysis of phosphatidylinositol 4,5-bisphosphate are unclear.

ADENYLATE CYCLASES

Localization, Specificity, and Function

Adenylate cyclase catalyzes the formation of cAMP, which is an important intracellular second messenger in cells, including neurons in the central nervous system. The synthesis of cAMP is regulated by stimulatory receptors: β-adrenergic, dopamine D_1, serotonin 5-HT_4, and vasopressin V_2 (Boess and Martin 1994; Mørk et al. 1992) and by inhibitory receptors: α_2-adrenergic, dopamine D_2, 5-HT_{1A}, or muscarinic M_2 receptors) (Boess and Martin 1994; Mørk and Geisler 1990; Mørk et al. 1992). The receptor signals are transferred to the catalytic protein of adenylate cyclases via stimulatory (G_s) and inhibitory (G_i) guanine nucleotide binding proteins (G proteins) (Offermanns and Schultz 1994) (Figure 6–1).

There is now evidence for nine different types of adenylate cyclase having distinct regulatory characteristics (Defer et al. 1994; Krupinski 1991; Mons et al. 1995). Types I, III, and VIII adenylate cyclases are sensitive to calcium-calmodulin (Ca^{2+}-CaM) and are thus stimulated by low physiological concentrations of Ca^{2+} (Chetkovich and Sweatt 1993; Defer et al. 1994; Hanoune et al. 1997; Krupinski et al. 1991; Mons et al. 1995). On the other hand, it has been demonstrated that types V and VI adenylate cyclases are inhibited by physiological concentrations of Ca^{2+} (Mons and Cooper 1994; Wayman et al. 1995).

Several studies have demonstrated organ and brain region specificity of the adenylate cyclases. Thus, messenger RNA (mRNA) for type I adenylate cyclase, which is neuron specific, is found in the neocortex, hippocampus, olfactory system, and cerebellum (Mons et al. 1995; Xia et al. 1993). In situ hybridization has provided evidence that that type V adenylate cyclase is highly concentrated in the striatal neurons, expressing both G_s-linked $D_1$1 receptors and Ca^{2+}-linked M_1 receptors (Glatt and Snyder 1993; Mons and Cooper 1994). Thus, type V adenylate cyclase may be regulated by opposing regulatory effects from D_1 and M_1 receptors.

A study using polyclonal antibodies against adenylate cyclases has demonstrated that these enzymes are located in dendrites and axon terminals. In the CA1 region a dense immunolabeling was found in postsynaptic densities

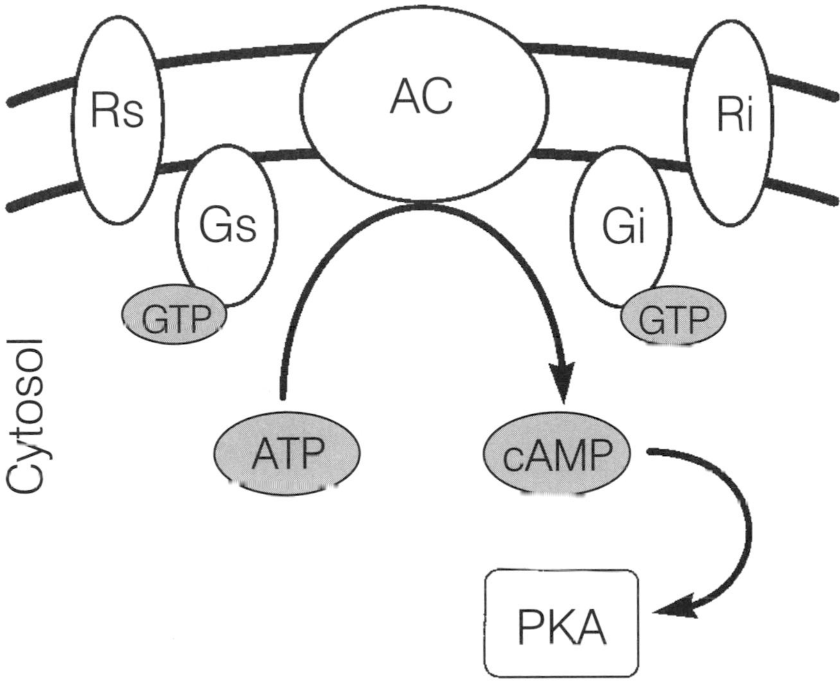

Figure 6–1. Schematic outline of the adenylate cyclase system. R_s = stimulatory receptor; R_i = inhibitory receptor; G_s = stimulatory guanine nucleotide binding protein; G_i = inhibitory guanine nucleotide binding protein; AC = catalytic protein of adenylate cyclase; GTP = guanosine triphosphate; ATP = adenosine triphosphate; cAMP = cyclic adenosine monophosphate; PKA = cAMP-dependent protein kinase.

(Mons et al. 1995). Presynaptic terminals were also labeled in accordance with the fact that cAMP is involved in modulation of neurotransmitter release (Chavez-Noriega and Stevens 1994).

Certain types of adenylate cyclases are also functionally coupled to *N*-methyl-D-aspartate (NMDA) receptors. The abundant amount of NMDA receptors in the CA1 region is associated with a substantial amount of adenylate cyclase in this area. Stimulation of NMDA receptors increases intracellular concentrations of Ca^{2+}, and this leads to activation of type I adenylate cyclase by Ca^{2+}-CaM (Chetkovich and Sweatt 1993; Mons et al. 1995; Tsuji et al. 1995; Yang et al. 1995). The cAMP produced facilitates the induction of long-term potentiation via cAMP-dependent protein kinase (Frey et al. 1993; Mons et al. 1995). Long-term potentiation seems to be important for learning, memory storage, and mood regulation (Kandel and Abel 1995).

Regulation of Adenylate Cyclases

As previously described, the activities of the adenylate cyclases are regulated by stimulatory and inhibitory receptors, G_s, G_i, and/or Ca^{2+}-CaM. The enzyme activities are also modulated by phosphorylation processes. Thus, receptor stimulation of adenylate cyclases leads to reversible desensitization of the cAMP response. However, adenosine A_2-receptor–induced desensitization of type I adenylate cyclase was not reversible in the presence of the phosphatase inhibitor okadaic acid, suggesting that protein kinases and phosphatases are involved in the regulation of adenylate cyclase activities (Chern et al. 1995).

Stress induces functional changes in receptors coupled to adenylate cyclase (Pandey et al. 1995). However, recent studies have also demonstrated that stress can induce changes in the levels of adenylate cyclase proteins. Thus, 12 hours intermittent stress induced increased cAMP production and enhanced levels of type II adenylate cyclase mRNA in rat frontal cortex (Morrill et al. 1993). Wolfgang et al. (1994) reported that chronic stress induced increased adenylate cyclase activity and increased levels of types I and II adenylate cyclase mRNA in rat hippocampus, indicating that functional alterations in the cAMP signaling system in the brain may also be due to changes in the protein levels of adenylate cyclases. Moreover, disruption of the gene for type I adenylate cyclase produced changes in behavior and decreased Ca^{2+}-CaM–stimulated cAMP production in the brain (Wu et al. 1995).

Increased forskolin (colforsin)-stimulated cAMP formation has been observed in postmortem brains from patients with bipolar affective illness (Young et al. 1993). Thus, the effects of lithium and other mood-stabilizing drugs on the cAMP signaling system may be involved in the therapeutic effects of these agents.

CYCLIC AMP–DEPENDENT PROTEIN KINASE

The most important known target for cAMP is cAMP-dependent protein kinase (PKA). PKA catalyzes the transfer of the terminal phosphate of adenosine triphosphate (ATP) to serine or threonine residues in specific regions of the substrates (reviewed by Francis and Corbin 1994). PKA consists of four subunits, two regulatory (R) and two catalytic (C) subunits arranged in the holoenzyme R_2-2C (Scott and Carr 1992). The PKAs are divided into two classes, type I and type II, based on the isoform of the R subunit (RI, RII). Until now four regulatory subunits (RIα, RIβ, RIIα, and RIIβ) and three catalytic subunits (Cα, Cβ, Cγ) have been identified in mammals as distinct gene products (Beebe 1994). The Cβ subunit is further divided into Cβ1 and Cβ2, but these subunits are thought to be products of alternative mRNA splicing. The activation of PKA is induced by binding of two molecules of cAMP to each R subunit. Following binding of cAMP, a conformational change of the holoenzyme causes release of the active C subunits, which then perform the phosphorylation (Francis and Corbin 1994).

The PKA isozymes are distributed region-specifically, with a high concentration of type Iβ and type IIβ in the brain. Type I is primarily located in the cytoplasm. In certain tissues, approximately 75% of type II is in a particulate form—for example, anchored to plasma membranes and cytoskeletal components. The anchoring is thought to involve the RII subunit and specific anchoring proteins. This colocalization of the kinases with the substrates ensures a local/specific and rapid action of the cAMP-induced phosphorylation. The anchoring proteins include MAP_2 and the p75/150 family (Scott and Carr 1992).

Alterations in cAMP-dependent phosphorylation in affective disorders have been reported. Recently, Perez et al. (1995) observed a significant change in the degree of phosphorylation of one PKA substrate in platelets from euthymic bipolar patients compared with control subjects. On the basis of the apparent molecular weight (22 kDa), the protein was suggested to be Rap 1b. Furthermore, chronic antidepressant treatments have been shown to affect substrates (Guitart and Nestler 1992; Perez et al. 1989), the amount of the RII subunit of PKA (Racagni et al. 1991), and the activity of PKA (Moyer et al. 1986; Nestler et al. 1989).

LITHIUM AND CYCLIC AMP FORMATION

Adenylate Cyclase System

Kanba et al. (1991) observed that the action of lithium on cAMP production in intact cells was potentiated by the sodium channel activator veratridine, indicating that intracellular levels of lithium are important for the action of lithium on second-messenger generation. When discussing the actions of lithium on the cAMP signaling system, it is important to be aware of the fact that magnesium (Mg^{2+}) regulates the activities of both G proteins and the catalytic unit of adenylate cyclases (Cech and Maguire 1982; Maguire 1982). Several studies suggest that lithium in situ (measured in vitro) affects the adenylate cyclase activities by counteracting the regulatory effect of Mg^{2+} on the catalytic protein of adenylate cyclases (Ebstein et al. 1987; Mørk and Geisler 1987a, 1987b; Wragg and MacNeil 1991). In 1987, Newman and Belmaker reported that the inhibitory effects of lithium in vitro on the adenylate cyclase activity stimulated by the GTP analogue guanylyl-5′-imidodiphosphate (Gpp(NH)p) and forskolin were competitive with Mg^{2+}. The Mg^{2+} site on G proteins may, however, also be of significance, since Mg^{2+} reverses lithium inhibition of β-adrenergic-receptor–induced and muscarinic-receptor–induced GTP binding in rat cerebral cortex (Avissar et al. 1991).

These lithium-Mg^{2+} interactions might explain the readily observed inhibition of neurotransmitter-stimulated adenylate cyclase in intact cells compared with membrane homogenates. For optimal adenylate cyclase activity in membrane homogenates, a high concentration of Mg^{2+} is usually present (2–5 mM), rendering the enzyme less sensitive to lithium. The intracellular concentrations of free Mg^{2+}, which is able to interact with adenylate cyclase, have been estimated as 0.3–1 mM (Maguire 1984; Vink et al. 1988). This is consistent with the observation that Mg^{2+} loading of intact renal cells abolishes the inhibitory effect of lithium (Goldberg et al. 1988). However, lithium does not influence all Mg^{2+} sites in the organism. This is in accordance with the fact that certain adenylate cyclase activities also respond differently to divalent ions (Cech and Maguire 1982; Hallcher and Sherman 1980).

Although many studies have demonstrated that lithium in vitro and ex vivo affects adenylate cyclase activities, there are differences in the experimental conditions when investigating the in vitro and chronic effects of lithium. Under the ex vivo conditions the concentrations of lithium in the brain tissue are far too small to produce an in vitro effect and, furthermore, the ex vivo effect of lithium does not seem to develop until after 2–4 weeks of treatment. A study by Mørk and Geisler (1989a) indicated that lithium exerts its in vitro and ex vivo effects on brain adenylate cyclase by distinct mechanisms, because 1) the sensitivity of adenylate cyclase activity to lithium in vitro was unaltered following chronic lithium treatment and the ex vivo and in vitro effects on this parameter were additive, 2) increasing concentrations of Mg^{2+} did not antagonize the effect of lithium ex vivo on adenylate cyclase activity, and 3) the lithium inhibition of the enzyme activity was persistent after the membranes were washed.

Achievement of the therapeutic action of lithium in the treatment of bipolar disorder requires days to weeks of administration. The chronic effect of lithium is thus generally considered more relevant than the in vitro effect. However, the in vitro effect of lithium may be relevant too, because the chronic effect of lithium must have been preceded by earlier effects, which generate the chronic effect. On the other hand, the delay in clinical response could be due partially to the pharmacokinetics of lithium, because reduction in psychopathology was evident within 2–3 days of high-dose lithiumization at the onset of therapy (Moscovich et al. 1992).

The existence of CaM-sensitive adenylate cyclases (types I, III, and VIII) (Defer et al. 1994; Krupinski 1991; Mons et al. 1995) allows Ca^{2+} in the presence of CaM to selectively activate the cAMP synthesis and mediate neurotransmitter-regulated cAMP accumulation in cells expressing the CaM-sensitive adenylate cyclases.

Lithium inhibits both manganese-calmodulin (Mn^{2+}-CaM)–stimulated and Ca^{2+}-CaM–stimulated adenylate cyclase activity in rat cerebral cortex (Mørk and Geisler 1987a, 1987b, 1995a; Mørk et al. 1990), confirming that lithium in vitro is able to inhibit the activity of the catalytic unit of adenylate cyclase, at least the CaM-sensitive forms. Thus, lithium-induced reduction in cAMP production in the stimulated cell is partially due to the effects of lithium on the CaM-sensitive adenylate cyclases. The substitution of Mn^{2+} for Mg^{2+} results in a Mn^{2+}-CaM stimulation of the enzyme (Mørk and Geisler 1987a). The effect of lithium on Mn^{2+}-stimulated cAMP formation (Andersen and Geisler 1984; Newman and Belmaker 1987) may thus be due to CaM, because lithium does not influence Mn^{2+}-stimulated adenylate cyclase in CaM-depleted membranes (Mørk and Geisler 1987b). The inhibitory action of lithium on Ca^{2+}-CaM–stimulated activity of isolated catalytic units of adenylate cyclase, furthermore, supports the hypothesis that lithium in vitro is able to interact directly with the enzyme.

Forskolin has been widely used in the study of adenylate cyclase activity. It has been suggested that forskolin interacts directly with the catalytic unit of adenylate cyclase, since it stimulates cAMP formation in the absence of functional G_s. Because of the observation that forskolin potentiates the action of preactivated G_s on cAMP formation (Krall and Jamgotchian 1987; Schimmer et al. 1987), studies involving forskolin have been interpreted differently; some authors have regarded forskolin as an activator of G_s. However, it has been demonstrated that the high-affinity binding of [^{3}H]forskolin to membranes in which G_s has been preactivated is presumably due to an increased binding of forskolin to the active α^{GTP}-catalytic unit complex (Alousi et al. 1991; Mollner and Pfeuffer 1988). Thus, the inhibitory effects of lithium in vitro on forskolin-stimulated adenylate cyclase activity may be due to effects on the catalytic unit.

Ca^{2+}-CaM–stimulated brain adenylate cyclase activity was found to be altered following chronic lithium treatment (Mørk and Geisler 1987b; Mørk et al. 1990), yielding serum lithium levels within the therapeutic range (0.5–1.0 mM). The reduced Ca^{2+}-CaM stimulation of adenylate cyclase activity in rat cerebral cortex demonstrates that the decreased cAMP synthesis in the cortex during lithium treatment is partially due to an effect of lithium on the CaM-sensitive adenylate cyclase. The existence of an effect of lithium on the catalytic unit of adenylate cyclase is supported by findings that lithium ex vivo reduces forskolin-stimulated (Andersen and Geisler 1984; Newman and Belmaker 1987) and Mn^{2+}-stimulated cortical adenylate cyclase activity (Mørk and Geisler 1989d; Newman and Belmaker 1987).

G Proteins Coupled to Adenylate Cyclase

Chronic lithium treatment decreases the degree of stimulation of cAMP formation by noradrenaline in the living brain of anesthetized rats (Masana et al. 1991) and in freely moving rats (Mørk and Geisler 1995b). Most studies support the assumption that lithium does not affect the number of α- and β-adrenergic receptors (Gross and Hanft 1990; Gross et al. 1988; Plenge et al. 1992), indicating that its actions on noradrenaline-mediated processes are due to effects distal to the receptor. Some studies have focused on the action of lithium on neurotransmitter-mediated receptor regulation of G proteins, because activation of cAMP formation is due to receptor-induced GTP stimulation of G_s (Offermanns and Schultz 1994). This process can be investigated by measuring receptor-induced GTP stimulation/inhibition of adenylate cyclase and GTP-stimulated enzyme activity.

Chronic lithium treatment decreased isoprenaline-induced GTP stimulation of adenylate cyclase activity in the cerebral cortex (Mørk and Geisler 1989b).This inhibition was observed only in the presence of small concentrations of added GTP. Lithium ex vivo did not affect the cortical enzyme activity stimulated by GTP alone. In the hippocampus, chronic lithium treatment decreased the inhibition of Ca^{2+}-CaM–stimulated adenylate cyclase by 5-HT. Lithium ex vivo also attenuated 5-HT–induced GTP inhibition of the enzyme activity, indicating that chronic lithium treatment decreases the function of G_i (Mørk and Geisler 1989c). In agreement with this observation, Newman et al. (1990) reported that lithium ex vivo decreased the degree of inhibition of forskolin-stimulated adenylate cyclase by 5-HT in rat hippocampus. An attenuation of the function of G_i in hippocampus may explain the enhanced Ca^{2+}-CaM–stimulated enzyme activity in this brain region (Mørk and Geisler 1989c). Hsiao et al. (1992) observed an increased pertussis toxin–stimulated ADP ribosylation in human platelet membranes after lithium treatment. The increased ADP ribosylation in the absence of changes in the level of G_i (the α_i immunoblotting was unchanged) could indicate a lithium-induced shift in G_i

in favor of its inactive form. Moreover, inactivation of G_i with pertussis toxin increased dialysate cAMP in rat prefrontal cortex. This pertussis toxin effect was abolished by chronic lithium treatment (Masana et al. 1992). An inhibitory effect of lithium on the function of G_i in tissues/brain regions in which this G protein exerts a major inhibitory action on the adenylate cyclase (e.g., in the rat hippocampus) may thus lead to enhanced enzyme activity.

The assumption that lithium affects the regulation of G proteins is supported by the fact that lithium is able to block isoprenaline- and carbachol-induced GTP binding in rat cerebral cortex (Avissar and Schreiber 1992; Avissar et al. 1988). However, Ellis and Lenox (1991) did not observe any effects of lithium on the ability of Gpp(NH)p to modulate the binding of oxotremorine to muscarinic receptors in the rat hippocampus and brain stem. Furthermore, Volonté (1988) reported that lithium in vitro enhanced GTP binding in membranes of PC12 cells. Thus, lithium does not seem to interfere equally with the receptor–G protein coupling in all systems.

High-affinity and low-affinity states for the β-adrenergic receptor have been determined in human lymphocytes and rat frontal cortex. Lithum ex vivo was found to increase the ratio between the dissociation constants for low- and high-affinity binding (K_L/K_H) (Risby et al. 1991), suggesting an increased coupling between the β-adrenergic receptor and G_s. Agonist binding to the receptor results in the formation of a ternary agonist–receptor–G protein complex, and this puts the receptor in a high-affinity state. This complex is short-lived, because GTP rapidly binds to G_s, leading to dissociation of the complex and formation of active α^{GTP}. Reversal of the lithium inhibition ex vivo of β-adrenoceptor function by GTP (Mørk and Geisler 1989b), lithium inhibition in vitro and ex vivo of β-adrenoceptor–induced GTP binding (Avissar and Schreiber 1992; Avissar et al. 1988), and the lithium-generated deficiency of the β-adrenoceptor to change hysteretic stimulation by Gpp(NH)p (Mørk and Geisler 1991) could indicate that lithium treatment impairs the coupling between the β-adrenoceptor and G_s. However, the ability of lithium to "lock" the β-adrenergic receptor into a high-affinity state while simultanously decreasing the cAMP formation may suggest that lithium prevents neurotransmitter-induced GTP stimulation of G_s by influencing the GTP-dependent conversion of G_s from its inactive to its active form.

The molecular mechanisms by which lithium exerts these effects are unknown. One possibility is that lithium induces phosphorylation of some protein components of the second-messenger systems and thereby reduces the receptor–G protein coupling or the stimulation of the G protein. An important role for phosphorylation/dephosphorylation in regulation of the cAMP signaling system has been suggested (Chern et al 1995; Choi et al. 1988; Yamashita et al. 1988).

OTHER MOOD-STABILIZING DRUGS

During recent years, alternatives to lithium have been introduced. Agents such as carbamazepine, valproic acid, and verapamil have been demonstrated to be effective in treatment of affective disorder (Höschl 1991; Lepkifker et al. 1995; Post and Chuang 1991).

The best responders to lithium treatment and prophylaxis are patients with a classic picture of affective disorder, whereas carbamazepine benefits patients with atypical forms of affective disorders (e.g., rapid-cycling) (Blumer et al. 1988; Rybakowski 1992). Moreover, combinations of lithium and carbamazepine may be used in the treatment of affective disorders when prophylactic monotherapy is unsatisfactory (Rybakowski 1992). Verapamil has an antimanic efficacy that is comparable to traditional therapies, and it appears that responders among depressed patients are mostly bipolar patients (Höschl 1991). Valproic acid has been reported to be efficient in rapid-cycling patients and may, furthermore, be used in patients who cannot tolerate lithium (Lepkifker et al. 1995).

With regard to the neurochemical effects, carbamazepine mimics lithium by in vitro inhibition of noradrenaline-stimulated cAMP production in the rat brain (Lewin and Bleck 1977). As reported for lithium (Gross et al. 1988), the number of β-adrenoceptors is unaffected by chronic carbamazepine (Marangos et al. 1985), suggesting that the effects on cAMP production are exerted distal to the receptor.

To compare the effects of these agents on agonist-induced cAMP production in the brain, rats were treated with these drugs for 4 weeks. The choice of doses was based on previous studies in the literature. Male Wistar rats were fed standard chow containing 40 mM/kg LiCl for 2 weeks, followed by chow containing 60 mM/kg LiCl for 2 weeks (yielding plasma lithium levels of about 0.7 mM). The lithium-treated rats had free access to NaCl. The carbamazepine-treated rats were fed chow containing 5.0 g/kg carbamazepine (yielding plasma carbamazepine levels of about 20 μM). The intraperitoneal dosages of verapamil and valproic acid were 4 mg/kg/day and 250 mg/kg/day, respectively. Control rats received the standard diet with no further addition and intraperitoneal injections with saline.

Figure 6–2 shows unstimulated cAMP production in cerebral cortex and hippocampus following 4 weeks of treatment. As regards lithium treatment, there was a trend toward increased activity in the cerebral cortex; a 40% increase was observed (although not significant). Increased unstimulated cAMP production was observed after treatment with verapamil, suggesting that chronic treatment with calcium antagonists may induce enhanced basal intracellular levels of cAMP in the cortex. Treatment with carbamazepine reduced the unstimulated cAMP production in this brain region. In the hippocampus, no significant changes were observed following the treatments (Figure 6–2).

Lithium, valproic acid, and carbamazepine reduced noradrenaline-stimulated cAMP production in the cerebral cortex following 4 weeks of treatment (Figure 6–3). The lack of effect of verapamil on receptor agonist stimulation might be due to the increased unstimulated cAMP production. In the hippocampus, chronic treatment with lithium and valproic acid reduced noradrenaline-stimulated cAMP production. In contrast to the effect in cortex, no effect of chronic carbamazepine on noradrenaline-stimulated cAMP production was observed in the hippocampus, indicating region specificity of this drug. Carbamazepine was reported (Van Calker et al. 1991) to have selective antagonistic action on adenosine A_1 receptors; no action on adenosine A_{2a} receptors was observed.

The present data demonstrate that some mood-stabilizing agents have lithium-like actions on the cAMP signaling system. These effects could be involved in their similar profile efficacy in affective illness.

BEHAVIOR AND cAMP

Several attempts to demonstrate a possible relation between formation of cAMP and behavior have been made, and experiments manipulating the levels

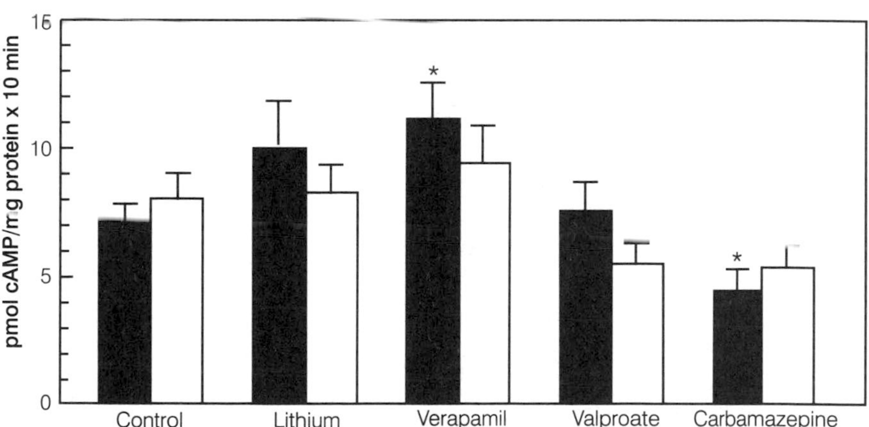

Figure 6–2. Effects of chronic treatment with lithium, verapamil, valproate, and carbamazepine on unstimulated cyclic adenosine monophosphate (cAMP) production in slices from rat cerebral cortex (filled bars) and hippocampus (open bars). *Note.* $^*P < 0.05$ (significantly different from control).

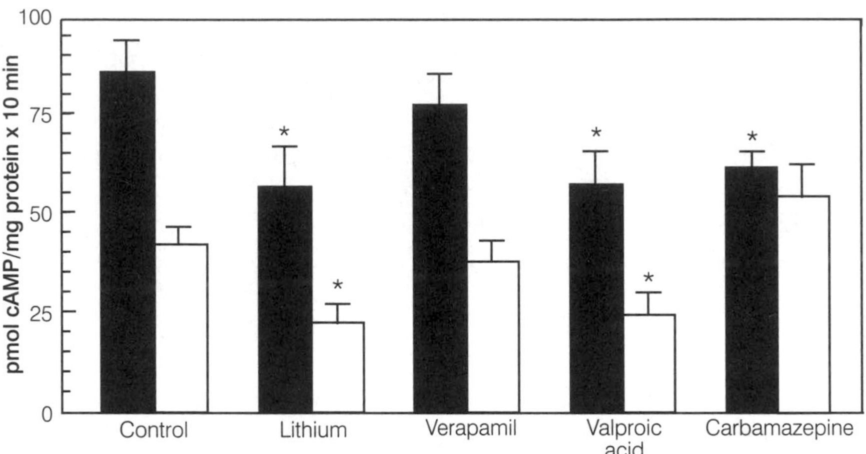

Figure 6–3. Effects of chronic treatment with lithium, verapamil, valproic acid, and carbamazepine on noradrenaline (100 μM)–stimulated cyclic adenosine monophosphate (cAMP) production in slices from rat cerebral cortex (filled bars) and hippocampus (open bars). $^*P < 0.05$ (significantly different from control).

of cAMP have indeed shown a potential relation to behavioral changes. Compounds affecting the cAMP level, such as lithium, forskolin, and phosphodiesterase inhibitors, are capable of inducing behavioral changes in animals. These changes includes hypoactivity and altered frequencies of grooming and head twitches.

The β-adrenergic agonist clenbuterol induces hypoactivity in rats, possibly mediated by central β_2-adrenergic receptors (Givant et al. 1990). Skolnick and Daly (1974) used different rat strains to investigate a potential correlation between spontaneous activity and the magnitude of noradrenaline-induced cAMP accumulation in the rat brain. They found a negative correlation in the cerebral cortex and a positive correlation in the midbrain-striatum. Using different mouse strains, Hamburger-Bar et al. (1986) also found a significant inverse correlation between spontaneous activity and noradrenaline-induced cAMP accumulation in the cortex. However, both studies failed to show any significant correlations between spontaneous behavioral activity and cAMP accumulation induced by adenosine. A region- and pathway-specific action of cAMP accumulation may be important in relation to behavior.

A significant lithium-induced depression of behavioral activity has been reported (Belmaker et al. 1990; Lerer et al. 1984). Furthermore, Hamburger-Bar et al. (1986) reported that lithium significantly reversed amphetamine-induced hyperactivity. In contrast, some studies have reported that lithium has no effect on behavioral activity (Givant et al. 1990; Kofman et al. 1991; Mattia et al. 1986).

Wachtel and Löschmann (1986) reported that intracerebroventricular forskolin significantly lowered activity in rats. Furthermore, Barraco et al. (1985) found that intracerebroventricular forskolin induced a dose-related depression of spontaneous locomotor activity in mice. Recently, Mørk and Geisler (1995b) reported that infusion of forskolin or noradrenaline into the dorsal hippocampus increased the behavioral activity of freely moving rats. This study may reflect an effect due to local stimulation rather than an overall brain effect, as may occur using intracerebroventricular injection. Following chronic treatment, lithium significantly reversed forskolin-induced hyperactivity (Mørk and Geisler 1995b). This lithium-forskolin interaction may involve the cAMP signaling system.

Phosphodiesterase inhibitors were reported to have antidepressant effects in humans (Horowski and Sastre Y-Hernandez 1985), and these substances were reported to be able to induce behavioral depression in rodents (Barraco et al. 1985; Givant et al. 1990; Smith 1990; Wachtel 1982). Behavioral depression induced by phosphodiesterase inhibitors was mimicked by the cAMP analogue dibutyryl-cAMP, but not the cyclic guanosine monophosphate (cGMP) analogue dibutyryl-cGMP (Wachtel 1982). This indicates that the cAMP-generating system may be more important than the cGMP-generating system in relation to behavioral changes. Chronic lithium treatment attenuates rolipram-induced hypoactivity in rodents (Smith 1990).

At present, it is not possible to state whether a connection between cAMP levels and changes in behavior is relevant in relation to humans. For example, the dramatic behavioral alterations induced by lithium-cholinergic interaction, the limbic seizures, seem to be limited to rodents (Cooney and Dinan 1995; Oppenheimer et al. 1988).

The studies discussed above demonstrate that lithium is able to normalize behavioral changes induced by manipulation of the adenylate cyclase cascade at various levels.

SUMMARY

At present, nine different types of adenylate cyclase are known. These enzyme systems are specific to tissue and brain region. They transform extracellular signals from receptors coupled to G_s and G_i to intracellular responses. Furthermore, types I, III, and VIII of adenylate cyclase are regulated by Ca^{2+}-CaM and are thus regulated by the Ca^{2+} signaling pathway.

Manipulation of the cAMP levels in the brain has been shown to provoke behavioral changes, underlining the importance to brain function of these widely distributed signaling systems. However, we do not yet have substantial knowledge about the roles of the different types of adenylate cyclases in behavior.

The marked effects of lithium on adenylate cyclase activities may indicate that this signaling system is involved in the therapeutic action of lithium. Lithium reduces neurotransmitter-induced GTP regulation of G proteins coupled to adenylate cyclases and affects Ca^{2+}-CaM–sensitive adenylate cyclases. These effects on the levels of cAMP result in changes in PKA-mediated protein phosphorylation. These interactions may be involved in lithium's stabilization of abnormal oscillations in neurotransmitter function. Other mood-stabilizing drugs—for example, valproic acid and carbamazepine— have lithium-like effects on the cAMP-generating system. This action could be the basis for the similar clinical profile of these drugs.

REFERENCES

Alousi AA, Jasper JR, Insel PA: Stoichiometry of receptor-G_S-adenylate cyclase interactions. FASEB J 5:2300–2303, 1991

Andersen PH, Geisler A: Lithium inhibition of forskolin-stimulated adenylate cyclase. Neuropsychobiology 12:1–3, 1984

Austin M-PV, Souza FGM, Goodwin GM: Lithium augmentation in antidepressant-resistant patients: a quantitative analysis. Br J Psychiatry 159:510–514, 1991

Avissar S, Schreiber G: The involvement of guanine nucleotide binding proteins in the pathogenesis and treatment of affective disorders. Biol Psychiatry 31:435–459, 1992

Avissar S, Schreiber G, Danon A, et al: Lithium inhibits adrenergic and cholinergic increases in GTP binding in rat cortex. Nature 331:440–442, 1988

Avissar S, Murphy DL, Schreiber G: Magnesium reversal of lithium inhibition of β-adrenergic and muscarinic receptor coupling to G proteins. Biochem Pharmacol 41:171–175, 1991

Barraco RA, Phillis JW, Altman HJ: Depressant effect of forskolin on spontaneous locomotor activity in mice. Gen Pharmacol 16:521–524, 1985

Batty IH, Downes CP: The inhibition of phosphoinositide synthesis and muscarinic-receptor-mediated phospholipase C activity by Li^+ as secondary, selective consequences of inositol depletion in 1321N1 cells. Biochem J 297:529–537, 1994

Beebe SJ: The cAMP-dependent protein kinases and cAMP signal transduction. Semin Cancer Biol 5:285–294, 1994

Belmaker RH, Livne A, Agam G, et al: Role of inositol-1-phosphatase inhibition in the mechanism of action of lithium. Pharmacol Toxicol 66:76–83, 1990

Blumer D, Helbronn M, Himmelhoch J: Indications for carbamazepine in mental illness: atypical psychiatric disorder or temporal lobe syndrome? Compr Psychiatry 29:108–122, 1988

Boess FG, Martin IL: Molecular biology of 5-HT receptors. Neuropharmacology 33: 275–317, 1994

Cade JFJ: Lithium salts in the treatment of psychotic excitement. Med J Aust 2:349–352, 1949

Cech SY, Maguire ME: Magnesium regulation of the beta-receptor-adenylate cyclase complex, I: effects of manganese on receptor binding and cyclase activation. Mol Pharmacol 22:267–273, 1982

Chavez-Noriega LE, Stevens CF: Increased transmitter release at excitatory synapse produced by direct activation of adenylate cyclase in rat hippocampal slices. J Neurosci 14:310–317, 1994

Chern Y, Chiou J-Y, Lai H-S, et al: Regulation of adenylyl cyclase type VI activity during desensitization of the A2a adenosine receptor-mediated cyclic AMP response: role for protein phosphatase 2A. Mol Pharmacol 48:1–8, 1995

Chetkovich DM, Sweatt JD: NMDA receptor activation increases cyclic AMP in area CA1 of the hippocampus via calcium/calmodulin stimulation of adenylyl cyclase. J Neurochem 61:1933–1942, 1993

Choi EJ, Toscano WA Jr: Modulation of adenylate cyclase in human keratinocytes by protein kinase C. J Biol Chem 263:17167–17172, 1988

Cooney JM, Dinan TG: The effect of lithium on cholinergically mediated GH responses in healthy volunteers. Human Psychopharmacology 10:333–337, 1995

Defer N, Marinx O, Stengel D, et al: Molecular cloning of the human type VIII adenylyl cyclase. FEBS Lett 351:109–113, 1994

Ebstein RP, Moscovich D, Zeevi S, et al: Effect of lithium in vitro and after chronic treatment on human platelet adenylate cyclase activity: postreceptor modification of second messenger signal amplification. Psychiatric Research 21:221–228, 1987

Ellis J, Lenox RH: Receptor coupling to G proteins: interactions not affected by lithium. Lithium 2:141–147, 1991

Francis SH, Corbin JD: Structure and function of cyclic nucleotide-dependent protein kinases. Annu Rev Physiol 56:237–272, 1994

Frey U, Huang Y-Y, Kandel ER: Effects of cAMP stimulate a late stage of LTP in hippocampal CA1 neurons. Science 260:1661–1664, 1993

Givant Y, Zohar J, Lichtenberg P, et al: Chronic lithium attenuates clenbuterol-induced hypoactivity. Lithium 1:183–185, 1990

Glatt CE, Snyder SH: Cloning and expression of an adenylyl cyclase localized to the corpus striatum. Nature 361:536–538, 1993

Goldberg H, Clayman P, Skorecki K: Mechanism of Li inhibition of vasopressin-sensitive adenylate cyclase in cultured renal epithelial cells. Am J Physiol 255: F995-F1002, 1988

Gross G, Hanft G: Does lithium in vitro and ex vivo alter the release of [^{3}H]noradrenaline from brain tissue and the sensitivity of presynaptic autoreceptors? Neuropharmacology 29:831–835,1990

Gross G, Dodt C, Hanft G: Effect of chronic lithium administration on adrenoceptor binding and adrenoceptor regulation in rat cerebral cortex. Naunyn Schmiedebergs Arch Pharmacol 337:267–272, 1988

Guitart X, Nestler EJ: Chronic administration of lithium or other antidepressants increases levels of DARPP-32 in rat frontal cortex. J Neurochem 59:1164–1167, 1992

Hallcher LM, Sherman WR: The effects of lithium ion and other agents on the activity of myo-inositol-1-phosphatase from bovine brain. J Biol Chem 255:10896–10901, 1980

Hamburger-Bar R, Robert M, Newman M, et al: Interstrain correlation between behavioral effects of lithium and effects on cortical cyclic AMP. Pharmacol Biochem Behav 24:9–13, 1986

Hanoune J, Pouille Y, Tzavara E, et al: Adenylyl cyclases: structure, regulation and function in an enzyme superfamily. Mol Cell Endocrinol 128(1–2):179–194, 1997

Horowski R, Sastre-Y-Hernandez M: Clinical effects of the neurotropic selective cAMP phosphodiesterase inhibitor rolipram in depressed patients: global evaluation of the preliminary reports. Current Therapy Research 38:23–29, 1985

Höschl C: Do calcium antagonists have a place in the treatment of mood disorders? Drugs 42:721–729, 1991

Hsiao JK, Manji HK, Chen G, et al: Lithium administration modulates platelet G_i in humans. Life Sci 50:227–233, 1992

Jope RS, Williams MB: Lithium and brain signal transduction systems. Biochem Pharmacol 47:429–441, 1994

Kanba S, Yagi G, Nakaki T, et al: Potentiation by a sodium channel activator of effects of lithium ion on cyclic AMP, cyclic GMP and inositol phosphates. Neuropharmacology 30:497–500, 1991

Kandel E, Abel T: Neuropeptides, adenylyl cyclase, and memory storage. Science 268: 825–826, 1995

Kofman O, Belmaker RH, Grisaru N, et al: Myo-inositol attenuates two specific behavioral effects of acute lithium in rats. Psychopharmacol Bull 27:185–190, 1991

Krall JF, Jamgotchian N: Forskolin refractoriness: exposure to the diterpene alters guanine nucleotide-dependent adenylate cyclase and calcium-uptake activity of cells cultured from the rat aorta. Biochem J 241:463–467, 1987

Krupinski J: The adenylyl cyclase family. Mol Cell Biochem 104:73–79, 1991

Lenox RH, Watson DG, Ellis J: Muscarinic receptor regulation and protein kinase C: sites for the action of chronic lithium in the hippocampus. Psychopharmacol Bull 27:191–197, 1991

Lepkifker E, Iancu I, Dannon R, et al: Valproic acid in ultrarapid cycling: a case report. Clin Neuropharmacol 18:72–75, 1995

Lerer B, Globus M, Brik E, et al: Effect of treatment and withdrawal from chronic lithium in rats on stimulated responses. Neuropsychobiology 11:28–32, 1984

Lewin E, Bleck V: Cyclic AMP accumulation in cerebral cortical slices: effect of carbamazepine, phenobarbital, and phenytoin. Epilepsia 18:237–242, 1977

Maguire ME: Magnesium regulation of the beta-receptor-adenylate cyclase complex, II: Sc^{3+} as a Mg^{2+} antagonist. Mol Pharmacol 22:274–280, 1982

Maguire ME: Hormone-sensitive magnesium transport and magnesium regulation of adenylate cyclase. Trends Pharmacol Sci 5:73–77, 1984

Marangos PJ, Weiss SRB, Montgomery P, et al: Chronic carbamazepine treatment increases brain adenosine receptors. Epilepsia 26:493–498, 1985

Masana MI, Bitran JA, Hsiao JK, et al: Lithium effects on noradrenergic-linked adenylate cyclase activity in intact rat brain: an in vivo microdialysis study. Brain Res 538:333–336, 1991

Masana MI, Bitran JA, Hsiao JK, et al: In vivo evidence that lithium inactivates G_i modulation of adenylate cyclase in brain. J Neurochem 59:200–205, 1992

Mattia A, El-Fakahany EE, Moreton JE: Behavioral and receptor binding studies of phencyclidine (PCP) and lithium interaction in rat. Life Sci 38:975–984, 1986

Mollner S, Pfeuffer T: Two different adenylyl cyclases in brain distinguished by monoclonal antibodies. Eur J Biochem 171:265–271, 1988

Mons N, Cooper DMF: Selective expression of one Ca^{2+}-inhibitable adenylyl cyclase in dopaminergically innervated rat brain regions. Brain Res Mol Brain Res 22: 236–244, 1994

Mons N, Harry A, Dubourg P, et al: Immunohistochemical localization of adenylyl cyclase in rat brain indicates a highly selective concentration at synapses. Proc Natl Acad Sci U S A 92:8473–8477, 1995

Mørk A, Geisler A: Mode of action of lithium on the catalytic unit of adenylate cyclase from rat brain. Pharmacol Toxicol 60:241–248, 1987a

Mørk A, Geisler A: Effects of lithium on calmodulin-stimulated adenylate cyclase activity in cortical membranes from rat brain. Pharmacol Toxicol 60:17–23, 1987b

Mørk A, Geisler A: The effects of lithium in vitro and ex vivo on adenylate cyclase in brain are exerted by distinct mechanisms. Neuropharmacology 28:307–311, 1989a

Mørk A, Geisler A: Effects of GTP on hormone-stimulated adenylate cyclase activity in cerebral cortex, striatum and hippocampus from rats treated chronically with lithium. Biol Psychiatry 26:279–288, 1989b

Mørk A, Geisler A: Effects of lithium ex vivo on the GTP-mediated inhibition of calcium-stimulated adenylate cyclase activity in rat brain. Eur J Pharmacol 168:347–354, 1989c

Mørk A, Geisler A: Lithium inhibition of adenylate cyclase activity: site of action and interaction with divalent cations, in New Directions in Affective Disorders. Edited by Lerer B, Gershon S. New York, Springer-Verlag, 1989d, pp 123–125

Mørk A, Geisler A: 5-Hydroxytryptamine receptor agonists influence calcium-stimulated adenylate cyclase activity in the cerebral cortex and hippocampus of the rat. Eur J Pharmacol 175:237–244, 1990

Mørk A, Geisler A: Hysteretic activation of adenylate cyclase by guanylyl-5′-imidodiphosphate in rat cerebral cortex following chronic lithium treatment. Lithium 2:127–133, 1991

Mørk A, Geisler A: A comparative study on the effects of tetracyclines and lithium on the cyclic AMP second messenger system in rat brain. Prog Neuropsychopharmacol Biol Psychiatry 19:157–169, 1995a

Mørk A, Geisler A: Effect of chronic lithium treatment on agonist-enhanced extracellular concentrations of cyclic AMP in the dorsal hippocampus of freely moving rats. J Neurochem 65:134–139, 1995b

Mørk A, Klysner R, Geisler A: Effects of treatment with a lithium-imipramine combination on components of adenylate cyclase in the cerebral cortex of the rat. Neuropharmacology 29:261–267, 1990

Mørk A, Geisler A, Hollund P: Effects of lithium on second messenger systems in the brain. Pharmacol Toxicol 71 (suppl I):4–17, 1992

Morrill AC, Wolfgang D, Levine MA, et al: Stress alters adenylyl cyclase activity in the pituitary and frontal cortex in the rat. Life Sci 53:1719–1727, 1993

Moscovich DG, Shapira B, Lerer B: Rapid lithiumization in acute manic patients. Human Psychopharmacology 7:343–345, 1992

Moyer JA, Sigg EB, Silver PJ: Antidepressants and protein kinases: desipramine treatment affects pineal gland cAMP-dependent kinase activity. Eur J Pharmacol 121:57–64, 1986

Nestler EJ, Terwillinger RZ, Duman RS: Chronic antidepressant administration alters the subcellular distribution of cyclic AMP-dependent protein kinase in rat frontal cortex. J Neurochem 53:1644–1647, 1989

Newman ME: Lithium and the phosphoinositide hydrolysis second messenger system: a critical review of its therapeutic relevance. Lithium 2:187–194, 1991

Newman ME, Belmaker RH: Effects of lithium in vitro and ex vivo on components of the adenylate cyclase system in membranes from the cerebral cortex of the rat. Neuropharmacology 26:211–217, 1987

Newman ME, Drummer D, Lerer B: Single and combined effects of desipramine and lithium on serotonergic receptor number and second messenger function in rat brain. J Pharmacol Exp Ther 252:826–831, 1990

Offermanns S, Schultz G: Complex information processing by the transmembrane signaling system involving G proteins. Naunyn Schmiedebergs Arch Pharmacol 350:329–338, 1994

Oppenheimer G, Ebstein RP, Belmaker RH: Effect of lithium on the physostigmine-induced behavioral syndrome and plasma cyclic GMP. J Psychiatr Res 24:45–52, 1988

Pandey SC, Ren X, Sagen J, et al: β-Adrenergic receptor subtypes in stress-induced behavioral depression. Pharmacol Biochem Behav 51:339–344, 1995

Perez J, Tinelli D, Brunello N, et al: cAMP-dependent phosphorylation of soluble and crude microtuble fractions of rat cerebral cortex after prolonged desmethylimipramine treatment. Eur J Pharmacol [Molecular Pharmacology Section] 172:305–316, 1989

Perez J, Zanardi R, Mori S, et al: Abnormalities of cAMP-dependent endogenous phosphorylation in platelets from patients with bipolar disorder. Am J Psychiatry 152:1204–1206, 1995

Plenge P, Mellerup ET, Jørgensen OS: Lithium treatment regimens induce different changes in [^{3}H]paroxetine binding protein and other rat brain proteins. Psychopharmacology (Berl) 106:131–135, 1992

Post RM, Chuang D-M: Mechanism of action of lithium: comparison and contrast with carbamazepine, in Lithium and the Cell. Edited by Birch NJ. London, Academic Press, 1991, pp 199–241

Racagni G, Tinelli D, Bianchi E, et al: cAMP-dependent binding proteins and endogenous phosphorylation after antidepressant treatment, in 5-Hydroxytryptamine in Psychiatry: A Spectrum of Ideas. Edited by Sandler M, Coppen A, Harnett S. Oxford, UK, Oxford University Press, 1991, pp 116–123

Risby ED, Hsiao JK, Manji HK, et al: The mechanisms of action of lithium, II: Effects on adenylate cyclase activity and β-adrenergic receptor binding in normal subjects. Arch Gen Psychiatry 48:513–524, 1991

Rybakowski J: Mechanisms of psychotropic action of lithium and carbamazepine. Pharmacol Toxicol 71 (suppl I):30–41, 1992

Schimmer BP, Tsao J, Borenstein R: Forskolin-resistant Y1 mutants harbor defects associated with the guanyl nucleotide-binding regulatory protein, G_s. J Biol Chem 262:15521–15526, 1987

Schou M: Clinical aspects of lithium in psychiatry, in Lithium and the Cell: Pharmacology and Biochemistry. Edited by Birch NJ. London, Academic Press, 1991, pp 1–6

Scott JD, Carr DW: Subcellular localization of the type II cAMP-dependent protein kinase. American Physiology Society 7:143–148:1992

Skolnick P, Daly JW: Norepinephrine-sensitive adenylate cyclase in rat brain: relation to behavior and tyrosine hydroxylase. Science 184:175–177, 1974

Smith DF: Effects of lithium and rolipram enantiomers on locomotor activity in inbred mice: Pharmacol Toxicol 66:142–145, 1990

Tsuji K, Nakamura Y, Ogata T, et al: Transient increase of cyclic AMP induced by glutamate in cultured neurons from rat spinal cord. J Neurochem 65:1816–1822, 1995

Van Calker D, Steber R, Klotz K-N, et al: Carbamazepine distinguishes between adenosine receptors that mediate different second messenger responses. Eur J Pharmacol [Molecular Pharmacology Section] 206:285–290, 1991

Vink R, McIntosh TK, Demediuk P, et al: Decline in intracellular free Mg^{2+} is associated with irreversible tissue injury after brain trauma. J Biol Chem 263:757–761, 1988

Volonté C: Lithium stimulates the binding of GTP to the membranes of PC12 cells cultured with nerve growth factor. Neurosci Lett 87:127–132, 1988

Wachtel H: Characteristic behavioural alterations in rats induced by rolipram and other selective adenosine cyclic 3′,5′ - monophosphate phosphodiesterase inhibitors. Psychopharmacology (Berl) 77:309–316, 1982

Wachtel H, Löschmann PA: Effects of forskolin and cyclic nucleotides in animal models predictive of antidepressant activity: interaction with rolipram. Psychopharmacology (Berl) 90:430–435, 1986

Wayman GA, Impey S, Storm DR: Ca^{2+} inhibition of type III adenylyl cyclase in vivo. J Biol Chem 270:21480–21486, 1995

Wolfgang D, Chen I, Wand GS: Effects of restraint stress on components of adenylyl cyclase signal transduction in the rat hippocampus. Neuropsychopharmacology 11:187–193, 1994

Wragg MS, MacNeil S: Inhibitory effect of lithium on basal and agonist-stimulated cAMP accumulation in porcine thyroid tissue: a potential model of lithium-induced hypothyroidism. Lithium 2:1–10, 1991

Wu Z-L, Thomas SA, Villacres EC, et al: Altered behavior and long-term potentiation in type I adenylyl cyclase mutant mice. Proc Natl Acad Sci U S A 92:220–224, 1995

Xia Z, Choi E-J, Wang F, et al: Type I calmodulin-sensitive adenylyl cyclase is neural specific. J Neurochem 60:305–311, 1993

Yamashita A, Kurokawa T, Une Y, et al: Phorbol ester regulates stimulatory and inhibitory pathways of the hormone-sensitive adenylate cyclase system in rat reticulocytes. Eur J Pharmacol 151:167–175, 1988

Yang Z, Copolov DL, Lim AT: Glutamate enhances the adenylyl cyclase-cAMP system-induced beta-endorphin secretion and POMC mRNA expression in rat hypothalamic neurons in culture: NMDA receptor-mediated modulation. Brain Res 692:129–136, 1995

Young LT, Li PP, Kish SJ, et al: Cerebral cortex $G_s\alpha$ protein levels and forskolin-stimulated cyclic AMP formation are increased in bipolar affective disorder. J Neurochem 61:890–898, 1993

CHAPTER 7

REGULATION OF SIGNAL TRANSDUCTION PATHWAYS BY MOOD-STABILIZING AGENTS

Implications for the Pathophysiology and Treatment of Bipolar Disorder

Husseini K. Manji, M.D., F.R.C.P.C., Guang Chen, M.D., John K. Hsiao, M.D., Monica I. Masana, Ph.D., Gregory J. Moore, Ph.D., and William Z. Potter, M.D., Ph.D.

Bipolar disorder (manic-depressive illness) is a common (lifetime prevalence of 1.2%) (Weissman et al. 1988), severe, chronic, and life-threatening illness. The discovery of lithium's efficacy as a mood-stabilizing agent revolutionized the treatment of bipolar disorder. After more than two decades, lithium continues to be the mainstay of treatment for this disorder, both for the acute manic phase and as prophylaxis for recur-

The authors wish to acknowledge the invaluable assistance of all the members of the Neuropsychiatric Research Unit. Research support from the National Institute of Mental Health (RO1-MH57743, RO1-MH59107), the Theodore and Vada Stanley Foundation, NARSAD, and Joseph Young Sr. Research Foundation is gratefully acknowledged. Outstanding editorial assistance was provided by Ms. Celia Knobelsdorf.

rent manic and depressive episodes (Goodwin and Jamison 1990). The effect on the broader community is highlighted by one estimate that the use of lithium saved the United States $4 billion in the period 1969–1979, by reducing associated medical costs and restoring productivity (Reifman and Wyatt 1980). Despite lithium's role as one of psychiatry's most important treatments, the cellular and molecular basis for lithium's antimanic and mood-stabilizing actions remains to be fully elucidated (Manji et al. 1995b). Furthermore, increasing evidence suggests that a significant number of patients respond poorly to lithium therapy, with several studies reporting that 20%–40% of patients do not show an adequate antimanic response to lithium, whereas many others are helped but continue to experience significant morbidity (Chou 1991; see Bowden, Chapter 16, and Post et al., Chapter 10, in this volume).

The recognition of the significant morbidity and mortality of the severe mood disorders, as well as the growing appreciation that a significant percentage of patients respond poorly to existing treatments, has made the task of discovering new therapeutic agents that work quickly, potently, specifically, and with fewer side effects increasingly important. This has led to extensive investigation of other pharmacological agents for both the treatment of acute mania and the long-term prophylaxis of bipolar disorder, and considerable evidence has shown that the anticonvulsants valproate (VPA) and carbamazepine (CBZ) are efficacious. Several double-blind studies have reported that VPA can work as effectively as lithium in the treatment of acute mania and, with oral loading, may bring about a more rapid remission of manic symptoms than does lithium (McElroy et al. 1996). Although to date the body of data from controlled studies is small, the preponderance of the evidence suggests that VPA also is effective in the long-term prophylaxis of bipolar disorder (see Bowden, Chapter 16, in this volume). Considerable evidence has also shown that CBZ is an alternative or adjunctive treatment to lithium, for both acute manic episodes and long-term prophylaxis in bipolar disorder (Post et al. 1984).

In addition to representing much-needed additions to our therapeutic armamentarium, the recognition of the therapeutic efficacy of these structurally very dissimilar compounds (see Figure 7–1) offers the potential for the elucidation of the targets both common to, and unique among, the different agents and may help to help identify the biochemical substrates predisposing individuals to bipolar disorder. To date, however, the molecular mechanisms underlying the therapeutic actions of lithium, VPA, and CBZ have not fully been elucidated. This is perhaps partially because, in contrast to other effective psychopharmacological drugs (such as antidepressants and antipsychotics), these agents do not consistently affect the density of most neurotransmitter

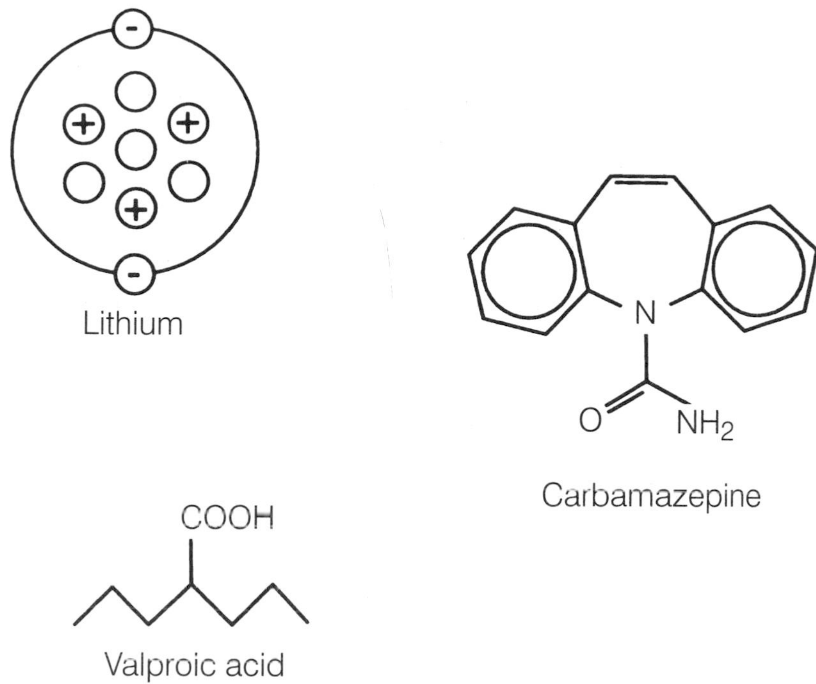

Figure 7–1. Structures of antimanic and mood-stabilizing agents. This figure depicts the structural dissimilarities among the three commonly used antimanic and mood-stabilizing agents, lithium, valproic acid, and carbamazepine.
Source. Reprinted from Manji HK, Chen G, Hsiao JK, et al.: "Regulation of Signal Transduction Pathways by Mood-Stabilizing Agents: Implications for the Delayed Onset of Therapeutic Efficacy." *Journal of Clinical Psychiatry* 57 (suppl 13):34–46, 1996b. Used with permission.

receptors (Manji et al. 1995b; Rogawski and Porter 1990; see Post et al., Chapter 10, in this volume). In addition, although several acute in vitro effects of these agents have been identified, their therapeutic effects in the treatment of bipolar disorder are seen only after chronic administration, thereby precluding any simple mechanistic interpretations based on acute biochemical effects. The search for the mechanisms of action of mood-stabilizing agents has been facilitated by the observations that rather than any single neurotransmitter system being responsible for depression or mania, multiple interacting and overlapping systems are involved in regulating mood (Hsiao et al. 1987, 1993; Manji 1992; Meltzer 1992; Risby et al. 1991) and that most effective drugs likely do not work on any particular neurotransmitter system in isolation but rather affect the functional balance between interacting systems (Hsiao et al. 1987, 1993; Manji 1992; Meltzer 1992; Risby et al. 1991).

Advances in our understanding of the cellular basis of neuronal communication have led to a reconceptualization of the mechanisms by which neuronal function is regulated, and it has become increasingly appreciated that in addition to regulating the levels of neurotransmitters per se, alterations in intracellular signaling can markedly regulate neurotransmitter *function* (Bourne and Nicoll 1993; Manji 1992; Ross 1989; Taylor 1990). In this context, signal transduction pathways are in a pivotal position in the central nervous system (CNS) and thus represent attractive targets to explain lithium's efficacy in treating multiple aspects of bipolar disorder (Bourne and Nicoll 1993; Hudson et al. 1993; Jope and Williams 1994; Lachman and Papolos 1991; Manji 1992; J. F. Wang et al. 1997). It is therefore not surprising that recent research aimed at the elucidation of the molecular and cellular events underlying the pathophysiology of bipolar disorder (Table 7–1) and the therapeutic effects of antimanic and mood-stabilizing agents (in particular, lithium) has focused on signal transduction pathways (see Jope et al., Chapter 8, and Post et al., Chapter 10, in this volume; Manji and Lenox, in press; Manji et al. 1995b). Although many of these studies have generally found that these mood-stabilizing agents affect the function of second-messenger generating systems in the brain, the attribution of *therapeutic relevance* to any observed biochemical effect must account for certain key features of the drugs when used clinically in the treatment of bipolar disorder (Lenox and Manji 1998; Manji et al. 1995b). As articulated already, one of the major considerations is that of the time course of the drug's actions; the antimanic effects of lithium appear to require days to weeks, whereas, with oral loading, those of VPA may be observed somewhat more rapidly (McElroy et al. 1996). In addition, at least for lithium, the long-term mood-stabilizing effect can continue indefinitely without tolerance

Table 7–1. Evidence for abnormalities in signal transduction pathways in bipolar disorder

Elevated levels of $G\alpha_s$ in peripheral circulating cells and perhaps postmortem brain
Elevated agonist-induced [^{3}H]Gpp(NH)p binding to mononuclear leukocytes
Elevated platelet membrane PKC activity in manic subjects
Blunted β- and α_2-adrenergic responses in peripheral circulating cells
Blunted growth hormone and prolactin responses to a variety of challenges in affective disorders (due to postreceptor abnormalities?)

Note. Gpp(NH)p = guanylyl-5′-imidodiphosphate; PKC = protein kinase C.
Source. Reprinted from Manji HK, Chen G, Hsiao JK, et al.: "Regulation of Signal Transduction Pathways by Mood-Stabilizing Agents: Implications for the Delayed Onset of Therapeutic Efficacy." *Journal of Clinical Psychiatry* 57 (suppl 13):34–46, 1996b. Used with permission.

and generally is not immediately reversed on discontinuation, although the risk of manic episodes may be significantly elevated after discontinuation (Goodwin and Jamison 1990; Suppes et al. 1991). Thus, any *relevant mechanism* postulated to explain the therapeutic actions of these drugs must account for this pattern of treatment response (i.e., changes induced during chronic administration that are likely to persist beyond abrupt discontinuation of treatment) (Lenox and Manji 1998; Manji et al. 1995b).

LITHIUM AND G PROTEINS

Abundant experimental evidence has shown that lithium attenuates receptor-mediated adenylyl cyclase (AC) activity and phosphatidylinositol (PI) turnover in rodents and in humans, in the absence of consistent changes in the density of the receptors themselves (reviewed in Lenox and Manji 1998; Manji et al. 1995b; Mørk and Jensen, Chapter 6, in this volume). The first direct evidence that guanine nucleotide binding proteins (G proteins) may be the targets of lithium's actions was provided by Avissar and colleagues (1988), who reported that lithium dramatically *eliminated* isoproterenol- and carbachol-induced increases in [^{3}H]guanosine triphosphate ([^{3}H]GTP) binding to various G proteins in rat cerebral cortical membranes. These effects were reported to occur both in vitro in the presence of 0.6 mM LiCl and in washed cortical membranes from rats treated with lithium carbonate for 2–3 weeks, suggesting that the function of several G proteins (e.g., stimulatory G protein [G_s], inhibitory G protein [G_i], $G_{q/11}$) might be modified by this mood-stabilizing drug. In animals withdrawn from lithium for 2 days, agonist-stimulated response ([^{3}H]GTP binding) returned. Although these studies have been of considerable heuristic interest and the preponderance of data *do* suggest an action of *chronic* lithium at the level of G proteins, such a *direct* action of lithium on G-protein function has been difficult to replicate (Ellis and Lenox 1991); moreover, the fact that routine assays of agonist-stimulated PI hydrolysis in brain slices are conducted in the presence of 10 mM LiCl suggests that the lithium ion does not *directly* exert any major effects on $G_{q/11}$ protein function. However, considerable evidence indicates that chronic lithium administration affects G-protein function (see Table 7–2), and numerous investigations have addressed the role of G proteins in the altered transmembrane signaling observed after chronic lithium administration in rodents and in humans (reviewed in Manji et al. 1995b; Mørk et al. 1992; Risby et al. 1991).

Our laboratory has used in vivo microdialysis measurements of cyclic adenosine monophosphate (cAMP) to assess lithium's effects on G proteins in

Table 7–2. Evidence for lithium's effects on G proteins

Attenuation of receptor-stimulated adenylyl cyclase activity
Attenuation of receptor-mediated and GTPγS-mediated PI turnover
Attenuation of agonist-induced [^{3}H]GTP binding
Reversal of the effects of lithium by increasing GTP
Increase in lymphocyte and rat brain β-adrenergic receptor K_L/K_H ratio
Increase in pertussis-toxin–catalyzed [^{32}P]ADP ribosylation in platelets and in rat brain
Reduction in $G\alpha_s$, $G\alpha_{i1}$, $G\alpha_{i2}$ mRNA in rat cortex

Note. GTP = guanosine triphosphate; PI = phosphatidylinositol; ADP = adenosine 5′ - diphosphate; mRNA = messenger RNA.
Source. Reprinted from Manji HK, Chen G, Hsiao JK, et al.: "Regulation of Signal Transduction Pathways by Mood-Stabilizing Agents: Implications for the Delayed Onset of Therapeutic Efficacy." *Journal of Clinical Psychiatry* 57 (suppl 13):34–46, 1996b. Used with permission.

the intact animal, because in previous in vitro and ex vivo studies, the particular tissue preparation affected the results obtained (reviewed in Masana et al. 1992). We found that chronic lithium treatment produced a significant increase in basal and postreceptor-stimulated (cholera toxin or forskolin [colforsin]) AC activity, while attenuating the β-adrenergic mediated effect in rat frontal cortex (Manji et al. 1991a; Masana et al. 1992). Interestingly, chronic lithium treatment resulted in an almost absent cAMP response to pertussis toxin (see Figure 7–2); taken together, these results suggest a lithium-induced attenuation of G_i function and of the β-adrenergic receptor–G_s interaction. To examine this more directly, we measured the levels of various G-protein α-subunits after chronic lithium administration. We were unable to identify any alterations in the amounts of α_s (52 kDa), α_s (45 kDa),α_{i1-3}, or α_o (Masana et al. 1992). However, lithium treatment resulted in a significant increase in pertussis-toxin–catalyzed [^{32}P]adenosine 5′ -diphosphate (ADP) ribosylation in both frontal cortex and hippocampus (see Figure 7–3). Because pertussis toxin selectively ADP-ribosylates the undissociated, inactive $\alpha\beta\gamma$ heterotrimeric form of G_i (Katada et al. 1986a, 1986b), these results suggest that lithium activates G_i via a stabilization of the inactive conformation (discussed in detail below) (see Figure 7–4).

To examine lithium's effects on the β-adrenergic receptor–G_s interactions in more detail, we measured the ratio of low- and high-affinity β-adrenergic receptor binding dissociation constants (K_L/K_H), which corresponds to the degree of stabilization of the high-affinity state. The attenuated functional responsiveness of the β-adrenergic receptor after chronic lithium treatment (reviewed in Mørk et al. 1992) was accompanied by an increase in

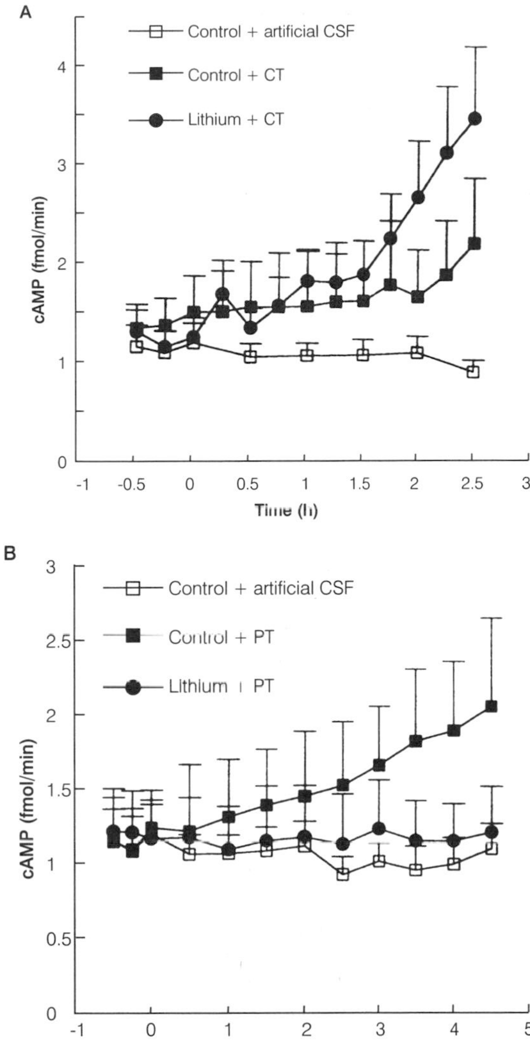

Figure 7–2. Effects of chronic lithium treatment on (A) cholera-toxin (CT)–induced or (B) pertussis-toxin (PT)–induced increases in cyclic adenosine monophosphate (cAMP) levels in prefrontal cortex. Rats were treated for 4–5 weeks with lithium (attaining serum levels similar to those observed in humans therapeutically). Toxins were injected adjacent to the microdialysis probe into the prefrontal cortex, and dialysate cAMP concentrations were determined with a radioimmunoassay kit. Chronic lithium treatment produced a significantly enhanced response to cholera toxin. By contrast, chronic lithium treatment resulted in a markedly attenuated (almost absent) response to pertussis toxin. *Note.* CSF = cerebrospinal fluid. *Source.* Reprinted with permission from Masana MI, Bitran JA, Hsiao JK, et al.: "In Vivo Evidence That Lithium Inactivates Gi Modulation of Adenylate Cyclase in Brain." *Journal of Neurochemistry* 59:200–205, 1992.

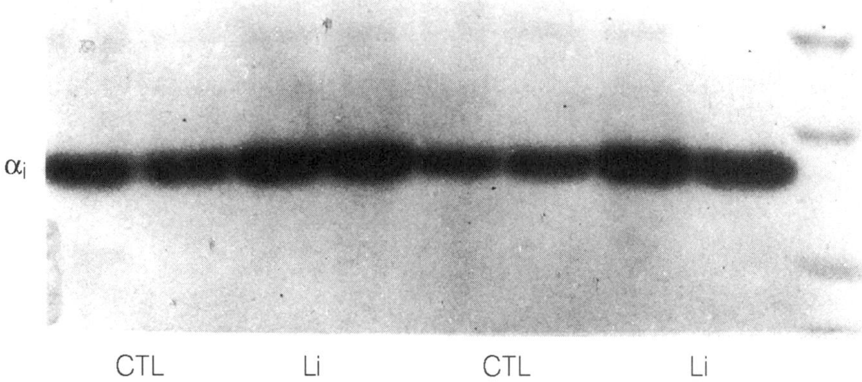

Figure 7–3A. Effects of chronic lithium on pertussis-toxin–catalyzed [^{32}P] adenosine 5′ -diphosphate ([^{32}P] ADP) ribosylation, rodent studies. Rats were treated with lithium for 3 weeks, achieving plasma levels similar to those attained during clinical treatment. Rat cortices were dissected and subjected to pertussis-toxin–catalyzed [^{32}P]ADP ribosylation. Samples were loaded in duplicate. *Note.* CTL = control; Li = lithium treated.
Source. Modified and reproduced from Masana MI, Bitran JA, Hsiao JK, et al.: "In Vivo Evidence That Lithium Inactivates Gi Modulation of Adenylate Cyclase in Brain." *Journal of Neurochemistry* 59:200–205, 1992. Used with permission.

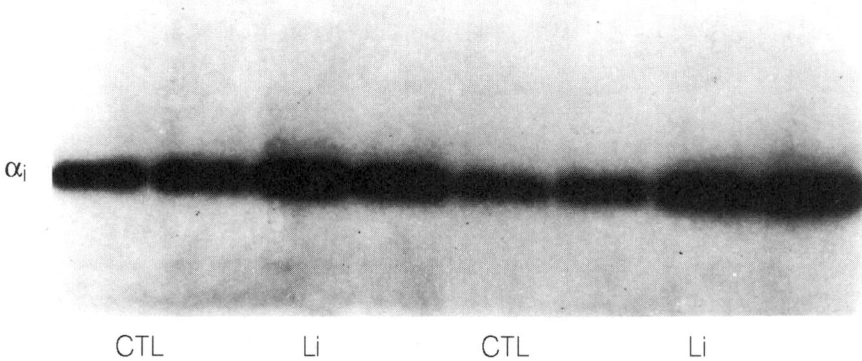

Figure 7–3B. Effects of chronic lithium on pertussis-toxin–catalyzed [^{32}P] adenosine 5′ -diphosphate ([^{32}P] ADP) ribosylation, human studies. Healthy volunteers were treated with lithium for 2 weeks, achieving plasma levels similar to those attained during clinical treatment. Platelets were isolated and subjected to pertussis-toxin–catalyzed [^{32}P]ADP ribosylation. Samples were loaded in duplicate. *Note.* CTL = healthy volunteer at baseline; Li = healthy volunteer after 2 weeks of lithium.
Source. Modified and reproduced from Hsiao JK, Manji HK, Chen GA, et al.: "Lithium Administration Modulates Platelet G_i in Humans." *Life Science* 50:227–233, 1992. Used with permission.

the K_L-to-K_H ratio for the β-adrenergic receptor (Turkka et al. 1992). Taken together, these results suggest that one of lithium's effects may be to stabilize the high-affinity ternary complex, perhaps by interfering with GTP binding. If dissociation of G-protein subunits were inhibited by lithium, β-adrenergic-stimulated AC activity could decrease and a relative stabilization of the receptor in a high-affinity state could be produced simultaneously.

Most studies of lithium's actions on G proteins (and indeed most of the current knowledge about its neurochemical effects) derive from animal and in

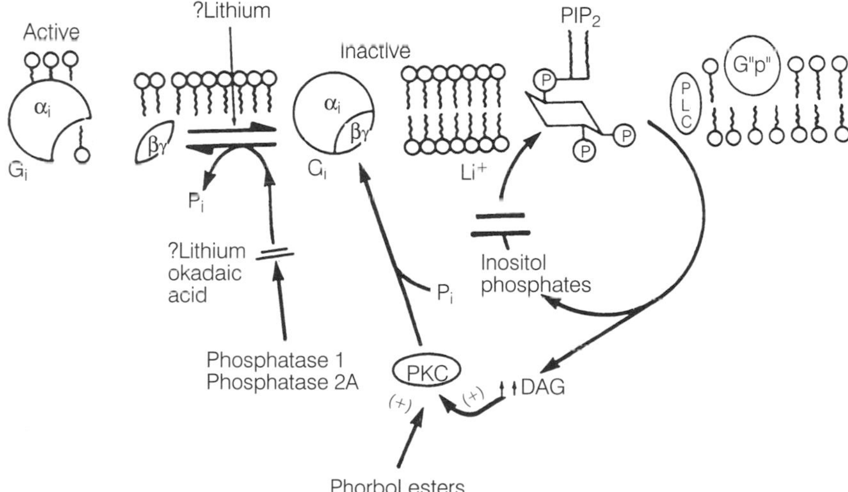

Figure 7–4. Inactivation of G_i by lithium: cross-talk with protein kinase C. The figure depicts the mechanisms by which chronic lithium may produce an inactivation of G_i. Activation of G_i shifts the equilibrium to the left toward the dissociated, active form of G_i. Chronic lithium treatment has been demonstrated to attenuate G_i function while increasing the pertussis-toxin (PT)–catalyzed [^{32}P]ADP ribosylation. Since PT selectively ADP-ribosylates the undissociated, inactive form of G_i, these results suggest that the effects of chronic lithium involve a stabilization of the inactive αβγ conformation of G_i. Activation of protein kinase C (PKC) by phorbol esters also inactivates G_i, and in several tissues, also leads to an increase in PT-catalyzed [^{32}P]ADP ribosylation. Thus, one possible mechanism for lithium's effects on G_i may be the modulation of the phosphorylation state of G_i. Lithium, via its inhibition of inositol 1-phosphatase, produces an elevation of diacylglycerol (DAG) levels, which may regulate the activity of PKC. Abbreviations: G_i, G protein mediating inhibition of adenylyl cyclase; PIP$_2$, phosphatidylinositol 4,5-bisphosphate; PLCβ, phospholipase C β isozyme; G′ ′ p′ ′ , G proteins coupled to stimulation of phosphoinositide turnover; Pi, inorganic phosphate; PKC, protein kinase C; DAG, diacylglycerol.

Source. Reprinted from Manji HK, Potter WZ, Lenox RH: "Signal Transduction Pathways: Molecular Targets for Lithium's Actions." *Archives of General Psychiatry* 52(7):531–543, 1995b. Used with permission.

vitro models. However, because lithium is clinically relevant only in humans, it is imperative to ascertain which of its actions in animals and in vitro generalize to humans. To overcome the potentially confounding significant effects of alterations in mood-state-dependent biochemical and neuroendocrine parameters, our studies have used healthy volunteers (Hsiao et al. 1992; Manji et al. 1991b; Risby et al. 1991). Any changes would presumably be a generalizable effect of lithium in humans (although the magnitude of the effect may depend on the preexisting set-point of the substrate).

In a series of clinical investigations, we examined the effects of 2 weeks of lithium administration at therapeutic levels to healthy volunteers on dynamic AC activity, G-protein measures, and β-adrenergic receptor binding parameters (Hsiao et al. 1992; Manji et al. 1991a, 1991b; Risby et al. 1991). A particularly striking, novel finding of the study was lithium's differential effects on AC activity in platelets and lymphocytes. Basal and postreceptor-stimulated AC activity was increased in platelets, but in the same subjects no significant effects were found in AC activity in lymphocytes (indeed, basal AC activity in lymphocytes tended to decrease) (Risby et al. 1991; see Figure 7–5). Because G_i appears to exert significant inhibitory effects on platelets but not on lymphocytes, these tissue-specific effects of lithium are compatible with an attenuation of G_i function. Similar to our findings in rat brain, we found no alterations in the levels of platelet G proteins (G_s or G_i) but observed a significant 40% increase in the pertussis-toxin–catalyzed [^{32}P]ADP ribosylation in platelet membranes following chronic lithium (Figure 7–3B; Hsiao et al. 1992), once again suggesting a stabilization of the inactive undissociated αβγ heterotrimeric form of G_i (see Figure 7–4 and Table 7–3). As observed in rat cortex and hippocampus, chronic lithium treatment produced a significant increase in the lymphocyte β-adrenergic receptor K_L-to-K_H ratio (Risby et al. 1991), in the absence of any alterations in the density for the receptor.

Modulation of G Proteins by Lithium: A Synthesis

The data suggest that chronic lithium does affect the signal-transducing G proteins in both humans and rodents (see Table 7–2). Interestingly, for both G_s and G_i, lithium's major effects appear to be a stabilization of the heterotrimeric, undissociated (αβγ) conformation of the G protein. The allosteric modulation of G proteins might explain lithium's long-term prophylactic efficacy in protecting susceptible individuals from spontaneous, stress- and drug (e.g., antidepressant, stimulant)-induced cyclic affective episodes. It also may be postulated that these effects on G proteins represent the mechanistic basis

Table 7–3. Lithium and G proteins

	Human platelets	Rat brain
Basal AC	↑	↑
Postreceptor AC	↑	↑
$G\alpha_{i2}$	0	0
$G\alpha_s$	0	0
Pertussis-toxin–catalyzed [^{32}P]ADPR	↑	↑
cAMP response to pertussis toxin	??	↓

Note. AC = adenylyl cyclase; ADPR = adenosine 5′-diphosphate ribosylation; cAMP = cyclic adenosine monophosphate.

Source. Reprinted from Manji HK, Chen G, Hsiao JK, et al.: "Regulation of Signal Transduction Pathways by Mood-Stabilizing Agents: Implications for the Delayed Onset of Therapeutic Efficacy." *Journal of Clinical Psychiatry* 57 (suppl 13):34–46, 1996b. Used with permission.

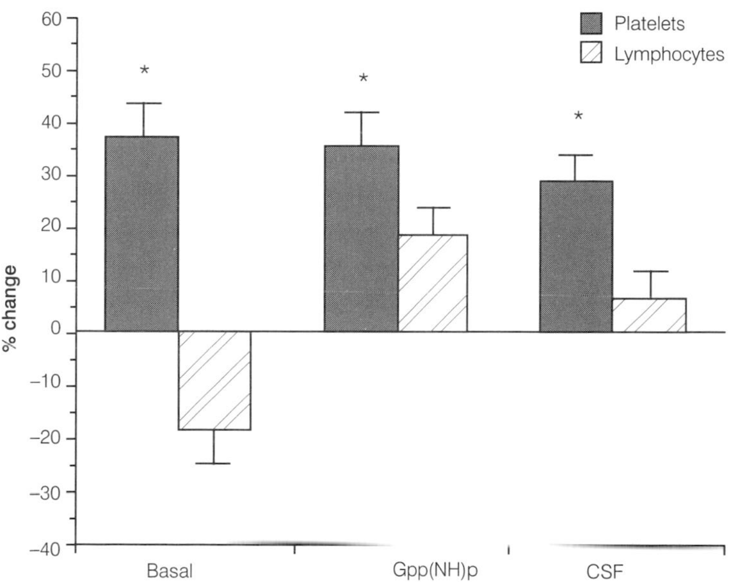

Figure 7–5. Effects of chronic lithium on adenylyl cyclase activity in healthy volunteers. Healthy volunteers were treated with lithium for 2 weeks, achieving plasma levels similar to those attained during clinical treatment. Platelets and lymphocytes were isolated, and basal and postreceptor-stimulated adenylyl cyclase activity was determined.

Note. Gpp(NH)p = guanylyl-5′-imidodiphosphate; CSF = cerebrospinal fluid. *$P < .05$ compared to baseline.

Source. Modified from Risby ED, Hsiao JK, Manji HK, et al.: "The Mechanisms of Action of Lithium." *Archives of General Psychiatry* 48:513–524, 1991. Used with permission.

by which chronic lithium administration blocks the development of supersensitive dopaminergic, adrenergic, and cholinergic receptors (Bunney and Garland-Bunney 1987; Lenox and Manji 1998). These supersensitive responses have been assayed by biochemical, electrophysiological, and behavioral studies; interestingly, most receptor binding studies generally have not shown lithium-induced alterations in the density of the receptors themselves, suggesting that lithium exerts its effects at postreceptor sites, in particular at the level of the signal-transducing G proteins. Such a contention is also supported by the observation that lithium's effects appear to involve different classes of receptors coupled to both AC and phospholipase C isozymes; however, lithium clearly exerts effects on additional intracellular targets, and these effects also probably contribute to the prevention of supersensitive receptor responses.

At present, the precise cellular mechanisms underlying lithium's effects on G proteins remain to be fully established. Some evidence suggests that lithium has acute in vitro effects on G proteins (Avissar et al. 1988; Greenwood and Jope 1994), but most of the effects of chronic lithium treatment persist after washing of the membranes and are therefore likely to be attributable to an indirect posttranslational modification of the G proteins (Jope and Williams 1994; Manji et al. 1995b). Because G-protein function has been postulated to be regulated by phosphorylation (Garcia-Sainz et al. 1989; Halenda et al. 1986; Houslay 1991; Jakobs et al. 1985; Lounsbury et al. 1991; Olianas and Onali 1986), and because considerable evidence has shown that lithium affects protein kinase C (PKC) (see next section), one potential mechanistic explanation for lithium's effects on G-protein subunit dissociation is phosphorylation by PKC. This does not imply that G_i is *directly* phosphorylated by PKC (see Figure 7–3). Thus, posttranslational modifications may underlie some of lithium's effects. Additionally, members of a recently discovered gene family, the regulators of G-protein signaling (RGS) family, have been shown to interact directly with G-protein α-subunits and to stimulate their GTPase activity (which would promote the reassociation of the heterotrimeric [$\alpha\beta\gamma$] form of the G protein; Berman et al. 1996). Furthermore, because RGS function has been shown to be dynamically modulated in the CNS (Ingi et al. 1998), the potential effects of lithium on RGS protein levels and activity are an exciting area for future research. Chronic lithium administration has been reported to reduce the messenger RNA (mRNA) levels of several G protein α-subunits in rat brain, including $G\alpha_{i1}$, $G\alpha_{i2}$, and $G\alpha_s$ (Colin et al. 1991; P. P. Li et al. 1991, 1993), suggesting that lithium produces complex transcriptional and posttranscriptional effects after chronic administration, many of which may be mediated via its effects on PKC. We now discuss the evidence for an effect of lithium on PKC isozymes.

LITHIUM AND PROTEIN KINASE C

Calcium-activated, phospholipid-dependent PKC is a ubiquitous enzyme, highly enriched in the brain, where it plays a major role in regulating pre- and postsynaptic aspects of neurotransmission (K. P. Huang 1989; Nishizuka 1992; Stabel and Parker 1991). PKC is one of the major intracellular mediators of signals generated on external stimulation of cells by a variety of neurotransmitter receptor subtypes that induce the hydrolysis of membrane phospholipids. PKC exists as a family of closely related subspecies, has a heterogeneous distribution in the brain (with particularly high levels in presynaptic nerve terminals), and plays a major role in the regulation of neuronal excitability, neurotransmitter release, and long-term alterations in gene expression and plasticity (K. P. Huang 1989; Nishizuka 1992; Stabel and Parker 1991).

Accumulating evidence from various laboratories has shown that lithium exerts significant effects on PKC in several cell systems, including the brain (Jope 1999b; Jope and Williams 1994; Lenox et al., Chapter 9, in this volume; Manji and Lenox 1994; Manji et al. 1995b) (see Table 7–4). The preponderance of the data suggests that chronic lithium exposure results in an attenuation of phorbol ester–mediated responses, which may be accompanied by a downregulation of PKC isozymes (Jope and Williams 1994; Manji and Lenox 1994, in press; Manji et al. 1995b) (see Table 7–4). Interestingly, this pattern of effects is seen both in cultured cells in vitro and in brain in vivo. Biochemical studies have found that chronic (3-week) lithium treatment at therapeutic levels attenuates both the phorbol ester–induced cytosol-to-membrane PKC

Table 7–4. Evidence for lithium's effects on protein kinase C

Biphasic effects on phorbol ester–mediated neurotransmitter release in rat hippocampus
Cross-desensitization with the effects of phorbol esters
Reduced in vitro PKC-mediated phosphorylation of major PKC substrates (80 kDa, 43 kDa)
Reduced [^{3}H]PDBu binding in hippocampal structures, notably CA1 and subiculum
Reduced phorbol ester–mediated Na^+/H^+ exchange in cultured cells
Reduced immunolabeling of PKCα and PKCε in rat brain and cultured cells

Note. PKC = protein kinase C; PDBu = phorbol 12,13-dibutyrate.
Source. Reprinted from Manji HK, Chen G, Hsiao JK, et al.: "Regulation of Signal Transduction Pathways by Mood-Stabilizing Agents: Implications for the Delayed Onset of Therapeutic Efficacy." *Journal of Clinical Psychiatry* 57 (suppl 13):34–46, 1996b. Used with permission.

translocation and the [^{3}H]serotonin release in the hippocampus (Anderson et al. 1988; H. Y. Wang and Friedman 1989). Activation of PKC facilitates the release of several neurotransmitters, although the precise mechanisms remain to be fully elucidated. It has been postulated, however, that the phosphorylation of myristoylated alanine-rich C kinase substrate (MARCKS) and growth associated protein (GAP-43) by PKC plays a key role in facilitating neurotransmitter release (DeGraan et al. 1990; Robinson 1991). In this context, it is noteworthy that the level of MARCKS, a protein implicated in synaptic transmission, was significantly reduced after chronic lithium exposure (Lenox et al. 1991, 1992; Lenox et al., Chapter 9, in this volume).

Manji and associates (1993) used quantitative autoradiographic techniques to show that chronic (5-week) lithium administration results in a significant decrease in membrane-associated PKC in several hippocampal structures, most notably the subiculum and CA1 region, with no significant changes in the other cortical and subcortical structures examined (Figure 7–6A). Furthermore, immunoblotting with monoclonal anti-PKCα antibodies has detected an isozyme-specific decrease in PKCα and PKCε, which have been implicated in facilitating neurotransmitter release (Ben-Schlomo et al. 1991; Oda et al. 1991); no significant alterations in PKCβ, PKCγ, PKCδ, or PKCζ were found (Manji and Lenox, in press; Manji et al. 1993) (Figure 7–6B).

The mechanisms by which lithium produces the isozyme-selective decreases in the immunolabeling of PKCα and PKCε and in the levels of MARCKS are unclear. Although PKC subspecies have subtle differences in their enzymatic properties, ligand binding, and substrate specificity in vitro, the isoforms show different tissue- and cell type–specific expression patterns in vitro, and they also differ in their susceptibility to degradation by phorbol esters (which potently cause activation and membrane insertion of the isozymes, thereby rendering them more susceptible to proteolytic degradation) (Borner et al. 1992; Isakov et al. 1990; Leli et al. 1993; S. Young et al. 1987). Interestingly, a study has also identified similar phorbol ester–induced subcellular distribution of PKCα and PKCε, compared with the subcellular distribution of PKCβ, PKCγ, PKCδ, PKCζ, or PKCη(Goodnight et al. 1995). It is also noteworthy that exposure of neuroblastoma cells (Leli and Hauser 1992) or PC12 cells (Jope et al., Chapter 8, in this volume; X. Li and Jope 1995) to 1 mM of lithium in vitro produces isozyme-selective decreases in PKCαand (in the case of PC12 cells) PKCε; these results are strikingly similar to the results we have observed in ex vivo (i.e., after chronic treatment in the animals) studies (Manji and Lenox, in press; Manji et al. 1993).

As a result of inositol depletion in the presence of lithium, metabolites within the phospholipid portion of the hydrolytic pathway, which include

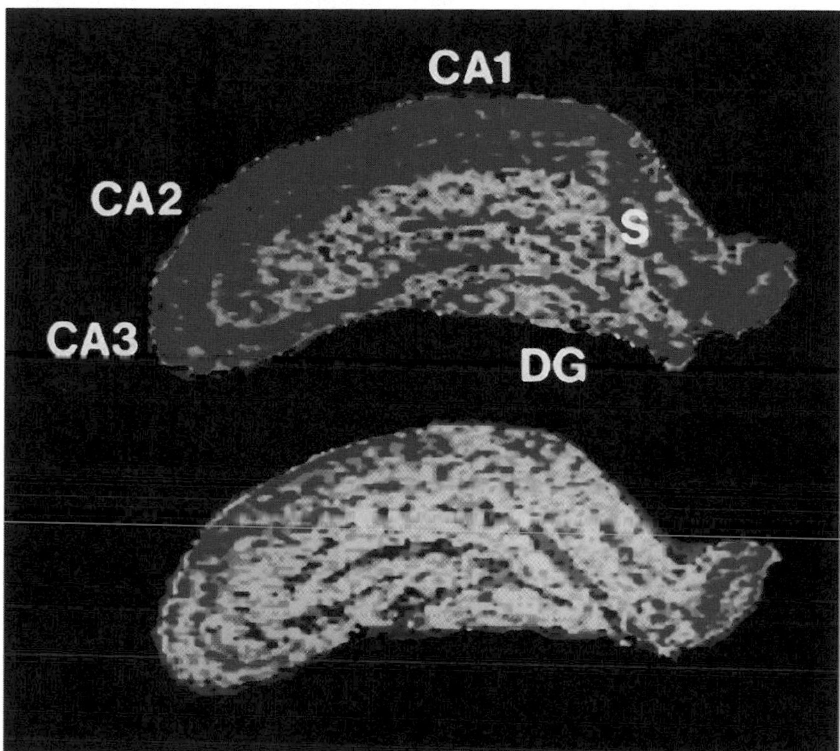

Figure 7–6A. Effects of chronic lithium on membrane-associated protein kinase C (PKC) in hippocampus. Rats were treated chronically with lithium for 4 weeks, and brain sections were incubated with [^{3}H] phorbol 12,13-dibutyrate (PDBu). Sections were analyzed every 100 μm throughout various regions of interest. Chronic lithium treatment produced significant decreases in [^{3}H]PDBu in the CA1 region and subiculum. Top, control rat; bottom, lithium-treated rat.
Note. CA1–CA3 = hippocampal subfields; S = subiculum; DG = dentate gyrus.
Source. Reprinted from Manji HK, Etcheberrigaray R, Chen G, et al.: "Lithium Decreases Membrane-Associated PKC in the Hippocampus: Selectivity for the Alpha Isozyme." *Journal of Neurochemistry* 61:2303–2310, 1993. Used with permission.

diacylglycerol (DAG), phosphatidic acid, and cytidine monophosphate phosphatidate, are significantly elevated; this effect can be prevented by the presence of high concentrations of inositol (Brami et al. 1991, 1993; Downes and Stone 1986; Drummond and Raeburn 1984; discussed in Manji and Lenox, in press). This result might be expected because the end metabolite in this pathway (i.e., cytidine monophosphate phosphatidate) requires free *myo*-inositol to resynthesize inositol phosphates for the regeneration of phosphatidylinositol 4,5-bisphosphate (PIP_2) (Fisher et. al. 1992; Rana and

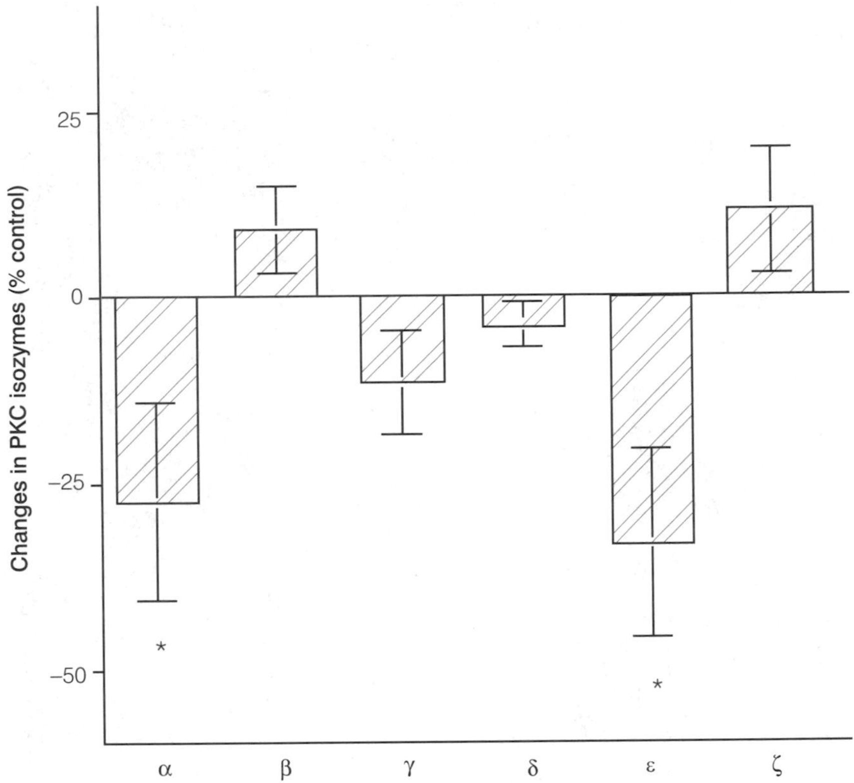

Figure 7–6B. Effects of chronic lithium on immunolabeling of protein kinase C (PKC) isozymes. Rats were treated with lithium for 5 weeks, attaining serum lithium levels of 0.78 ± 0.06 mM. Cytosolic and membrane fractions were prepared and subjected to Western blotting. Quantitation of the immunoblots was performed by densitometric scanning of the autoradiograms. Chronic lithium treatment resulted in a significant reduction in the immunolabeling of membrane-associated PKCα and membrane-associated PKCε, but did not affect the immunolabeling of any of the other PKC isozymes.
Note. α = PKC α isozyme; β = PKCβ (I/II) isozyme; γ = PKCγ isozyme; δ = PKCδ isozyme; ε = PKCε isozyme; ζ = PKC ζ isozyme.
*$P < .05$ compared to control animals.
Source. Reprinted from Manji HK, Chen G, Hsiao JK, et al.: "Regulation of Signal Transduction Pathways by Mood-Stabilizing Agents: Implications for the Delayed Onset of Therapeutic Efficacy." *Journal of Clinical Psychiatry* 57 (suppl 13):34–46, 1996b. Used with permission.

Hokin 1990). Because PKC activation is often followed by its rapid proteolytic degradation (S. Young et al. 1987), a prolonged increase in DAG levels by chronic lithium may lead to an increased membrane translocation and subsequent degradation and downregulation of PKC isozymes. Moreover, studies of fibroblasts have found that activation of PKC results in a significant reduction in the levels of both MARCKS protein and mRNA (Erusalimsky et al. 1991; Linder et al. 1992). Thus, the reduction in hippocampal MARCKS observed after chronic lithium administration (Lenox et al., Chapter 9, in this volume) may similarly be mediated by a lithium-induced increase in DAG levels and subsequent activation of PKC isozymes (Figure 7–7).

We have recently undertaken a series of studies to investigate the hypothesis that the action of chronic lithium on PKC isozymes and substrates may be secondary to its effect in inhibiting the recycling of inositol. In preliminary studies, we found that co-incubation of rat C6 glioma cells with 10 mM of *myo*-inositol markedly reduced the lithium-induced attenuation of the immunolabeling of particulate PKCα (see Figure 7–8). It is obviously imperative to ascertain whether such a mechanism is also operative in the CNS in vivo in order to ascribe any potential therapeutic relevance to it; a major obstacle in such an investigation, however, is that *myo*-inositol penetrates the blood-brain barrier poorly. To overcome this problem, we administered lithium to a group of rats for 3 weeks and coadministered *myo*-inositol or saline by twice-daily intracerebroventricular injections to other rats (Manji et al. 1996a). We found a significant interaction between chronic lithium and *myo*-inositol administration, with the chronic intracerebroventricular administration of *myo*-inositol attenuating lithium's effects on PKCα, PKCε, and pertussis-toxin–catalyzed [^{32}P]ADP ribosylation (Manji et al. 1996a). These results suggest that some of the effects of chronic lithium on signal transduction pathways may stem from its inhibition of inositol 1-phosphatase.

To determine whether such mechanisms may be operative in the *human* brain, our research group recently used proton magnetic resonance spectroscopy (MRS) in a series of studies. We sought to determine whether lithium *does* indeed reduce the levels of *myo*-inositol in critical brain regions of individuals with bipolar disorder and whether lithium-induced CNS *myo*-inositol reductions are associated with its therapeutic effects. After extensive validation of this method for in vivo measurement of regional brain *myo*-inositol concentration as well as careful determination that the 1.5 Tesla *myo*-inositol resonance is indeed predominantly *myo*-inositol (≥80%) (Moore et al., in press), we have begun to apply this methodology in our studies of patients with bipolar disorder. Following medication washout (≥2 weeks), MRS scans were performed in patients at baseline, after 5 days of lithium treatment, and after 4 weeks of lithium administration. We found that therapeutic administration of lithium *does* indeed produce significant reductions in *myo*-inositol levels in patients with bipolar disorder in brain regions that previously have been implicated in the pathophysiology of bipolar disorder (Moore et al., in press). However, the major lithium-induced *myo*-inositol reductions are observed

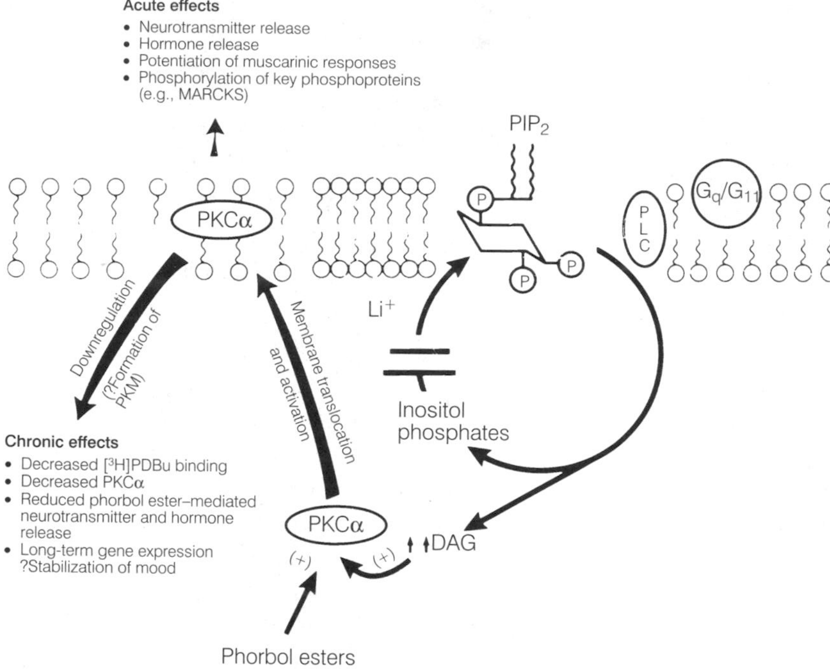

Figure 7–7. Acute and chronic effects of lithium mediated via protein kinase C (PKC). This figure depicts a number of potential sites at which lithium, via its effects on PKC, may affect synaptic function. Inhibition of inositol 1-phosphatase by lithium may result in an elevation of diacylglycerol (DAG) levels, leading to an activation of PKC. Activation of PKC isozymes exerts both immediate and long-term effects on the regulation of synaptic function and neuronal excitability; only some of these effects are depicted here. PKC also exerts long-term effects by transcriptional and posttranscriptional effects on gene expression, which likely play a role in long-term stabilization of mood. MARCKS = myristoylated alanine-rich C kinase substrate; PIP_2 = phosphatidylinositol 4,5-bisphosphate; G_q/G_{11} = G proteins coupled to phosphoinositide turnover; P = phosphate; PLC = phospholipase C; Li, = lithium; PKCα = protein kinase C α isozyme; PKM = protein kinase M; PDBu = phorbol 12,13-dibutyrate.
Source. Reprinted from Manji HK, Chen G, Hsiao JK, et al.: "Regulation of Signal Transduction Pathways by Mood-Stabilizing Agents: Implications for the Delayed Onset of Therapeutic Efficacy." *Journal of Clinical Psychiatry* 57 (suppl 13): 34–46, 1996b. Used with permission.

only after 5 days of lithium administration, *at a time when the bipolar disorder patients' clinical state is completely unchanged.* Consequently, we have shown that although lithium *does* produce a reduction in *myo*-inositol levels, as has been articulated by Jope and Williams (1994), reducing *myo*-inositol levels per se is

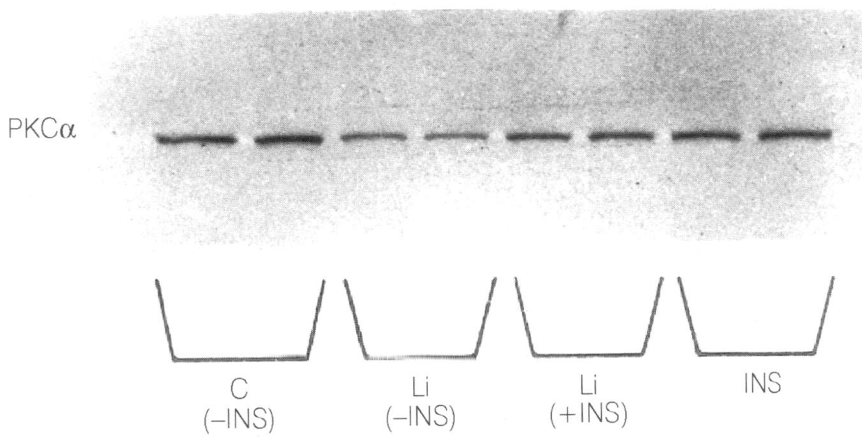

Figure 7–8. Effects of chronic lithium on immunolabeling of membrane-associated protein kinase C α isozyme (PKCα) in rat C6 glioma cells. C6 glioma cells were grown in inositol-free medium in the absence or presence of lithium (1 mM) and supplemental *myo*-inositol (10 mM). Membrane fractions were prepared and subjected to sodium dodecyl sulfate–polyacrylamide gel electrophoresis (SDS-PAGE) on 10% polyacrylamide gels. Blots were incubated overnight with anti-PKC isozyme antibodies. *Note.* Li = lithium-treated; C = control; INS = *myo*-inositol.

not associated with therapeutic response. Thus, although the inositol depletion hypothesis, as originally articulated, does not receive support from our study, it remains an attractive working hypothesis that some of the initial actions of lithium may occur with a relative depletion of *myo*-inositol (Manji et al. 1995b, Moore et al., in press); this relative depletion of *myo*-inositol may initiate a cascade of secondary changes at different levels of the signal transduction process and gene expression in the CNS, effects that are ultimately responsible for lithium's therapeutic efficacy (Jope and Williams 1994; Manji et al. 1995b). Studies are currently under way to determine whether the lithium-induced reductions in *myo*-inositol levels are associated with components of ultimate therapeutic response.

Do these ex vivo effects of lithium on PKC isozymes translate into any functional effects in vivo? To address this question, we used in vivo microdialysis measurements of cAMP because although considerable evidence now indicates that lithium affects both major transmembrane signaling systems, most studies to date have investigated lithium's effects on these systems in isolation. However, it has become clear in recent years that the various signal transduction pathways expressed in cells modulate one another's activity at multiple levels and that these interactions between distinct second-messenger generating systems represent a fine-tuned cellular network that regulates the neurons' responses to numerous extracellular signals, thereby playing a crucial role in the integrative functions of the CNS (Bourne and Nicoll 1993; Ross 1989; Taylor 1990). A growing body of evidence suggests that the PKC isozymes play a major role in mediating the intracellular cross-talk with the cAMP generating system; these effects have been postulated to occur at the level of receptors (Houslay 1991; Huganir and Greengard 1990), G proteins (Bell and Brunton 1986; Houslay 1991; Sagi-Eisenberg 1989), and the catalytic subunits of ACs (Iyengar 1993; Yoshimasa et al. 1987; Yoshimura and Cooper 1993). The net effect of the various potential interactions probably depends on quantitative and qualitative (e.g., conformational states) differences among subtypes of G proteins, ACs, and PKC isozymes. Our in vivo microdialysis measurements indicated that chronic lithium treatment attenuated the cAMP efflux in response to phorbol 12,13-dibutyrate (PDBu) infusion in the prefrontal cortex and the hippocampus. These results are similar to the attenuated cAMP responses to pertussis toxin that we observed after chronic lithium (Masana et al. 1992) and are suggestive of an effect of chronic lithium on a PKC/G_i interaction. In this context, it is also noteworthy that the modulation of AC by phorbol esters in SK-N-MC cells has been postulated to be specifically mediated by PKCα (Zhou et al. 1994), one of the isozymes that was most affected by chronic lithium in both frontal cortex and hippocampus.

Do these effects of lithium on MARCKS and PKC have any clinical relevance? The decrease in the levels of MARCKS, PKCα, and PKCε after chronic lithium administration may be one mechanism by which chronic lithium attenuates the release of catecholamines and, with its effects on receptor/G-protein coupling, may be relevant to lithium's protective effects against spontaneous, stress- and drug (e.g., stimulant)-induced manic episodes. Indeed, given the key role(s) of these PKC isozymes in the regulation of neuronal excitability and neurotransmitter release, the possibility that inhibition of PKC isozymes represents the therapeutically relevant biochemical effect of lithium responsible for its antimanic effects is a heuristic and testable hypothesis (discussed in more detail in "Are PKC Inhibitors Effective in the Treatment of Acute Mania?" later in this chapter).

A major problem inherent in neuropharmacological research is the difficulty in attributing therapeutic relevance to any observed biochemical finding. One approach we have been using is to identify common biochemical targets that are modified by drugs that are in the same therapeutic class (e.g., antimanic agents) but that have distinct chemical structures (e.g., lithium and VPA) when these drugs are administered in a therapeutically relevant paradigm (i.e., effects that are observed after chronic drug administration and that persist beyond abrupt drug discontinuation). In this context, increasing recent evidence has shown that the branched fatty acid anticonvulsant VPA is an effective antimanic agent. In view of lithium's significant effects on PKC outlined earlier in this chapter, we investigated the effects of VPA on various aspects of PKC functioning.

EFFECTS OF VALPROIC ACID ON PROTEIN KINASE C PATHWAYS

VPA is a potent broad-spectrum antiepileptic (Bourgeois 1989). In recent years, VPA also has been shown to have antimanic properties in the treatment of bipolar disorder (Bowden, Chapter 16, in this volume; Bowden et al. 1994; McElroy et al. 1992), which are observed only after several days of drug administration. VPA has acute effects on inhibitory and excitatory amino acid systems and membrane-associated ion channels in the CNS; these effects may underlie the rapid anticonvulsant properties of the drug (Loscher 1993; Rogawski and Porter 1990). However, the biochemical basis for VPA's antimanic actions is unknown to date (Post et al., Chapter 10, in this volume; Post et al. 1992).

Because both the clinical antimanic effects of VPA (Bowden et al. 1994; McElroy et al. 1992) and the effects of lithium on PKC (Casebolt and Jope 1991; Lenox et al. 1992; Manji and Lenox 1994; Manji et al. 1993) require chronic treatment, we investigated the effects of VPA on PKC activity and levels after several days of treatment. Exposure of C6 cells to VPA for 6–7 days resulted in significantly lower PKC activity in both membrane (52%) and cytosolic (35%) fractions (see Figure 7–9); VPA itself had no effect on PKC activity at concentrations of up to 5 mM. We used Western blot analysis and found that chronic exposure of C6 cells to 0.5 mM of VPA selectively decreased the levels of PKCα and PKCε in both cytosolic and membrane fractions (Figure 7–9). To determine the time course of VPA's effects on the PKC levels, we focused on the α isozyme, and we observed decreases as early as 3 days in membrane fraction and after 5 days in cytosolic fraction. The mechanisms by which chronic administration of VPA produces these isozyme-specific effects are currently under investigation. Whatever the underlying mechanisms, it is intriguing that the structurally highly dissimilar antimanic agents lithium and VPA, when administered in a therapeutically relevant paradigm, produce strikingly similar effects on the PKC signaling pathway (Table 7–5). Do these effects of lithium and VPA on PKC isozymes and substrates have any clinical relevance? Given the key role(s) of these PKC isozymes in the regulation of neuronal excitability, and neurotransmitter release, the possibil-

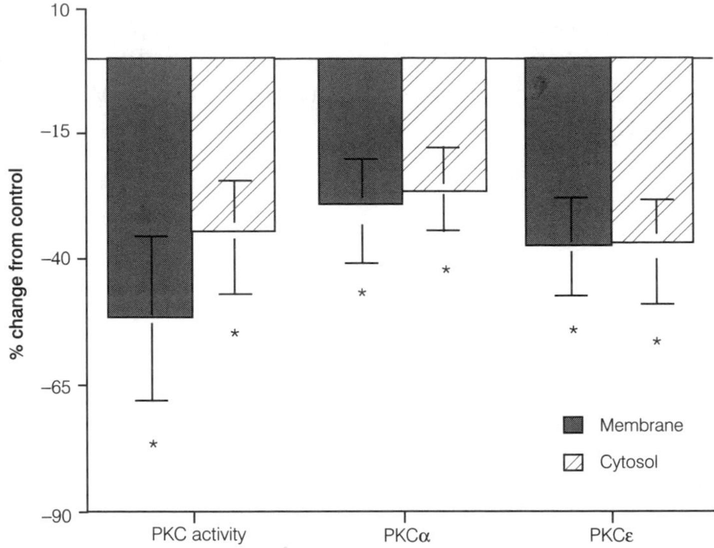

Figure 7–9. Effects of chronic valproic acid (VPA) on the activity and immunolabeling of protein kinase C (PKC) isozymes in rat C6 glioma cells. C6 glioma cells were incubated with VPA for 5–7 days. Membrane and cytosolic fractions were prepared and assayed for PKC activity as well as for immunolabeling of PKC isozymes. PKCα = PKCα isozyme immunolabeling; PKCε = PKCε isozyme immunolabeling.
*$P < 0.05$ compared with control.
Source. Modified with permission from Chen G, Manji HK, Hawver DB, et al: "Chronic Sodium Valproate Selectively Decreases Protein Kinase C α and ε In Vitro." *Journal of Neurochemistry* 63:2361–2364, 1994.

Table 7–5. Effects of lithium and valproic acid on protein kinase C isozymes and substrates

	Lithium	VPA
PKC activity	↓	↓
PKCα	↓	↓
PKCε	↓	↓
MARCKS levels	↓	↓
AP-1 binding activity	↑	↑
Inositol responsive	+	-

Note. VPA = valproic acid; PKC = protein kinase C; MARCKS = myristoylated alanine-rich C kinase substrate; AP-1 = activator binding protein-1.
Source. Reprinted from Manji HK, Chen G, Hsiao JK, et al.: "Regulation of Signal Transduction Pathways by Mood-Stabilizing Agents: Implications for the Delayed Onset of Therapeutic Efficacy." *Journal of Clinical Psychiatry* 57 (suppl 13):34–46, 1996b. Used with permission.

ity that inhibition of PKC isozymes represents the biochemical effect most therapeutically relevant for lithium's antimanic effects is a heuristic and testable hypothesis.

ARE PKC INHIBITORS EFFECTIVE IN THE TREATMENT OF ACUTE MANIA?

In view of the pivotal role of the PKC signaling pathway in the regulation of neuronal excitability, neurotransmitter release, and long-term synaptic events, we postulated that the attenuation of PKC activity may play a major role in the antimanic effects of lithium and VPA. Thus, an investigation of the efficacy of PKC inhibitors in the treatment of mania was clearly needed. Only one relatively selective PKC inhibitor is currently available for human use—tamoxifen. Tamoxifen, a synthetic nonsteroidal antiestrogen, has been widely used in the treatment of breast cancer (Catherino and Jordan 1993; Jordan 1994). Several of its effects are the result of estrogen receptor antagonism (Jordan 1994), but it has become clear that it is also a potent PKC inhibitor at therapeutically relevant concentrations (Couldwell et al. 1993). We therefore initiated a pilot study investigating the efficacy of tamoxifen in the treatment of acute mania (Bebchuk et al., in press). We found that tamoxifen does indeed possess antimanic efficacy (Bebchuk et al., in press). Clearly, these results must be considered preliminary because of the small sample size thus far. Nevertheless, the significant (and in some cases rapid and striking) results we observed are intriguing and support the hypothesis that the antimanic effects of lithium and VPA may be mediated, in large part, by PKC inhibition. In view of the preliminary data suggesting the involvement of the PKC signaling system in the pathophysiology of bipolar disorder (Friedman et al. 1993; H. Y. Wang and Friedman 1996), these results suggest that PKC inhibitors may be very useful agents in the treatment of bipolar disorder. Larger double-blind, placebo-controlled studies of tamoxifen and of novel selective PKC inhibitors in the treatment of mania are clearly warranted.

EFFECTS OF CARBAMAZEPINE ON THE CYCLIC ADENOSINE MONOPHOSPHATE GENERATING SYSTEM

Considerable evidence has also shown that CBZ (an atypical anticonvulsant) is an alternative or adjunctive treatment to lithium for both acute manic episodes and long-term prophylaxis in bipolar disorder (Post et al. 1984). Despite the widespread clinical use of CBZ, the molecular mechanisms underlying its anticonvulsant and mood-stabilizing effects have not been identified (Post et al. 1992; Rogawski and Porter 1990).

The cAMP generating system plays a major role in the regulation of neuronal excitability and has been postulated to play a role in the pathophysiology of both seizure disorders (Ludvig and Moshe 1989; Ludvig et al. 1992; Purpura and Shofer 1972) and bipolar disorder (Hudson et al. 1993; Warsh et al., Chapter 13, in this volume). Thus, intracerebral injection of dibutyryl-cAMP (a cell-membrane-permeable analogue of cAMP) into the cortex, amygdala, hypothalamus, and hippocampus causes convulsions in rats and cats (Gessa et al. 1970; Kuriyama and Kakita 1980; Ludvig and Moshe 1989; Ludvig et al. 1992; Purpura and Shofer 1972). Repeated injection of subconvulsive doses of cAMP into rat amygdala induces chemical kindling (Yokoyama et al. 1989). With respect to bipolar disorder, studies have reported elevated levels of forskolin-stimulated AC activity in areas of postmortem brain (L. T. Young et al. 1993); these effects may be the result of elevated levels of $G\alpha_s$ that occur in both brain and peripheral cells in bipolar disorder (Table 7–1; Manji et al. 1995a; Mitchell et al. 1997; Warsh et al., Chapter 13, in this volume; L. T. Young et al. 1994).

In view of the evidence of the involvement of the cAMP generating system described in this section, it is noteworthy that CBZ decreases the basal concentrations of cAMP in mouse cerebral cortex and cerebellum (Palmer 1979), as well as in rabbit cerebrospinal fluid (Myllyla 1976). CBZ also reduces cAMP production induced by norepinephrine (Palmer 1979; Palmer et al. 1979), adenosine (Elphick et al. 1990; Palmer 1979; Van Calker et al. 1991), and the epileptogenic compounds ouabain (Lewin and Bleck 1977; Palmer 1979) and veratridine (Ferrendelli and Kinscherf 1979) in brain slices. In manic patients, CBZ decreased elevated cerebrospinal fluid levels of cAMP (Post et al. 1982). Studies have also reported that CBZ inhibits forskolin-induced *c-fos* (an immediate-early gene) expression in cultured pheochromocytoma (PC-12) cells (Divish et al. 1991). Thus, overall, considerable evidence indicates that CBZ inhibits cAMP formation, but the mechanism underlying these effects has not been elucidated. Interestingly, lithium (the prototypic antimanic agent) inhibits AC activity (Manji et al. 1995b; Mørk and Jensen, Chapter 6, in this volume; Mørk et al. 1992), suggesting that inhibition of AC activity plays a role in the antimanic efficacy of these agents.

We therefore investigated the possible mechanisms by which CBZ inhibits the cAMP generating system. We found that CBZ, at therapeutically relevant concentrations, inhibited both basal AC and forskolin-stimulated cAMP accumulation in C6 glioma cells (G. Chen et al. 1996). Within the clinical therapeutic range (50 μM), CBZ inhibited basal cAMP levels by 10%–20% and forskolin-stimulated cAMP production by 40%–60%. Together, these data indicate that CBZ is more effective in inhibiting the activated AC system, although the possibility of "floor effects" (i.e., an inability to lower basal cAMP levels beyond certain levels in this system) cannot be ruled out.

To further characterize the mechanisms by which CBZ attenuates basal and forskolin-stimulated cAMP, we investigated G_i. In most systems, AC activity is regulated in concert by G_s and G_i. Thus, a CBZ-induced activation of G_i might underlie the decreases in basal and forskolin-stimulated cAMP that we observed in the present study. Such a contention receives additional support from the data suggesting that CBZ interacts with adenosine A_1 receptors (reviewed in Rogawski and Porter 1990), which are coupled to G_i. Although it is unknown whether rat C6 glioma cells contain adenosine A_1 receptors, we used pertussis toxin to investigate whether CBZ activates G_i. Pertussis toxin catalyzes the ADP ribosylation of G_i and G_o and thereby inactivates these G proteins and uncouples them from receptors (Ui 1990). We found that incubation of C6 glioma cells with pertussis toxin for 24 hours resulted in a significant increase in both basal and forskolin-stimulated cAMP production, compatible with a removal of the tonic inhibitory effect of G_i. CBZ exerted its inhibitory effects on the cAMP generating system in pertussis-toxin–treated cells, similar to that in control cells, suggesting that the action of CBZ was likely mediated through a G_i-independent mechanism.

To further characterize the site at which CBZ exerts its inhibitory effects, we purified ACs from rat cerebral cortex with a forskolin affinity purification column. We found that similar to the situation observed in intact C6 cells, and in C6 cell membranes, CBZ inhibited both basal and forskolin-stimulated activity of purified AC (G. Chen et al. 1996; see Table 7–6). Taken together, the data suggest that CBZ inhibits cAMP production by acting directly on AC and/or through factors that are tightly associated with, and co-purify with, AC.

It is now well established that the antimanic effects of CBZ show a lag period of onset. In this context, it is noteworthy that Divish and colleagues (1991) showed that CBZ attenuates forskolin-induced *c-fos* expression in PC-12 cells. Because *c-fos* and other immediate-early genes are involved in mediating several long-term neuronal responses (Sheng and Greenberg 1990), these effects might be postulated to play a role in the delayed therapeutic effect of CBZ. We found that in C6 glioma cells, forskolin enhanced phosphorylation of cAMP response element binding protein (CREB) and that CBZ significantly inhibited forskolin-induced phosphorylation of CREB. These results are very consistent with the results of Divish and associates (1991) and suggest that the inhibitory effects of CBZ on AC can bring about

Table 7–6. Effects of carbamazepine on adenylyl cyclase activity

Basal activity	↓
Forskolin (colforsin) stimulated	↓
Cholera toxin stimulated	↓
Phosphodiesterases	0
Purified AC activity	↓
CREB phosphorylation	↓

Note. AC = adenylyl cyclase; CREB = cyclic adenosine monophosphate response element binding protein.
Source. Reprinted from Manji HK, Chen G, Hsiao JK, et al.: "Regulation of Signal Transduction Pathways by Mood-Stabilizing Agents: Implications for the Delayed Onset of Therapeutic Efficacy." *Journal of Clinical Psychiatry* 57 (suppl 13):34–46, 1996b. Used with permission.

long-term changes in gene expression and thereby regulate cellular function.

Preliminary data from our laboratory indicate that CBZ exerts a similar inhibitory effect on AC in rat frontal cortex in vivo (H. K. Manji and G. Chen, unpublished observations, January 1995). In view of the major role of the cAMP system in the regulation of neuronal excitability and neurotransmitter release, and the evidence for this system in the pathophysiology of seizure disorders and bipolar disorder, these effects may play a role in CBZ's therapeutic effects and are worthy of further study.

EFFECTS OF LITHIUM AND VALPROIC ACID ON TRANSCRIPTION FACTORS AND GENE EXPRESSION

As discussed earlier in this chapter, the therapeutic effects of mood stabilizers and antidepressants require chronic administration (days to weeks), a temporal profile that suggests the likelihood of alterations at the genomic level (Duman et al. 1997; Hyman and Nestler 1996; Jope 1999b; Manji et al. 1995b; J. F. Wang et al. 1997). In this context, it recently has been found that lithium, at therapeutically relevant concentrations, produces complex alterations in basal and stimulated DNA binding of 12-o-tetradecanoyl-phorbol 13-acetate (TPA) response element (TRE) to activator protein 1 (AP-1) transcription factors in human SH-SY5Y cells in vitro and in rat brain following chronic, in vivo administration (Asghari et al. 1998; Jope 1999a; Ozaki and Chuang 1997; Unlap and Jope 1997; Williams and Jope 1995; Yuan et al. 1998). AP-1 is a collection of homodimeric and heterodimeric complexes composed of products from two transcription factor families, Fos and Jun. These products bind to a common DNA site (known as TRE) in the regulatory domain of the gene and activate gene transcription (Hughes and Dragunow 1995; Karin and Smeal 1992). The genes known to be regulated by the AP-1 family of transcription factors in the brain include genes for various neuropeptides, neurotrophins, receptors, transcription factors, enzymes involved in neurotransmitter biosynthesis, and proteins that bind to cytoskeletal elements (Hughes and Dragunow 1995). Together, these data suggest that lithium, via its effects on the AP-1 family of transcription factors, may bring about strategic changes in gene expression in critical neuronal circuits, effects that may ultimately underlie its efficacy in the treatment of a very complex neuropsychiatric disorder (Asghari et al. 1998; Jope 1999b; Manji et al. 1995b; Ozaki and Chuang 1997; J. F. Wang et al. 1997). The mechanisms by which lithium regulates AP-1 DNA binding remain to be fully elucidated. However, several studies have shown that lithium treatment exerts complex, temporally specific effects on basal and stimulated *c-fos* mRNA levels and Fos protein (Asghari et al. 1998; Divish et al. 1991; Kalasapudi et al. 1990; Lee et al. 1999; Leslie et al. 1993; Miller and Mathe 1997; Moorman and Leslie 1998; Namima et al. 1998, 1999; Ozaki and Chuang 1997; Weiner et al. 1991). These effects of lithium on the Fos family of proteins have been postulated to involve PKC (Divish et al. 1991; Kalasapudi et al. 1990; Weiner et al. 1991) and likely play a role in mediating lithium's effects on AP-1.

We have undertaken a series of studies and have found that both lithium and VPA, at therapeutically relevant concentrations, produce a time- and concentration-dependent increase in AP-1 DNA binding activity in rat brain ex vivo and in cultured human neuroblastoma cell factors (G. Chen et al. 1997, 1999a; Yuan et al. 1998). We have further confirmed that these effects on AP-1 DNA binding activity do, in fact, translate into changes at the gene expression level. Effects of lithium on gene expression were first studied in cells transiently transfected with the pGL2-control vector. The reporter gene luciferase in the pGL2-control vector is driven by an SV40 promoter that has two characterized AP-1 sites. We used this reporter gene transfection system to attempt to further verify the role of AP-1 sites in mediating VPA's effects on gene expression by eliminating the AP-1 sites by mutagenesis. Lithium and VPA increased in a time- and concentration-dependent manner the expression of a luciferase reporter gene driven by an SV40 promoter that contained TREs (Figures 7–10 and 7–11) (G. Chen et al. 1997, 1999a; Yuan et al. 1998). Furthermore, mutations in the TRE sites of the reporter gene promoter markedly attenuated these effects. These data indicate that lithium and VPA may stimulate gene expression (at least in part) through the AP-1 transcription factor pathway, effects that may play an important role in its long-term clinical actions (G. Chen et al.1999a ; Yuan et al. 1998).

In order to ascribe any potential therapeutic relevance to the observed biochemical findings, it is obviously necessary to demonstrate that they do, in fact, also occur in critical regions of the CNS in vivo. It is well established that the expression of tyrosine hydroxylase is mediated in large part by the AP-1 family of transcription factors (Kumer and Vrana 1996). We therefore investigated the effects of acute and chronic lithium administration on the levels of tyrosine hydroxylase in three brain areas that have been implicated in the pathophysiology of mood disorders—frontal cortex, hippocampus, and striatum (Drevets et al. 1997; Goodwin and Jamison 1990; Ketter et al. 1997). We found that chronic lithium significantly increased the levels of tyrosine hydroxylase in all three brain areas (G. Chen et al. 1998). Future in situ hybridization studies or immunohistochemistry studies are clearly needed to determine whether lithium also increases the expression of tyrosine hydroxylase in brain areas known to contain the cell bodies of the major noradrenergic and dopaminergic systems, namely, the locus coeruleus, ventral tegmental area, and substantia nigra. These results clearly show that, in addition to increasing AP-1 DNA binding activity and the expression of the luciferase reporter gene in vitro, chronic lithium increases the tyrosine hydroxylase levels in areas of rat brain ex vivo. Importantly, an independent research group recently replicated these findings, demonstrating robust lithium-induced increases in tyrosine hydroxylase levels in cultured cells of human neuronal origin (Zigova et al. 1999).

A recent study was also undertaken to investigate lithium's effects on endothelial nitric oxide synthase (NOS) type 2 expression, because the NOS type 2 gene is known to be regulated by AP-1 sites; this study found that lithium also robustly increased NOS type 2 levels (Feinstein 1998). Together, these results suggest that lithium does indeed modulate endogenous genes known to be driven by AP-1 and that lithium has the potential to regulate complex patterns of gene expression in critical neuronal circuits (Boyle et al. 1991; Lin et al. 1993). In view of the key roles of these nuclear transcription regulatory factors in long-term neuronal plasticity and cellular responsiveness, and the potential to regulate patterns of gene expression in critical neuronal circuits (Boyle et al. 1991; Lin et al. 1993), these effects may play a major role in lithium's and VPA's therapeutic efficacy and are worthy of further study.

The mechanisms by which lithium regulates AP-1 DNA binding activity may involve effects on PKC isozymes (Jope 1999a; Manji and Lenox, in press). In addition, it is noteworthy that lithium, at clinically relevant concentrations, recently has been shown to inhibit the activity of glycogen synthase kinase-3β (GSK-3β) (Hedgepeth et al. 1997; Klein and Melton 1996; Stambolic et al.

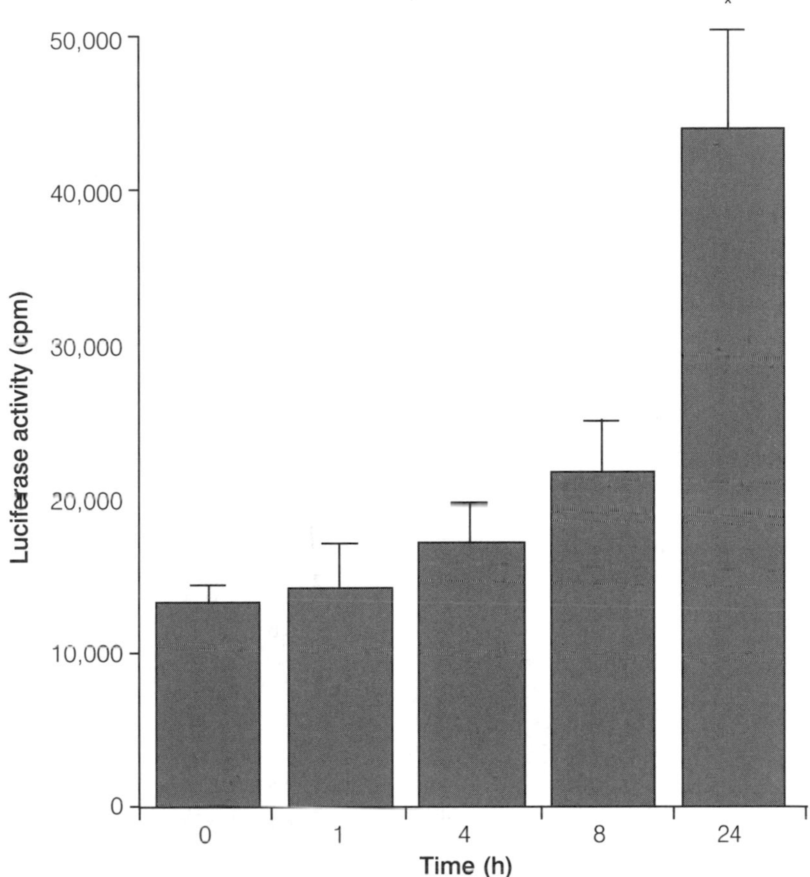

Figure 7–10. Effects of lithium on luciferase gene activity in C6 glioma cells. Rat C6 glioma cells were transfected with pGL-2-control vector. After 24 hours, the transfection mixture was replaced with fresh medium and the transfected cells were transferred to a 6-well dish and grown for 4 hours. Then the cells were exposed to 1 mM of lithium for the times indicated in the figure. The cells were washed with phosphate-buffered saline three times, and the luciferase activity was assayed with the luciferase assay system from Promega. Values are mean ±SE from four experiments. *$P < 0.05$ compared to 0-hour exposure.
Source. Reprinted from Manji HK, Chen G, Hsiao JK, et al.: "Regulation of Signal Transduction Pathways by Mood-Stabilizing Agents: Implications for the Delayed Onset of Therapeutic Efficacy." *Journal of Clinical Psychiatry* 57 (suppl 13):34–46, 1996b. Used with permission.

1996). GSK-3β is known to phosphorylate *c-jun* at three sites adjacent to the DNA binding domain, thereby reducing TRE binding (Lin et al. 1993; Stambolic et al. 1996).

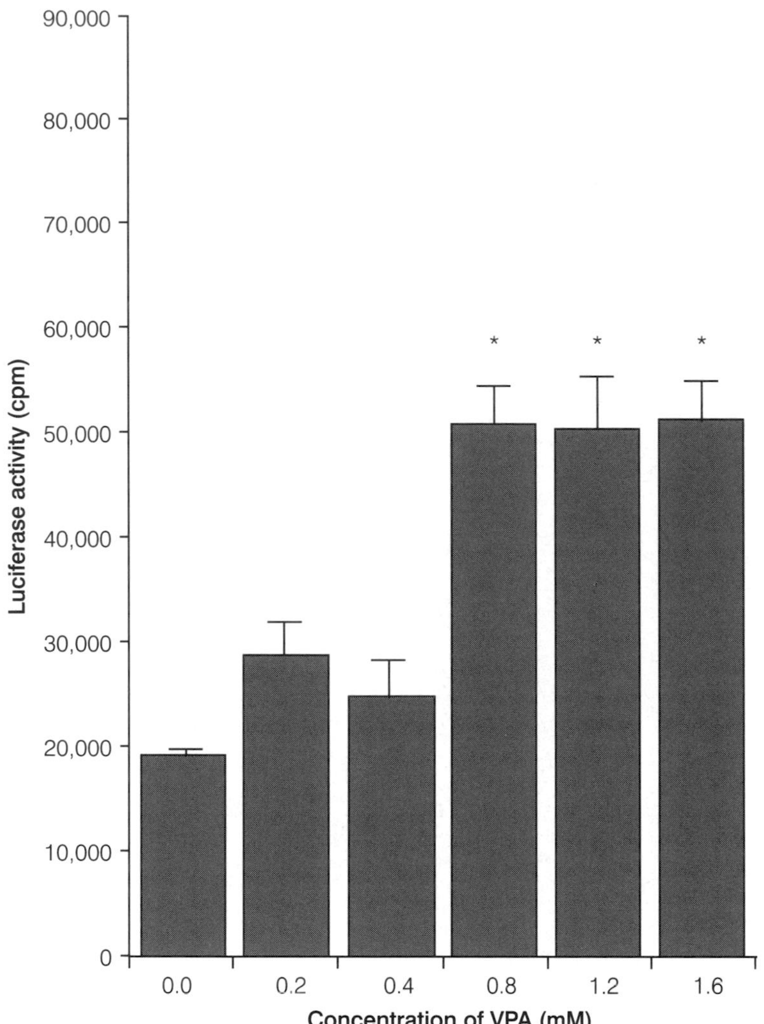

Figure 7–11. Effects of valproic acid (VPA) on luciferase gene activity in C6 glioma cells. Rat C6 glioma cells were transfected with pGL-2-control vector. After 24 hours, the transfection mixture was replaced with fresh medium, and the transfected cells were transferred to a 6-well dish and grown for 4 hours. Then the cells were exposed to different concentrations of VPA, indicated in the figure, for 20 hours. The cells were washed with phosphate-buffered saline three times, and the luciferase activity was assayed with the luciferase assay system from Promega. Values are mean ± SE from four experiments. *$P < 0.05$ compared to 0-hour exposure.
Source. Reprinted from Manji HK, Chen G, Hsiao JK, et al.: "Regulation of Signal Transduction Pathways by Mood-Stabilizing Agents: Implications for the Delayed Onset of Therapeutic Efficacy." *Journal of Clinical Psychiatry* 57 (suppl 13):34–46, 1996b. Used with permission.

IS GLYCOGEN SYNTHASE KINASE 3_β A THERAPEUTICALLY RELEVANT TARGET FOR MOOD-STABILIZING AGENTS?

Recently, a completely unexpected target for the action of lithium has been identified. Klein and Melton (1996) were the first to show that lithium, at therapeutically relevant concentrations, is an inhibitor of GSK3β. GSK3β, an evolutionarily highly conserved kinase, was originally identified as a regulator of glycogen synthesis. It is now known to play a critical role in the CNS by regulating various cytoskeletal processes via its effects on *tau* and synapsin I and long-term nuclear events via phosphorylation of *c-jun* and nuclear translocation of β-catenin (Jope 1999b; Klein and Melton 1996). However, lithium causes a variety of biochemical effects, and it is unclear if inhibition of GSK-3β represents a therapeutically relevant effect.

We have therefore undertaken a series of studies to determine whether VPA, like lithium, also regulates GSK-3α and GSK-3β. We found that VPA inhibits in a concentration-dependent manner both GSK-3α and GSK-3β, with significant effects observed at concentrations of VPA similar to those attained clinically (G. Chen et al. 1999b). Incubation of intact human neuroblastoma SH-SY5Y cells with VPA results in an increase in the subsequent in vitro recombinant GSK-3β-mediated [^{32}P] incorporation into two putative GSK-3 substrates (molecular weight ~ 85 kDa and 200 kDa), compatible with inhibition of endogenous GSK-3β by VPA. Incubation of SH-SY5Y cells with VPA also results in a significant time-dependent increase in both cytosolic and nuclear β-catenin levels. GSK-3β is a common target for both lithium and VPA; inhibition of GSK-3β in the CNS thus may underlie some of the long-term therapeutic effects of mood-stabilizing agents and represents an exciting area of future research.

LITHIUM, SIGNAL TRANSDUCTION, AND GENE EXPRESSION: THE IDENTIFICATION OF NOVEL TARGETS

It has become increasingly appreciated in recent years that the long-term treatment of complex neuropsychiatric disorders such as bipolar disorder likely involves the strategic regulation of signaling pathways and gene expression in critical neuronal circuits (Duman et al. 1997; Hyman and Nestler 1996; Jope 1999b; Manji et al. 1995b). As discussed above, lithium clearly exerts major effects on the AP-1 family of transcription factors; these effects have the potential to regulate the expression of several critical genes in the CNS. Although many genes that are the targets of long-term lithium treatment have been identified, it has been estimated that 10,000–15,000 genes may be expressed in a given cell at any time, and thus additional novel methodologies are clearly required to study the complex pattern of gene expression changes induced by chronic drug treatment (Jope 1999b; Manji et al., in press; Nestler 1998).

In recent years, new methodologies have evolved to identify the *differential expression* of multiple genes (e.g., in pathological vs. normal tissue, or in control vs. treated tissue); one such methodology that is being used increasingly is reverse transcription polymerase chain reaction mRNA differential display (RT-PCR DD; Liang et al. 1995). J. F. Wang and Young (1996) used this method and were the first to demonstrate that lithium increased 2′,3′-cyclic nucleotide 3′-phosphodiesterase mRNA levels in C6 glioma cells. To identify changes in gene expression likely to be associated with the *therapeutic efficacy* of mood stabilizers (Ikonomov and Manji, in press), we used RT-PCR DD to investigate the effects of lithium and VPA in the CNS, following chronic treatment of rodents in vivo (G. Chen et al. 1999c). Although these two structurally highly dissimilar agents likely do not exert their therapeutic effects by precisely the same mechanisms, identifying the genes that are regulated in concert by these two agents, when administered in a therapeutically relevant paradigm, may provide important leads about the molecular mechanisms underlying mood stabilization.

Inbred male Wistar Kyoto rats (selected to reduce potential false-positive results due to individual differences) were treated chronically with lithium, VPA, or saline. RNA was extracted from frontal cortices (FCx) to study gene expression with RT-PCR DD (Liang et al. 1995). The treatments markedly increased the expression of the transcription factor PEBP2β (polyoma virus enhancer binding protein, beta subunit) (GenBank Accession Number: AF087437, discussed in G. Chen et al. 1999c). In the absence of available antibodies to PEBP2β, we next sought to determine whether the treatments induced *functional changes* in PEBP2 transcription factor activity. Treatment with both lithium and VPA increased the DNA binding activity of PEBP2 α_β in FCx (G. Chen et al. 1999c). To determine whether these effects are specific for mood stabilizers, we investigated the effects of chronic *d*-amphetamine sulfate and chlordiazepoxide; neither of these treatments produced any detectable changes in PEBP2 α_β DNA binding activity. We therefore sought to investigate putative targets of the PEBP2 transcription factor that may be of therapeutic relevance in the treatment of bipolar disorder.

The promoter of the human B-cell lymphoma protein-2 (bcl-2) gene has a PEBP2 binding site, and this site clearly has been shown to increase the expression of a reporter gene driven by the bcl-2 promoter (Klampfer et al. 1996). A neuroprotective role for bcl-2 is well established, and constitutive expression of high levels of bcl-2 protein enhances the survival of cells when exposed to adverse stimuli (Jacobson and Raff 1995; Merry and Korsmeyer 1997). Additionally, the in vivo delivery of a *bcl-2* expression vector protects neurons against focal ischemia (Lawrence et al. 1996), and bcl-2 also has been shown to promote neuronal regeneration (D. F. Chen et al. 1997). In this context, it is noteworthy that recent studies have shown that mood disorders, including bipolar disorder, are associated with volumetric changes on magnetic resonance imaging (MRI) and computed tomography (CT) scans suggestive of neuronal atrophy or loss (Drevets et al. 1997; Ketter et al. 1997; Rajkowska et al. 1999). Furthermore, both brain imaging studies and postmortem morphometric 3-D cell counting studies have implicated the FCx as a site of neuronal atrophy or loss in bipolar disorder (Drevets et al. 1997; Ketter et al. 1997; Ongur et al. 1998; Rajkowska et al. 1999).

We therefore next sought to determine whether the treatment-induced increase in PEBP2αβ DNA binding activity in FCx was accompanied by changes in the levels of the neuroprotective protein bcl-2. We found that chronic lithium treatment in rats resulted in a *doubling* of bcl-2 levels in FCx, accompanied by a marked increase in the number of bcl-2 immunoreactive cells in layers II and III of FCx. Interestingly, the importance of neurons in layers II to IV of the FCx in mood disorders has recently been emphasized, because primate studies have indicated that these sites are important for connections with other cortical regions and are major targets for subcortical input (discussed in Rajkowska et al. 1999). Subsequent studies have shown that chronic lithium treatment also produces a marked increase in the number of bcl-2 immunoreactive cells in the dentate gyrus and striatum (Manji et al., in press).

To determine whether lithium also increases bcl-2 levels in human cells of neuronal origin, human neuroblastoma SH-SY5Y cells were treated with 1.0 mM of lithium for 6 days. Similar to the situation observed in rat brain in vivo, lithium produced a marked increase in bcl-2 levels in SH-SY5Y cells. Interestingly, lithium has recently also been shown to increase bcl-2 levels in rat cerebellar granule cells (Chen and Chuang 1999), a model system in which it has been found to exert protective effects against a variety of insults (discussed below and in Post et al., Chapter 10, in this volume). Moreover, lithium has recently been reported to *reduce* the levels of the *pro*-apoptotic protein p53 both in cerebellar granule cells (Chen and Chuang 1999) and in SH-SY5Y cells (Lu et al. 1999). Thus, the data clearly show that chronic lithium robustly increases bcl-2 levels in areas of the FCx, hippocampus, and striatum and in cells of human neuronal origin; furthermore, at least in cultured cell systems, lithium has been shown to reduce the levels of p53.

Lithium's robust effects on bcl-2 in the mature CNS suggest that this cation, at therapeutically relevant concentrations, also may have significant neuroprotective properties. Indeed, although the effects of lithium on bcl-2 have been observed very recently, several earlier studies had identified neuroprotective properties of lithium (reviewed in Manji et al., in press). More recently, a growing body of evidence is convincingly demonstrating that lithium *does* exert neuroprotective effects both in vitro and in vivo. The protective effects of lithium have been investigated in some in vitro studies that used rat cerebellar granule cells. When switched to nondepolarizing medium after maturation in vitro, cerebellar granule cells have undergone massive apoptotic cell death. Lithium robustly protects against the toxic effects of various insults, including glutamate, *N*-methyl-D-aspartate receptor activation, low potassium, and toxic concentrations of anticonvulsants (Nonaka et al. 1998a, 1998b; Post et al., Chapter 10, in this volume). A number of studies have also investigated lithium's neuroprotective effects in vivo (discussed in Manji et al., in press; Post et al., Chapter 10, in this volume). These results suggesting potential neuroprotective effects of lithium follow the exciting findings demonstrating that chronic administration of a variety of antidepressants increases the expression of neurotrophic factors (Duman et al. 1997; Smith et al. 1995); these observations have led to a heuristic molecular and cellular hypothesis of depression (Duman et al. 1997). Together, the results suggest that antidepressants and lithium may exert *some* of their long-term beneficial effects via underappreciated neurotrophic/neuroprotective effects and represent an exciting area for future medication development (Nestler 1998).

Does long-term lithium treatment actually retard disease- or affective episode–induced cell loss or atrophy? The distinction between disease progression and affective episodes per se is an important one, because it is quite possible that the cytoprotective effects of lithium may be independent of its ability to treat or prevent affective episodes. We are not aware of any current longitudinal studies that can adequately address this question, but this is clearly a very important and fundamental issue worthy of investigation. Thus, longitudinal studies comparing the long-term beneficial effects (using serial volumetric MRI scans, for example) of lithium and anticonvulsants that do not share lithium's effects on bcl-2 are clearly warranted. Similarly, the data suggest that the potential protective effects of lithium in conditions associated with high glucocorticoid levels such as Cushing's disease also may be worthy of investigation. The robust increases in bcl-2 levels and the clear evidence for neuroprotective effects suggest that the potential efficacy of lithium in the long-term treatment of various neurodegenerative disorders should be investigated (Manji et al., in press).

CONCLUSION

The mood-stabilizing agents lithium, VPA, and CBZ are very effective in the treatment of mania and in the reduction of the frequency and severity of recurrent affective episodes, but, despite extensive research, the underlying biological basis for their therapeutic efficacy is unknown. In recent years, however, there has been considerable progress in the identification of signal transduction pathways as targets for their actions. Regulation of signal transduction within critical regions of the brain by lithium affects the intracellular signal generated by multiple neurotransmitter systems; these effects are attractive targets for their therapeutic efficacy because the behavioral and physiological manifestations of bipolar disorder are complex and are likely mediated by a network of interconnected neurotransmitter pathways.

There have been significant advances in our understanding of the long-term action of lithium and VPA on PKC-mediated events, in particular, the inhibitory effects on PKCα, PKCε, and MARCKS. Nevertheless, much remains to be explained to translate these biochemical findings into improved therapeutic options for patients (Ikonomov and Manji, in press). For example, do the effects of chronic lithium administration on signal transduction pathways and gene expression stem exclusively from its demonstrated efficacy as an inhibitor of inositol monophosphatase and resultant changes in the DAG pathway, or does lithium under therapeutic conditions have other, more direct effects? The data showing the attenuation of lithium's effects on key signaling elements by the coadministration of *myo*-inositol suggest that this may be a major initial site of action but do not, in any way, preclude other, more direct effects of lithium. Studies currently under way to examine the effects of other inositol monophosphatase inhibitors (with no structural similarity to lithium) should soon yield important clues and offer insights into new drug development. In contrast, it is clear that the very similar biochemical effects of VPA do not depend on the regulation of inositol levels, and the mechanisms by which VPA regulates PKC isozymes and MARCKS levels remain to be elucidated. Nevertheless, the complex but strikingly similar effects of lithium and VPA on PKC isozymes and MARCKS represent both attractive and heuristic mechanisms by which the expression of various proteins involved in neuronal plasticity and cellular response is modulated, thereby causing long-term changes in neuronal excitability. Current studies of the long-term lithium-induced changes in the PKC signaling pathway (including PKC isozyme regulation, posttranslational modification of key phosphoproteins, and PKC-mediated alterations in gene and protein expression) are a most promising avenue for future investigation.

The recent advances in the identification of signal transduction pathways as targets for mood-stabilizing agents are also leading to new concepts for the development of effective pharmacotherapies for mood disorders. It is becoming increasingly clear that for many patients, new drugs simply mimicking the "traditional" drugs that directly or indirectly alter neurotransmitter levels and those that bind to cell-surface receptors may be of limited benefit (Manji and Potter 1995; Nestler 1998). This is because such strategies implicitly assume that the target receptors are functionally intact and that altered synaptic activity thus will be transduced to modify the postsynaptic "throughput" of the system. However, the existence of putative abnormalities in signal transduction pathways suggests that for patients refractory to conventional medications, improved therapeutic drugs may be obtained only by the direct targeting of postreceptor sites.

Recent findings concerning a variety of mechanisms involved in the formation and inactivation of second messengers offer the promise of the development of novel pharmacological agents designed to "site specifically" target signal transduction pathways. Compounds designed to affect second messengers must be lipophilic (to gain entry into the cell) or must use active processes to pass across membranes. Contrary to previous expectations, pharmacological agents may selectively affect second-messenger systems because they are quite heterogeneous at the molecular and cellular level, are linked to receptors in various ways, and are expressed in different stoichiometries in distinct cell types. In addition, given the extensive cross-talk between signaling systems, normal cells may adequately compensate for signal transduction manipulations, whereas diseased tissue may not, resulting in targeted potency of effects. It is now well known that different combinations of G-protein subunits have different affinities for individual receptors and effectors. These combinatorial relations can selectively serve to regulate the association between receptors and G proteins because when each receptor is transiently activated, it will interact with the subset of combinations for which it has the highest intrinsic activity.

Similarly, because signal transduction pathways have certain unique characteristics depending on their activity state (e.g., rate of guanine nucleotide exchange, G-protein conformational states, GTP hydrolysis, cytosol-to-membrane translocation of PKC isozymes and receptor kinases), they offer built-in targets for relative specificity of action, depending on the set-point of the substrate. The information in the preceding sections suggests that G proteins may be an important site of action of neuropsychiatric drugs. In addition to the modifications observed with chronic lithium or antidepressant administration described in this chapter, an increasing number of new drugs that directly affect G proteins are being developed. Among the most interesting of these are the amphipathic polyanionic agents (which appear to intercalate into an amphipathic α-helix at the receptor/G-protein interface) (Mousli et al. 1990) and the benzimidazole derivatives (which reversibly modulate guanine nucleotide exchange and show some degree of G-protein specificity) (R. R. Huang et al. 1990). The wasp venom peptide mastoparan directly promotes guanine nucleotide exchange and G-protein activation (Higashijima et al. 1990). This activity of mastoparan is apparently related to its structure, an amphipathic helix that allows it to mimic an intracellular region of a 7-transmembrane receptor and interact with the carboxyl terminus of the α-subunit (Higashijima et al. 1988, 1990). Other peptides such as substance P and the polyamine mast cell activator 48/80 may produce similar effects on other G proteins in a receptor-independent manner and offer promise for drug development.

Reports also have identified a novel class of agents that serve as allosteric enhancers and stabilize the high-affinity agonist-preferring conformation of the receptor (Bruns and Fergus 1990). The concept of allosteric enhancers is appealing because such agents may serve to effectively re-equilibrate dysregulated neuronal systems (which are likely to be involved in mood disorders) without the commonly encountered phenomena of tachyphylaxis (receptor downregulation) and supersensitivity. Other intracellular CNS-specific proteins may also modulate G-protein function; investigators have found (Strittmatter et al. 1990) that GAP-43 (an intracellular neuronal protein associated with the growth cone at the tip of elongating dendrites and axons) is a weak promoter of guanine nucleotide exchange on G_0, the major CNS G protein (which is believed to play a crucial role in regulating neuronal firing and neurotransmitter release). These effects of GAP-43 on G_0 raise the intriguing possibility that the activity of certain G proteins can be modulated directly by other proteins whose activity is regulated by phosphorylation and dephosphorylation. Thus, CNS-specific phosphoproteins such as GAP-43 are attractive targets for the development of drugs designed to selectively modulate G-protein function in the CNS. A novel family of proteins, termed *RGS proteins* (for regulators of G-protein signaling), recently have been identified. They may play a critical role in the tissue-specific regulation of G-protein function and thus represent very attractive targets for CNS-specific drug development. Some of the potential developments in the designing of pharmacological agents targeting signal transduction pathways are listed in Table 7–7.

In summary, an increasing number of avenues is emerging by which transmembrane signal transduction can be modulated (Chahdi et al. 1998; Freissmuth et al. 1999; Gelb et al. 1998; Glazer 1998; Skaper and Walsh 1998; Souroujon and Mochly-Rosen 1998), and the growing body of evidence impli-

Table 7–7. Developments in the designing of drugs targeting G protein–coupled signal transduction pathways

Allosteric induction of conformational change in receptor mimicking occupancy by agonists/antagonists
Receptor–G protein coupling receptor peptides
Dissociation of heterotrimer
Activation of effector by α and/or βγ
GTP hydrolysis
Regulation of the activity of RGSs
Modulation of rate and extent of desensitization via βARK-like agents

Note. GTP = guanosine triphosphate; RGS = regulators of G-protein signaling; βARK = beta-adrenergic receptor kinase.
Source. Reprinted from Manji HK, Chen G, Hsiao JK, et al.: "Regulation of Signal Transduction Pathways by Mood-Stabilizing Agents: Implications for the Delayed Onset of Therapeutic Efficacy." *Journal of Clinical Psychiatry* 57 (suppl 13):34–46, 1996b. Used with permission.

cating signal transduction pathways in the pathophysiology of mood disorders suggests that compounds with potent effects distal to the receptor are worthy of study in the treatment of mood disorders. The challenge for the next era in neuropsychopharmacology is to transform the knowledge gained from advances in neurobiology, cellular physiology, and molecular pharmacology into clinical use.

The rapid technological advances in both biochemistry and molecular biology have greatly enhanced our ability to understand the complexities of the regulation of neuronal function; these advances hold much promise for the development of novel improved therapeutic drugs for mood disorders, as well as for our understanding of the pathophysiology of bipolar disorder.

REFERENCES

Anderson SMP, Godfrey PP, Grahame-Smith DG: The effects of phorbol esters and lithium on 5-HT release in rat hippocampal slices (abstract). Br J Pharmacol 93:96P, 1988

Asghari V, Wang JF, Reiach JS, et al: Differential effects of mood stabilizers on Fos/Jun proteins and AP-1 DNA binding activity in human neuroblastoma SH-SY-5Y cells. Mol Brain Res 58:95–102, 1998

Avissar S, Schreiber G, Danon A, et al: Lithium inhibits adrenergic and cholinergic increases in GTP binding in rat cortex. Nature 331:440–442, 1988

Bebchuk JM, Arfken CL, Dolan-Manji S, et al: A preliminary investigation of a protein kinase C inhibitor (tamoxifen) in the treatment of acute mania. Arch Gen Psychiatry (in press)

Bell JD, Brunton LL: Enhancement of adenylate cyclase activity in S49 lymphoma cells by phorbol esters: withdrawal of GTP-dependent inhibition. J Biol Chem 261: 12036–12041, 1986

Ben-Schlomo H, Sigmund O, Stabel S, et al: Preferential release of catecholamine from permeabilized PC12 cells by α- and β-type protein kinase C subspecies. Biochem J 280:65–69, 1991

Berman DM, Wilkie TM, Gilman AG: GAIP and RGS4 are GTPase-activating proteins for the Gi subfamily of G protein α subunits. Cell 86:445–452, 1996

Borner C, Guadagno SN, Fabbro D, et al: Expression of four protein kinase C isoforms in rat fibroblasts: distinct subcellular distribution and regulation by calcium and phorbol esters. J Biol Chem 267:12892–12899, 1992

Bourgeois BFD: Valproate: clinical use, in Antiepileptics, 3rd Edition. Edited by Levy R, Mattson R, Meldrum B, et al. New York, Raven, 1989, pp 633–641

Bourne HR, Nicoll R: Molecular machines integrate coincident synaptic signals. Cell 72 (suppl):65–75, 1993

Bowden CL, Brugger AM, Swann AC, et al: Efficacy of divalproex vs. lithium and placebo in the treatment of mania. JAMA 271:918–924, 1994

Boyle WJ, Smeal T, Defize LH, et al: Activation of protein kinase C decreases phosphorylation of c-Jun at sites that negatively regulate its DNA-binding activity. Cell 64:573–584, 1991

Brami BA, Leli U, Hauser G: Influence of lithium on second messenger accumulation in NG108-15 cells. Biochem Biophys Res Commun 174:606–612, 1991

Brami BA, Leli U, Hauser G: Elevated phosphatidyl-CMP is not the source of diacylglycerol accumulation induced by lithium in NG108–15 cells. J Neurochem 60:1137–1142, 1993

Bruns RF, Fergus JH: Allosteric enhancement of adenosine A1 receptor binding and function by 2-amino-3-benzoylthiophenes. Mol Pharmacol 38:939–949, 1990

Bunney WE, Garland-Bunney BL: Mechanisms of lithium in affective illness: basic and clinical implications, in Psychopharmacology: The Third Generation of Progress. Edited by Meltzer HY. New York, Raven, 1987, pp 553–565

Casebolt TL, Jope RS: Effects of chronic lithium treatment on protein kinase C and cyclic AMP-dependent protein phosphorylation. Biol Psychiatry 29:233–243, 1991

Catherino WH, Jordan VC: A risk-benefit assessment of tamoxifen therapy. Drug Saf 8:381–397, 1993

Chahdi A, Daeffler L, Gies JP, et al: Drugs interacting with G protein alpha subunits: selectivity and perspectives. Fundam Clin Pharmacol 12(2):121–132, 1998

Chen RW, Chuang DM: Long term lithium treatment suppresses p53 and Bax expression but increases Bcl-2 expression: a prominent role in neuroprotection against excitotoxicity. J Biol Chem 274 (10):6039–6042, 1999

Chen DF, Schneider GE, Martinou JC, et al: Bcl-2 promotes regeneration of severed axons in mammalian CNS. Nature 385:434–439, 1997

Chen G, Manji HK, Hawver DB, et al: Chronic sodium valproate selectively decreases protein kinase C α and ε in vitro. J Neurochem 63:2361–2364, 1994

Chen G, Hawver D, Wright C, et al: Attenuation of adenylyl cyclases by carbamazepine in vitro. J Neurochem 67:2079–2086, 1996

Chen G, Yuan PX, Hawver DB, et al: Increase in AP-1 transcription factor DNA binding activity by valproic acid. Neuropsychopharmacology 16:238–245, 1997

Chen G, Yuan PX, Jiang Y, et al: Lithium increases tyrosine hydroxylase levels both in vivo and in vitro. J Neurochem 70:1768–1771, 1998

Chen G, Yuan PX, Jiang Y, et al: Valproate robustly enhances AP-1 mediated gene expression. Mol Brain Res 64:52–58, 1999a

Chen G, Huang LD, Jiang YM, et al: The mood stabilizing agent valproate inhibits the activity of glycogen synthase kinase 3. J Neurochem 72:1327–1330, 1999b

Chen G, Zeng WZ, Jiang L, et al: The mood stabilizing agents lithium and valproate robustly increase the expression of the neuroprotective protein bcl-2 in the CNS. J Neurochem 72:879–882, 1999c

Chou JC: Recent advances in treatment of acute mania. J Clin Psychopharmacol 11(1): 3–21, 1991

Colin SF, Chang HC, Mollner S, et al: Chronic lithium regulates the expression of adenylate cyclase and G_I-protein alpha subunit in rat cerebral cortex. Proc Natl Acad Sci U S A 88:10634–10637, 1991

Couldwell WT, Weiss MH, DeGiorgio CM, et al: Clinical and radiographic response in patients with recurrent malignant gliomas treated with high-dose tamoxifen. Neurosurgery 32:485–489, 1993

DeGraan PN, Schrama LH, Heemskerk FM, et al: The role of protein kinase C substrate B-50 (GAP-43) in neurotransmitter release and long-term potentiation. Adv Exp Med Biol 268:347–358, 1990

Divish MM, Sheftel G, Boyle A, et al: Differential effect of lithium on fos protooncogene expression mediated by receptor and postreceptor activators of protein kinase C and cyclic adenosine monophosphate: model for its antimanic action. J Neurosci Res 28:40–48, 1991

Downes CP, Stone MA: Lithium-induced reduction in intracellular inositol supply in cholinergically stimulated parotid gland. Biochem J 234:199–204, 1986

Drevets WC, Price JL, Simpson JR Jr, et al: Subgenual prefrontal cortex abnormalities in mood disorders. Nature 386:824–827, 1997

Drummond AH, Raeburn CA: The interaction of lithium with thyrotropin releasing hormone-stimulated lipid metabolism in GH3 pituitary tumor cells. Biochem J 224:129–136, 1984

Duman RS, Heninger GR, Nestler EJ: A molecular and cellular theory of depression. Arch Gen Psychiatry 54:597–606, 1997

Ellis J, Lenox RH: Receptor coupling to G proteins: interactions not affected by lithium. Lithium 2:141–147, 1991

Elphick M, Taghavi Z, Powell T, et al: Chronic carbamazepine down-regulates adenosine A2 receptors: studies with the putative selective adenosine antagonists PD 115, 199 and PD 116, 948. Psychopharmacology (Berl) 100:522–529, 1990

Erusalimsky JD, Brooks SF, Herget T, et al: Molecular cloning and characterization of the acidic 80-kDa protein kinase C substrate from rat brain. J Biol Chem 266: 7073–7080, 1991

Feinstein DL: Potentiation of astroglial nitric oxide synthase type-2 expression by lithium chloride. J Neurochem 71:883–886, 1998

Ferrendelli JA, Kinscherf DA: Inhibitory effects of anticonvulsant drugs on cyclic nucleotide accumulation in brain. Ann Neurol 5:533–538, 1979

Fisher SK, Heacock AM, Agranoff BW: Inositol lipids and signal transduction in the nervous system: an update. J Neurochem 58:18–38, 1992

Freissmuth M, Waldhoer M, Bofill-Cardona E, et al: G protein antagonists. Trends Pharmacol Sci 20:237–245, 1999

Friedman E, Hoau YW, Levinson D, et al: Altered platelet protein kinase C activity in bipolar affective disorder, manic episode. Biol Psychiatry 33:520–525, 1993

Garcia-Sainz JA, Gutierrez VG: Activation of protein kinase C alters the interaction of alpha 2-adrenoceptors and the inhibitory GTP-binding protein (Gi) in human platelets. FEBS Lett 257:427–430, 1989

Gelb MH, Scholten JD, Sebolt-Leopold JS: Protein prenylation: from discovery to prospects for cancer treatment. Curr Opin Chem Biol 2(1):40–48, 1998

Glazer RI: The protein kinase ABC's of signal transduction as targets for drug development. Current Pharmaceutical Design 4(3):277–290, 1998

Goodnight J, Mischak H, Kolch W, et al: Immunocytochemical localization of eight protein kinase C isozymes overexpressed in NIH 3T3 fibroblasts. J Biol Chem 270:9991–10001, 1995

Goodwin FK, Jamison KR: Manic-Depressive Illness. New York, Oxford University Press, 1990

Greenwood AF, Jope RS: Brain G-protein proteolysis by calpain: enhancement by lithium. Brain Res 636:320–326, 1994

Halenda SP, Volpi M, Zavoico GB, et al: Effects of thrombin, phorbol myristate acetate, and prostaglandin D2 on 40–41 kDa protein that is ADP ribosylated by pertussis toxin in platelets. FEBS Lett 204:341–346, 1986

Hedgepeth CM, Conrad LJ, Zhang J, et al: Activation of the Wnt signaling pathway: a molecular mechanism for lithium action. Dev Biol. 185:82–91, 1997

Higashijima T, Uzu S, Nakajima T, et al: Mastoparan, a peptide toxin from wasp venom, mimics receptors by activating GTP-binding regulatory proteins (G proteins). J Biol Chem 263:6491–6494, 1988

Higashijima T, Burnier J, Ross EM: Regulation of Gi and Go by mastoparan, related amphiphilic peptides, and hydrophobic amines: mechanism and structural determinants of activity. J Biol Chem 265:14176–14186, 1990

Houslay MD: 'Crosstalk': a pivotal role for protein kinase C in modulating relationships between signal transduction pathways. Eur J Biochem 195:9–27, 1991

Hsiao JK, Argen H, Bartko JJ, et al: Monoamine neurotransmitter interactions and the prediction of antidepressant response. Arch Gen Psychiatry 44:1078–1083, 1987

Hsiao JK, Manji HK, Chen GA, et al: Lithium administration modulates platelet G_I in humans. Life Sci 50:227–233, 1992

Hsiao JK, Colison J, Bartko JJ, et al: Monoamine neurotransmitter interactions in drug-free and neuroleptic-treated schizophrenics. Arch Gen Psychiatry 50:606–614, 1993

Huang KP: The mechanism of protein kinase C activation. Trends Neurosci 12:425–432, 1989

Huang RR, Dehaven RN, Cheung AH, et al: Identification of allosteric antagonists of receptor-guanine nucleotide-binding protein interactions. Mol Pharmacol 37: 304–310, 1990

Hudson CJ, Young LT, Li PP, et al: CNS signal transduction in the pathophysiology and pharmacotherapy of affective disorders and schizophrenia. Synapse 13:278–293, 1993

Huganir RL, Greengard P: Regulation of neurotransmitter receptor desensitization by protein phosphorylation. Neuron 5:555–567, 1990

Hughes P, Dragunow M: Induction of immediate-early genes and the control of neurotransmitter-regulated gene expression within the nervous system. Pharmacol Rev 47:133–178, 1995

Hyman SE, Nestler EJ: Initiation and adaptation: a paradigm for understanding psychotropic drug action. Am J Psychiatry 153:151–162, 1996

Ikonomov O, Manji J: Molecular mechanisms underlying nood-stabilization in manic-depressive illness: the phenotype challenge. Am J Psychiatry (in press)

Ingi T, Krumins AM, Chidiac P, et al: Dynamic regulation of RGS2 suggests a novel mechanism in G-protein signaling and neuronal plasticity. J Neurosci 18:7178–7188, 1998

Isakov N, McMahon P, Altman A: Selective post-transcriptional down-regulation of protein kinase C isoenzymes in leukemic T cells chronically treated with phorbol ester. J Biol Chem 265:2091–2097, 1990

Iyengar R: Molecular and functional diversity of mammalian Gs-stimulated adenylyl cyclases. FASEB J 7(9):768–775, 1993

Jacobson MD, Raff M: Programmed cell death and Bcl-2 protection in very low oxygen. Nature 374:814–816, 1995

Jakobs KH, Bauer S, Watanabe Y: Modulation of adenylate cyclase of human platelets by phorbol ester: impairment of the hormone-sensitive inhibitory pathway. Eur J Biochem 151:425–430, 1985

Jope RS: A bimodal model of the mechanism of action of lithium. Mol Psychiatry 4: 21–25, 1999a

Jope R.S: Anti-bipolar therapy: mechanism of action of lithium. Mol Psychiatry 4: 117–128, 1999b

Jope RS, Williams MB: Lithium and brain signal transduction systems. Biochem Pharmacol 47:429–441, 1994

Jope RS, Song L, Li PP, et al: The phosphoinositide signal transduction system is impaired in bipolar affective disorder brain. J Neurochem 66(6):2402–2409, 1996

Jordan VC: A current view of tamoxifen for the treatment of breast cancer. Br J Pharmacol 110:507–517, 1994

Kalasapudi VD, Sheftel G, Divish MM, et al: Lithium augments fos protoonocogene expression in PC12 pheochromocytoma cells: implications for therapeutic action of lithium. Brain Res 521:47–54, 1990

Karin M, Smeal T: Control of transcription factors by signal transduction pathways: the beginning of the end. Trends Biochem Sci 17:418–422, 1992

Katada T, Oinuma M, Ui M: Two guanine nucleotide-binding proteins in rat brain serving as the specific substrate of islet-activating protein, pertussis toxin: interaction of the alpha-subunits with beta gamma-subunits in development of their biological activities. J Biol Chem 261:8182–8191, 1986a

Katada T, Oinuma M, Ui M: Mechanisms for inhibition of the catalytic activity of adenylate cyclase by the guanine nucleotide-binding proteins serving as the substrate of islet-activating protein, pertussis toxin. J Biol Chem 261:5215–5221, 1986b

Ketter TA, George MS, Kimbrell TA, et al: Neuroanatomical models and brain imaging studies, in Bipolar Disorder: Biological Models and Their Clinical Application. Edited by Joffe RT, Young LT. New York, Marcel Dekker, 1997, pp 179–217

Klampfer L, Zhang J, Zelenetz AO, et al: The AML1/ETO fusion protein activates transcription of Bcl-2. Proc Natl Acad Sci U S A 26:14059–14064, 1996

Klein PS, Melton DA: A molecular mechanism for the effect of lithium on development. Proc Natl Acad Sci U S A 93:8455–8459, 1996

Kumer SC, Vrana KE: Intricate regulation of tyrosine hydroxylase activity and gene expression. J Neurochem 67:443–461, 1996

Lachman HM, Papolos DF: Abnormal signal transduction: a hypothetical model for bipolar affective disorder. Life Sci 45:1413–1426, 1991

Lawrence MS, Ho DY, Sun GH, et al: Overexpression of Bcl-2 with herpes simplex virus vectors protects CNS neurons against neurological insults in vitro and in vivo. J Neurosci 16:486–496, 1996

Lee Y, Hamamura T, Ohashi K, et al: The effect of lithium on methamphetamine-induced regional Fos protein expression in the rat brain. Neuroreport 10:895–900, 1999

Leli U, Hauser G: Lithium modifies diacylglycerol levels and protein kinase C in neuroblastoma cells (Z187F), in Abstracts of the 8th International Conference on Second Messengers and Phosphoproteins, Glasgow, Scotland, September 1992

Leli U, Shea TB, Cataldo A, et al: Differential expression and subcellular localization of protein kinase C α, β, γ, δ, and ε isoforms in SH-SY5Y neuroblastoma cells: modifications during differentiation. J Neurochem 60:289–298, 1993

Lenox RH, Manji HK: Lithium, in American Psychiatric Press Textbook of Psychopharmacology, 2nd Edition. Edited by Nemeroff CB, Schatzberg AF. Washington, DC, American Psychiatric Press, 1998, pp 379–430

Lenox RH, Watson DG, Ellis J: Muscarinic receptor regulation and protein kinase C: sites for the action of chronic lithium in the hippocampus. Psychopharmacol Bull 27:191–199, 1991

Lenox RH, Watson DG, Patel J, et al: Chronic lithium administration alters a prominent PKC substrate in rat hippocampus. Brain Res 570 (1):333–340, 1992

Leslie RA, Moorman JM, Grahame-Smith DG: Lithium enhances 5-HT2A receptor-mediated c-fos expression in rat cerebral cortex. Neuroreport 5:241–244, 1993

Lewin E, Bleck V: Cyclic AMP accumulation in cerebral cortical slices: effect of carbamazepine, phenobarbital, and phenytoin. Epilepsia 18:237–242, 1977

Li PP, Tam YK, Young LT, et al: Lithium decreases Gs, Gi-1 and Gi-2 alpha-subunit mRNA levels in rat cortex. Eur J Pharmacol 206:165–166, 1991

Li PP, Sibony D, Green MA, et al: Lithium modulation of phosphoinositide signaling system in rat cortex: selective effect on phorbol ester binding. J Neurochem 61: 1722–1730, 1993

Li X, Jope RS: Selective inhibition of the expression of signal transduction proteins by lithium in nerve growth factor-differentiated PC12 cells. J Neurochem 65:2500–2508, 1995

Liang P, Bauer D, Averboukh L, et al: Analysis of altered gene expression by differential display. Methods Enzymol 254:304–321, 1995

Lin A, Smeal T, Binetruy B, et al: Control of AP-1 activity by signal transduction cascades. Adv Second Messenger Phosphoprotein Res 28:255–260, 1993

Linder D, Gschwendt M, Marks F: Phorbol ester-induced down-regulation of the 80-kDa myristoylated alanine-rich C-kinase substrate-related protein in Swiss 3T3 fibroblasts. J Biol Chem 267:24–26, 1992

Loscher W: Effects of the antiepileptic drug valproate on metabolism and function of inhibitory and excitatory amino acids in the brain. Neurochem Res 18:485–502, 1993

Lounsbury KM, Casey PJ, Brass LF, et al: Phosphorylation of Gz in human platelets: selectivity and site of modification. J Biol Chem 266(32):22051–22056, 1991

Lu R, Song L, Jope RS: Lithium attenuates p53 levels in human neuroblastoma SH-SH-SY5Y cells. Neuroreport 10:1123–1125, 1999

Ludvig N, Moshe SL: Different behavioral and electrographic effects of acoustic stimulation and dibutyryl cyclic AMP injection into the inferior colliculus in normal and in genetically epilepsy-prone rats. Epilepsy Res 3:185–190, 1989

Ludvig N, Mischra PK, Yan QS, et al: The combined EEG-intracerebral microdialysis technique: a new tool for neuropharmacological studies on freely behaving animals. J Neurosci Methods 43:129–137, 1992

Manji HK: G proteins: implications for psychiatry. Am J Psychiatry 149:746–760, 1992

Manji HK, Lenox RH: Long-term action of lithium: a role for transcriptional and post-transcriptional factors regulated by protein kinase C. Synapse 16:11–28, 1994

Manji HK, Lenox RH: Protein kinase C signaling in the brain: molecular transduction of mood stabilization in the treatment of manic-depressive illness. Ziskind-Somerfeld Award Paper. Biol Psychiatry (in press)

Manji HK, Potter WZ: Emerging strategies in affective disorders, in Emerging Strategies in Neurotherapeutics. Edited by Pullan L, Patel J. Totowa, NJ, Humana Press, 1995, pp 35–83

Manji HK, Bitran JA, Masana MI, et al: Signal transduction modulation by lithium: cell culture, cerebral microdialysis and human studies. Psychopharmacol Bull 27:199–208, 1991a

Manji HK, Hsiao JK, Risby ED, et al: The mechanisms of action of lithium. Arch Gen Psychiatry 48:505–512, 1991b

Manji HK, Etcheberrigaray R, Chen G, et al: Lithium decreases membrane-associated PKC in the hippocampus: selectivity for the alpha isozyme. J Neurochem 61: 2303–2310, 1993

Manji HK, Chen G, Shimon H, et al: Guanine nucleotide-binding proteins in bipolar affective disorder: effects of long-term lithium treatment. Arch Gen Psychiatry 52:135–144, 1995a

Manji HK, Potter WZ, Lenox RH: Signal transduction pathways: molecular targets for lithium's actions. Arch Gen Psychiatry 52(7):531–543, 1995b

Manji HK, Bersudsky Y, Chen G, et al: Regulation of PKC isozymes and substrates by lithium: the role of myo-inositol. Neuropsychopharmacology 15:370–382, 1996a

Manji HK, Chen G, Risby ED, et al: Regulation of signal transduction pathways by mood stabilizing agents: implications for the delayed onset of therapeutic efficacy. J Clin Psychiatry 57 (suppl):34–46, 1996b

Manji HK, Moore GJ, Chen G: Lithium at 50: have the neuroprotective effects of this unique cation been overlooked ? Biol Psychiatry 46:929–940, 1999

Masana MI, Bitran JA, Hsiao JK, et al: In vivo evidence that lithium inactivates Gi modulation of adenylate cyclase in brain. J Neurochem 59:200–205, 1992

McElroy SL, Keck JPE, Pope JHG, et al: Valproate in the treatment of bipolar disorder: literature review and clinical guidelines. J Clin Psychopharmacol 12:42S–52S, 1992

McElroy SL, Keck PE, Stanton SP, et al: A randomized comparison of divalproex oral loading versus haloperidol in the initial treatment of acute psychotic mania. J Clin Psychiatry 57:142–146, 1996

Meltzer HY: The importance of serotonin-dopamine interactions in the action of clozapine. Br J Psychiatry 17 (suppl):22–29, 1992

Merry DE, Korsmeyer SJ: Bcl-2 gene family in the nervous system. Annu Rev Neurosci 20:245–267, 1997

Miller JC, Mathe AA: Basal and stimulated C-fos mRNA expression in the rat brain: effect of chronic dietary lithium. Neuropsychopharmacology 16:408–418, 1997

Mitchell PB, Manji HK, Chen G, et al: Increased levels of Gα_s in platelets of euthymic bipolar affective disorder patients. Am J Psychiatry 154:218–223, 1997

Moore GJ, Bebchuk JM, Parrish JK, et al: Temporal dissociation between lithium-induced CNS myo-inositol changes and clinical response in manic-depressive illness. Am J Psychiatry (in press)

Moorman JM, Leslie RA: Paradoxical effects of lithium on serotonergic receptor function: an immunocytochemical, behavioural and autoradiographic study. Neuropharmacology 37:357–374, 1998

Mørk A, Geisler A, Hollund P: Effects of lithium on second messenger systems in the brain. Pharmacol Toxicol 71 (suppl 1):4–17, 1992

Mousli M, Bueb JL, Bronner C, et al: G protein activation: a receptor-independent mode of action for cationic amphiphilic neuropeptides and venom peptides. Trends Pharmacol Sci 11(9):358–362, 1990

Myllyla VV: Effects of convulsions and anticonvulsive drugs on cerebrospinal fluid cyclic AMP in rabbit. Eur Neurol 14:97–107, 1976

Namima M, Sugihara K, Okamoto K: Lithium inhibits the reverse tolerance and the c-Fos expression induced by methamphetamine in mice. Brain Res 782:83–90, 1998

Namima M, Sugihara K, Watanabe Y, et al: Quantitative analysis of the effects of lithium on the reverse tolerance and the c-Fos expression induced by methamphetamine in mice. Brain Res Brain Res Protoc 4:11–18, 1999

Nestler EJ: Antidepressant treatments in the 21st century. Biol Psychiatry 44:526–533, 1998

Nishizuka Y: Intracellular signaling by hydrolysis of phospholipids and activation of protein kinase C. Science 258:607–614, 1992

Nonaka S, Hough CJ, Chuang DM: Chronic lithium treatment robustly protects neurons in the central nervous system against excitotoxicity by inhibiting N-methyl-D-aspartate receptor-mediated calcium influx. Proc Natl Acad Sci U S A 95:2642–2647, 1998a

Nonaka S, Katsube N, Chuang DM: Lithium protects rat cerebellar granule cells against apoptosis induced by anticonvulsants, phenytoin and carbamazepine. J Pharmacol Exp Ther 286:539–547, 1998b

Oda T, Shearman MS, Nishizuka Y: Synaptosomal protein kinase C subspecies, B: down-regulation promoted by phorbol ester and its effect on evoked norepinephrine release. J Neurochem 56:1263–1269, 1991

Olianas MC, Onali P: Phorbol esters increase GTP-dependent adenylate cyclase activity in rat brain striatal membranes. J Neurochem 7:890–897, 1986

Ongur D, Drevets WC, Price JL: Glial reduction in the subgenual prefrontal cortex in mood disorders. Proc Natl Acad Sci U S A 95:13290–13295, 1998

Ozaki N, Chuang DM: Lithium increases transcription factor binding to AP-1 and cyclic AMP-responsive element in cultured neurons and rat brain. J Neurochem 69:2336–2344, 1997

Palmer GC: Interactions of antiepileptic drugs on adenylate cyclase and phosphodiesterases in rat and mouse cerebrum. Exp Neurol 63:322–335, 1979

Palmer GC, Jones DJ, Medina MA, et al: Anticonvulsant drug actions on in vitro and in vivo levels of cyclic AMP in the mouse brain. Epilepsia 20:95–104, 1979

Post RM, Ballenger JC, Uhde TW, et al: Effect of carbamazepine on cyclic nucleotides in CSF of patients with affective illness. Biol Psychiatry 17:1037–1045, 1982

Post RM, Ballenger JC, Uhde TW, et al: Efficacy of carbamazepine in manic-depressive illness: implications for underlying mechanisms, in Neurobiology of Mood Disorders. Edited by Post RM, Ballenger JC. Baltimore, MD, Williams & Wilkins, 1984, pp 777–816

Post RM, Leverich GS, Altshuler L, et al: Lithium-discontinuation-induced refractoriness: preliminary observations. Am J Psychiatry 149:1727–1729, 1992

Purpura DP, Shofer RJ: Excitatory action of dibutyryl cyclic adenosine monophosphate on immature cerebral cortex. Brain Res 38:179–181, 1972

Rajkowska G, Miguel-Hidalgo JJ, Wei J, et al: Morphometric evidence for neuronal and glial prefrontal cell pathology in major depression Biol Psychiatry 45:1085–1098, 1999

Rana RS, Hokin LE: Role of phosphoinositides in transmembrane signaling. Physiol Rev 70:115–164, 1990

Reifman A, Wyatt RJ: Lithium: a brake in the rising cost of mental illness. Arch Gen Psychiatry 37:385–388, 1980

Risby ED, Hsiao JK, Manji HK, et al: The mechanisms of action of lithium. Arch Gen Psychiatry 48:513–524, 1991

Robinson PJ: The role of protein kinase C and its neuronal substrates dephosphin, B-50, and MARCKS in neurotransmitter release. Mol Neurobiol 5:87–130, 1991

Rogawski MA, Porter RJ: Antiepileptic drugs: pharmacological mechanisms and clinical efficacy with consideration of promising development stage compounds. Pharmacol Rev 42:223–286, 1990

Ross EM: Signal sorting and amplification through G protein-coupled receptors. Neuron 3:141–152, 1989

Sagi-Eisenberg R: GTP-binding proteins as possible targets for protein kinase C action. Trends Biochem Sci 14:355–357, 1989

Sheng M, Greenberg ME: The regulation and function of c-fos and other immediate early genes in the nervous system. Neuron 4:477–485, 1990

Skaper SD, Walsh FS: Neurotrophic molecules: strategies for designing effective therapeutic molecules in neurodegeneration. Mol Cell Neurosci 12(4/5):179–193, 1998

Smith MA, Makino S, Altemus M, et al: Stress and antidepressants differentially regulate neurotrophin 3 mRNA expression in the locus coeruleus. Proc Natl Acad Sci U S A 92:8788–8792, 1995

Souroujon MC, Mochly Rosen D: Peptide modulators of protein-protein interactions in intracellular signaling. Nat Biotechnol 16(10):919–924, 1998

Stabel S, Parker PJ: Protein kinase C. Pharmacol Ther 51:71–95, 1991

Stambolic V, Ruel Laurent R, Woodgett JR: Lithium inhibits glycogen synthase kinase-3 activity and mimics wingless signalling in intact cells. Curr Biol 6:1664–1668, 1996

Strittmatter SM, Valenzuela D, Kennedy TE, et al: Go is a major growth cone protein subject to regulation by GAP-43. Nature 344(6269):836–841, 1990

Suppes T, Baldessarini RJ, Faedda GL, et al: Risk of recurrence following discontinuation of lithium treatment in bipolar disorder. Arch Gen Psychiatry 48:1082–1088, 1991

Taylor CW: The role of G proteins in transmembrane signaling. Biochem J 272:1–13, 1990

Turkka J, Bitran JA, Manji HK, et al: Effects of chronic lithium on agonist and antagonist binding to β adrenergic receptors of rat brain. Lithium 3:43–47, 1992

Ui M: Pertussis toxin as a valuable probe for G protein involvement in signal transduction, in ADP-Ribosylation Toxins and G Proteins. Edited by Moss J, Vaughn M. Washington, DC, American Society for Microbiology, 1990

Unlap MT, Jope RS: Lithium attenuates nerve growth factor-induced activation of AP-1 DNA binding activity in PC12 cells. Neuropsychopharmacology 17:12–17, 1997

Van Calker D, Steber R, Klotz K, et al: Carbamazepine distinguishes between adenosine receptors that mediate different second messenger responses. Eur J Pharmacol Mol Pharmacol Sect 206:285–290, 1991

Wang HY, Friedman E: Lithium inhibition of protein kinase C activation-induced serotonin release. Psychopharmacology (Berl) 99:213–218, 1989

Wang HY, Friedman E: Enhanced protein kinase C activity and translocation in bipolar affective disorder brains. Biol Psychiatry 40:568–575, 1996

Wang JF, Young LT: Differential display PCR reveals increased expression of 2',3'-cyclic nucleotide 3'-phosphodiesterase by lithium. FEBS Lett 386:225–229, 1996

Wang JF, Young LT, Li PP, et al: Signal transduction abnormalities in bipolar disorder, in Bipolar Disorder: Biological Models and their Clinical Application. Edited by Joffe RT, Young LT. New York, Marcel Dekker, 1997, pp 41–79

Weiner ED, Kalasapudi VD, Papolos DF, et al: Lithium augments pilocarpine-induced fos gene expression in rat brain. Brain Res 553 (1):117–122, 1991

Weissman MM, Leaf PJ, Tischler GL, et al: Affective disorders in five United States communities. Psychol Med 18:141–153, 1988

Williams MB, Jope RS: Circadian variation in rat brain AP-1 DNA binding activity after cholinergic stimulation: modulation by lithium. Psychopharmacology 122:363–368, 1995

Yokoyama N, Mori N, Kumashiro H: Chemical kindling induced by cAMP, transfer to electrical kindling. Brain Res 492:158–162, 1989

Yoshimasa T, Sibley DR, Bouvier M, et al: Cross-talk between cellular signalling pathways suggested by phorbol-ester-induced adenylate cyclase phosphorylation. Nature 327:67–70, 1987

Yoshimura M, Cooper DM Type-specific stimulation of adenylylcyclase by protein kinase C. J Biol Chem 268(7):4604–4607, 1993.

Young LT, Li PP, Kish SJ, et al: Cerebral cortex G_s a protein levels and forskolin-stimulated cyclic AMP formation are increased in bipolar affective disorder. J Neurochem 61:890–898, 1993

Young LT, Li PP, Kamble A, et al: Mononuclear leukocyte levels of G proteins in depressed patients with bipolar disorder or major depressive disorder. Am J Psychiatry 151:594–596, 1994

Young S, Parker PJ, Ullrich A, et al: Down-regulation of protein kinase C is due to an increased rate of degradation. Biochem J 24:775–779, 1987

Yuan PX, Chen G, Huang, LD, et al: Lithium stimulates gene expression through the AP-1 transcription factor pathway. Mol Brain Res 58:225–230, 1998

Zhou XM, Curran P, Baumgold J, et al: Modulation of adenylyl cyclase by protein kinase C in human neurotumor SK-N-MC cells: evidence that the α isozyme mediates both potentiation and desensitization. J Neurochem 63:1361–1370, 1994
Zigova T, Willing AE, Tedesco EM, et al: Lithium chloride induces the expression of tyrosine hydroxylase in hNT neurons. Exp Neurol 157:251–258, 1999

CHAPTER 8

MODULATION OF NEURONAL SIGNAL TRANSDUCTION SYSTEMS BY LITHIUM

Richard S. Jope, Ph.D., Mary B. Williams, Ph.D.,
Xiaohua Li, M.D., Ph.D., Ling Song, M.D.,
Carol A. Grimes, B.S., M. Tino Unlap, Ph.D., and
Mary A. Pacheco, Ph.D.

As exemplified by the many notable findings eloquently reported in recent years, there is much evidence that lithium influences signal transduction systems in the brain (reviewed in Jope 1999b; Jope and Williams 1994; Manji and Lenox 1994). If such sites represent therapeutic targets of action of lithium for the treatment of affective disorders, then they represent objectives for the development of new therapies, and the possibility arises that altered activities of signal transduction systems may contribute to the etiology of affective disorders. Therefore, it is vital to understand more precisely the regulatory processes that influence the activity of signal transduction systems and the modulatory mechanisms of action of lithium.

To address these issues, a variety of experimental strategies and techniques must be applied to test individual hypotheses concerning potential actions of lithium. Our laboratory has addressed these points, with an emphasis

This chapter was supported by grants from the National Institutes of Health (MH 38752) and the Theodore and Vada Stanley Foundation. Collaboration with Drs. C. A. Stockmeier, J. J. Warsh, P. P. Li, L. T. Young, and S. J. Kish in the studies of phosphoinositide hydrolysis in postmortem brain is gratefully acknowledged.

on the phosphoinositide signal transduction system, by examining 1) the in vivo effects of lithium administration to rats on responses to receptor-selective drugs, 2) the effects of lithium on signaling systems in cultured cells and transcription factor activation, and 3) the activity of the phosphoinositide second-messenger system in postmortem human brain from subjects with affective disorders and matched control subjects. In this chapter, we focus on recent results that are related to each of these three topics of investigation.

IN VIVO EFFECTS OF LITHIUM IN RATS

Because many in vitro actions of lithium have been described, to help to discriminate which may have therapeutic relevance, we thought that it would be useful to determine which of these actions were expressed and could be examined in vivo in rats that were treated with lithium. One approach adopted was to use electroencephalographic (EEG) recordings to determine whether lithium treatment altered in vivo responses to selective neurotransmitter receptor agonists. This strategy could provide information about the influence of lithium on receptor subtype–mediated signal transduction stimulation.

In rats, the in vivo administration of lithium potentiated responses to all cholinomimetics that were tested, including pilocarpine, the most widely studied agonist in this paradigm; acetylcholinesterase inhibitors; and other agonists (Jope 1993). These potentiated responses were quantitated with EEG detection of paroxysmal spikes, spike trains, and seizures. For example, lithium-treated rats given a dose of pilocarpine (30 mg/kg) much below that which causes seizures in lithium-naive rats develop paroxysmal spikes approximately 20 minutes after pilocarpine administration (Figure 8–1). Within a few minutes, the spikes evolve into spike trains and then to status epilepticus, which is generalized to all brain regions that have been examined and which continues unabated for several hours and is lethal. Although seizure activity is used as an experimentally identifiable endpoint, lithium would be expected to have the same potentiating effect on in vivo responses with endogenous neurotransmitters, which would be much below the level of response that causes seizures. Especially noteworthy are the findings that potentiation of the response to pilocarpine by lithium was observed even with a lithium dose as low as 0.75 mmol/kg, much below the widely used dose range of 2–5 mmol/kg, and that chronic lithium treatment at a dose (0.85 mM) that produced a therapeutically relevant plasma concentration was as effective as, or more effective than, acute lithium treatment (Morrisett et al. 1987). No effects of lithium pretreatment on responses to agonists of several other receptor subtypes, including kainate, *N*-methyl-D-aspartate, pentylenetetrazol, and bicuculline, were detectable (Ormandy et al. 1991). This selectivity in the potentiating action of lithium led to the suggestion that this in vivo effect of lithium was caused by a specific interaction with the cholinergic system (Jope 1993). However, we recently confirmed that this was not the case because lithium potentiated the in vivo response to DOI (2,5-dimethoxy-4-iodoprenyl-2-aminopropane), an agonist at serotonin 5-HT_2/5-HT_{1C} receptors (Williams and Jope 1994b, 1995b). Because these serotonin receptors are coupled to phosphoinositide hydrolysis, as are many cholinergic receptors, and because much other evidence has indicated that the phosphoinositide system is a target of lithium (Jope and Williams 1994), we hypothesized that the in vivo effects of lithium detected with these methods are the result of modulation of phosphoinositide signal transduction systems that were influenced by lithium in vivo (Williams and Jope 1995b).

Evidence linking the in vivo agonist-potentiating effects of lithium to the phosphoinositide system was first reported by Sherman's group (reviewed in Sherman et al. 1986). Among their findings was the result that lithium greatly

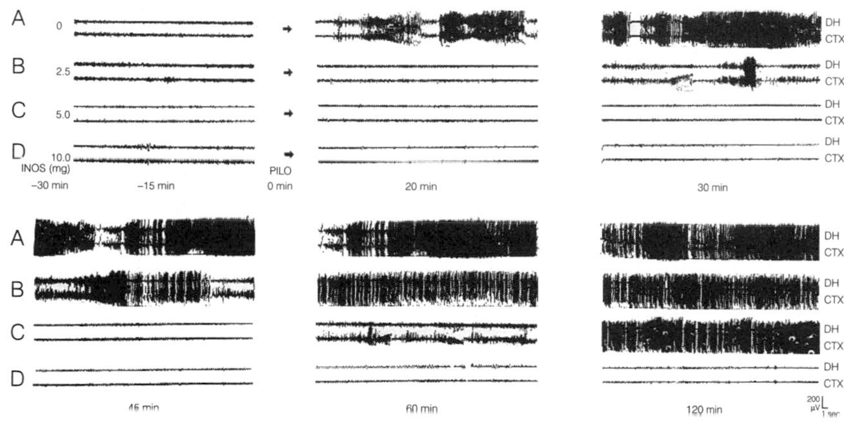

Figure 8–1. Electroencephalographic (EEG) recordings demonstrating the seizures induced by administration of pilocarpine (PILO) to lithium-pretreated rats and the attenuation caused by infusion of *myo*-inositol (INOS). Rats were pretreated with acute lithium (3 mmol/kg; intraperitoneally; 20 hours prior), followed by (A) 0, (B) 2.5, (C) 5.0, or (D) 10.0 mg of INOS (intraventricularly in 40 µL of artificial cerebrospinal fluid) 30 minutes prior to PILO (30 mg/kg; subcutaneously in saline). EEG recordings were obtained from depth electrodes implanted in the dorsal hippocampus (DH) and from cortical electrodes (CTX).
Source. Reprinted from Williams MB, Jope RS: "Modulation by Inositol of Cholinergic and Serotonergic-Induced Seizures in Lithium-Treated Rats." *Brain Research* 685:169–178, 1995. Used with permission.

potentiated pilocarpine-induced inositol monophosphate accumulation in rat brain, indicating increased activation of phosphoinositide hydrolysis. However, results from Tricklebank's laboratory (Tricklebank et al. 1991) indicated that lithium's interactions with pilocarpine-induced responses may consist of decreased phosphoinositide signaling. They found that centrally administered *myo*-inositol, which had been hypothesized to be depleted by lithium treatment (Berridge et al. 1982), attenuated seizures induced by pilocarpine in lithium-treated mice (Tricklebank et al. 1991). Belmaker and colleagues confirmed and extended those findings in rats in a comprehensive series of behavioral studies (Kofman and Belmaker 1993). Our EEG measurements indicated that intraventricular *myo*-inositol administration attenuated seizures induced by lithium plus pilocarpine in rats (Williams and Jope 1995b). The effective doses ranged from 2.5 mg (14 μmol) of *myo*-inositol, which slightly retarded the initiation of seizures, to 10 mg (55.5 μmol), which completely blocked all seizure activity (Figure 8–1). However, we were concerned that intraventricular infusions of a large volume (40 μL, necessitated by inositol's solubility limit) and a high *myo*-inositol concentration (1.4 M) may have affected processes other than those associated with the phosphoinositide second-messenger system or may have altered this system by a mechanism other than by providing a source of *myo*-inositol for phosphoinositide synthesis. Also difficult to reconcile with the phosphoinositide-repletion hypothesis were the findings that *myo*-inositol was not very effective in attenuating seizures induced by DOI after lithium pretreatment and that *myo*-inositol was less effective after chronic, compared with acute, lithium pretreatment (Williams and Jope 1995b). These concerns were substantiated by our finding that seizures induced by acute lithium plus pilocarpine were effectively attenuated by *epi*-inositol, an isomer of inositol that is not used for phosphoinositide synthesis (Williams and Jope 1995b). This finding brings into question the hypothesis that the anticonvulsant effect of *myo*-inositol is solely the result of phosphoinositide repletion and suggests that it at least partly results from other actions that are also generated by *epi*-inositol. At present, it appears most likely that centrally administered *myo*-inositol has multiple effects based on its many physiological roles. Substantiation of this conclusion may be inferred from the intriguing findings of Belmaker and his colleagues (1996) that *myo*-inositol has therapeutic properties with various psychiatric disorders, a line of investigation that has opened new vistas in affective disorder research.

In summary, the use of EEG recordings in rats treated with lithium and receptor agonists has provided a means to observe in vivo effects of therapeutically relevant doses of lithium and has implicated the phosphoinositide second-messenger system as a target of lithium. Lithium, at therapeutic levels, clearly selectively enhanced responses to cholinergic and serotonergic agonists that activate receptors coupled to the phosphoinositide signal transduction system. Nevertheless, the precise mechanism of action of lithium that potentiates responses to cholinergic and serotonergic agonists and the intriguing actions of inositol remain to be clarified.

LITHIUM'S EFFECTS ON SIGNALING SYSTEMS IN CULTURED CELLS AND RAT BRAIN

Much evidence indicates that lithium modulates the activity of guanine nucleotide binding protein (G-protein)–linked second-messenger systems and may directly affect the function and levels of G proteins (Hudson et al. 1993; Jope 1999b; Jope and Williams 1994; Manji 1992). To examine lithium's effects on G-protein expression, investigators have studied adult rat brain, which showed significant, but small, inhibitory effects of lithium (reviewed in Jope and Williams 1994). We hypothesized that the sensitivity for detecting the influence of lithium on G-protein expression might be increased by using a more dynamic model system in which G-protein levels were undergoing relatively large increases. PC12 cells subjected to nerve growth factor (NGF)–induced differentiation into a neuronal phenotype were found to be suitable for this purpose because several G-protein subtypes increased in concentration several-fold after NGF treatment compared with undifferentiated PC12 cells (X. Li et al. 1995). Chronic treatment (12 days) with a low concentration of lithium (1 mM) reduced the NGF-induced increases of $G\alpha_s$ (52 kD subtype) by 35%, $G\alpha_{i1}$ by 36%, $G\alpha_{o1}$ by 42%, and $G\alpha_{q/11}$ by 82%, whereas several other G-protein subunits were unaffected by 1 mM of lithium (X. Li and Jope 1995). The morphological differentiation of PC12 cells by NGF and the levels of several other proteins, including tubulin, three phospholipase C subtypes (β, δ, and γ), and two protein kinase C (PKC) subtypes (β and ζ), were unaltered by treatment with 1 mM of lithium, but the PKCα and PKCε subtypes were reduced. These results indicated that the levels of certain signal transduction– linked proteins are susceptible to modulation by a therapeutically relevant concentration of lithium and, furthermore, that modulation by lithium is limited to a select group of these proteins. The mechanism by which lithium modulates the levels of these signal transduction proteins and the repercussions on in vivo signaling systems remain to be investigated, but it is notable that only chronic, not acute, lithium treatment was effective in modulating signal transduction protein levels in PC12 cells (X. Li and Jope 1995). These findings provide further support for the hypothesis that G-protein–linked signal transduction systems are susceptible to regulation by therapeutic concentrations of lithium.

The selective effect of lithium in reducing the levels of PKCα and PKCε is especially intriguing. Since we first reported that chronic lithium treatment selectively reduced PKC-mediated phosphorylation of specific proteins in rat brain (Casebolt and Jope 1991), increasing evidence supports the hypothesis that regulation of PKC activity is an important effect of lithium. For example, a selective downregulation of PKCα by lithium was identified in rat hippocampus (Manji et al. 1993); myristoylated alanine-rich C kinase substrate (MARCKS) protein was identified as a substrate whose phosphorylation by PKC was modulated by lithium (Lenox et al. 1992); and valproate, an alternative to lithium in the treatment of bipolar affective disorder, selectively reduced PKCα and PKCε in glioma cells (Chen et al. 1994). These findings indicate that PKCα and PKCε are selectively downregulated by lithium in PC12 cells, glioma cells, and rat brain. The cause of the selectivity of the effect of lithium on PKCα and PKCε is unknown, but it may be related to the recent finding that these two kinases share a common subcellular localization when stimulated that differs from other PKC subtypes (Goodnight et al. 1995). A critical issue to be clarified is determining if, and how, this is related to lithium's actions on the phosphoinositide signaling system, which is a major contributory factor in the regulation of PKC activity.

One mechanism by which lithium could reduce the levels of proteins associated with signal transduction processes is by inhibition of gene expression, and, indeed, lithium reduced G-protein messenger RNA (mRNA) levels in rat brain (Colin et al. 1991; P. P. Li et al. 1991). Interference with the activation of transcription factors by lithium could contribute to this effect. Unfortunately, the transcription factors that regulate G-protein expression have not been fully elucidated. However, lithium has been reported to modulate mRNA levels for *c-fos*, the protein product of which is a constituent of the activator protein 1 (AP-1) transcription factor (Arenander et al. 1989; Kalasapudi et al. 1990). Therefore, we sought to determine whether lithium modulated the stimulation of AP-1 DNA binding activity in cultured cells and in rat brain.

An early event in NGF-induced differentiation of PC12 cells is stimulation of AP-1 DNA binding activity. We determined the time course of NGF-induced AP-1 activity in PC12 cells, which was maximal 2 hours after application of NGF, and then tested whether lithium modulated this response. Acute treatment (24 hours) with a therapeutic concentration of lithium (1 mM) only slightly reduced NGF-induced AP-1, whereas chronic treatment (2 weeks) or a higher concentration (5 mM) of lithium resulted in a larger inhibition (Unlap and Jope 1997). Thus, these findings demonstrated that lithium can modulate transcription factor activation, providing a potential site that could mediate lithium's effects on the expression of proteins involved in signaling cascades.

We also examined whether stimulation of AP-1 activity in rat brain was modulated by lithium treatment. In rat brain after in vivo treatments, it was difficult to measure the effects of lithium on pilocarpine-induced AP-1 DNA binding activity for two reasons. First, seizures produced by cotreatment with lithium and pilocarpine undoubtedly were a major contributory factor to enhanced AP-1 activity, which could obscure the modulatory effects of lithium. Second, administration of a pilocarpine dose low enough not to cause seizures in lithium-treated rats barely induced the expression of the immediate-early genes (Williams and Jope 1994a). Nonetheless, we were able to identify a circadian variation in pilocarpine-induced AP-1 activity, and, within this cycle, chronic lithium treatment reduced the peak activation of AP-1 stimulated by pilocarpine (Williams and Jope 1995a). Pilocarpine-induced AP-1 DNA binding activity in rat cerebral cortex was increased twice as much when measured at 0800 h compared with 1600 h. In rats acutely pretreated with lithium, this time-of-day difference in the AP-1 response to pilocarpine was still evident (Figure 8–2), although the stimulation was greater because of the generation of seizures caused by coadministration of lithium and pilocarpine. However, after chronic lithium treatment, although pilocarpine administration still caused seizures, the peak AP-1 DNA binding activity measured at 0800 h was reduced to a level equal to that observed at 1600 h (Figure 8–2). Therefore, chronic, but not acute, lithium treatment reduced the maximal in vivo activation of AP-1 induced by pilocarpine in rat cortex (Williams and Jope 1995a).

The difficulty encompassed by seizures during in vivo studies of lithium's modulatory effects on the stimulation of AP-1 led us to continue further studies with human neuroblastoma SH-SY5Y cells. These cells endogenously express muscarinic M_3 receptors coupled to the phosphoinositide signal transduction system, and activation of this system with an agonist, such as carbachol, stimulates AP-1 DNA binding activity (Jope and Song 1997). Acute pretreatment with 1 mM of lithium inhibited carbachol-stimulated AP-1 DNA binding activity by 35%. Higher concentrations of lithium more completely inhibited carbachol-stimulated AP-1 DNA binding activity and also, in the absence of carbachol, increased basal AP-1 DNA binding, an effect likely due to the inhibition by lithium of glycogen synthase kinase-3β (Jope and Song 1997). In contrast to its inhibition of the response to carbachol, lithium did not inhibit activation of AP-1 in response to stimulation of PKC. This and other findings indicated that lithium may influence the calcium arm, rather than the PKC arm, of the phosphoinositide signal transduction system (Jope and Song 1997).

Carbamazepine and sodium valproate, in addition to lithium, are therapeutic for bipolar disorder, and each of these three agents must be adminis-

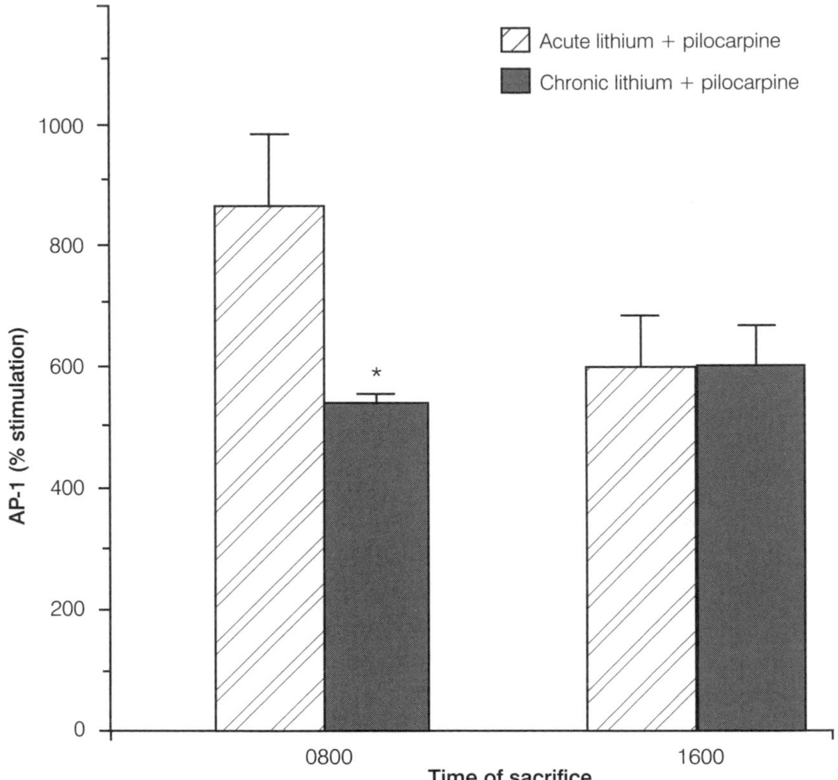

Figure 8–2. Activator protein 1 (AP-1) DNA binding activity in rat cerebral cortex. Rats were given pilocarpine (30 mg/kg, subcutaneous) after acute lithium (3 mmol/kg, intraperitoneal, 20 hours before pilocarpine), or chronic lithium (dietary, for 4 weeks). AP-1 binding was measured at 0800 h or 1600 h, as indicated in the figure, 2 hours after pilocarpine administration, as described in Williams and Jope (1995a). Data are expressed as percent stimulation above controls (untreated rats) obtained at the same time of sacrifice. Means ±SEM. $^{*}P < 0.05$.
Source. Reprinted with permission from Williams MB, Jope RS: "Circadian Variation in Rat Brain AP-1 DNA Binding Activity After Cholinergic Stimulation: Modulation by Lithium." *Psychopharmacology* 122:363–368, 1995a. Copyright 1995, Springer-Verlag.

tered chronically to obtain a therapeutic response. Therefore, further studies of transcription factors were carried out in SH-SY5Y cells by administering chronic, 7-day, treatments with each of the three drugs. In addition to AP-1, the DNA binding activity of early growth response-1 (Egr-1, also called zif268, krox 24, NGF1-A, and tis8) was examined because it is also activated in response to stimulation of muscarinic receptors coupled to the phosphoinositide signaling cascade. In these studies, chronic treatment with 1 mM of lithium or 0.05 mM of carbamazepine, but not 0.5 mM of valproate, inhibited carbachol-stimulated AP-1 DNA binding activity (Pacheco and Jope, in press). In contrast, chronic treatment with valproate, but not lithium or carbamazepine, inhibited Egr-1 DNA binding activity (Grimes and Jope, in press). Thus, all three drugs that are therapeutic for bipolar disorder modulate transcription factors activated by the phosphoinositide signaling cascade, but AP-1 and Egr-1 have differential sensitivities according to which drug is administered. It is interesting to speculate that these differences may contribute to some patients responding to one but not to another of these agents.

Taken together, current studies of the effects of lithium, as well as carbamazepine and sodium valproate, led to the development of a bimodal mechanism of action in their therapeutic effects on bipolar disorder (Jope 1999a). This model suggests that the comprehensive effect of lithium and other therapeutic agents on signaling systems is to dampen the magnitude of fluctuations in signaling activities. This appears to be accomplished, at least in some circumstances, by the therapeutic agents elevating basal activities of signaling systems and attenuating maximal activities. Through this mechanism, the activities of signaling systems may be stabilized, an effect that may contribute to the mood-stabilizing actions of these agents.

ACTIVITY OF THE PHOSPHOINOSITIDE SYSTEM IN POSTMORTEM HUMAN BRAIN

As discussed briefly earlier in this chapter, much evidence indicates that the activity of the phosphoinositide signal transduction system is a therapeutic target of lithium. This and other evidence suggests that the phosphoinositide system may be dysfunctional in patients with affective disorders. To address this issue directly, a method to measure the function of the phosphoinositide system in human brain would be of enormous utility. Until in vivo imaging techniques are developed for this purpose, development of methods that use postmortem brain from well-characterized subjects appears to be the most feasible strategy to pursue. Therefore, our laboratory applied to postmortem human brain methods that had been devised for measuring phosphoinositide hydrolysis in rat brain membranes (Claro et al. 1989) to examine whether such methods could be adapted to determine whether the function of the phosphoinositide system was altered in subjects with affective disorders.

We have reported the results of several studies characterizing the activity of the phosphoinositide system in postmortem human brain membranes with [^{3}H]phosphatidylinositol (PI) as the substrate (Greenwood et al. 1995; Jope et al. 1994a, 1994b, 1994c). Hydrolysis of [^{3}H]PI was stimulated by calcium, which directly activates phospholipase C; by guanosine triphosphate (GTP)γS and sodium fluoride (NaF), which activate G proteins coupled to phospholipase C; and by agonists for several neurotransmitter receptors. The response to each of these agents was stable in human brain obtained within the postmortem interval range of 5–21 hours (Greenwood et al. 1995). Selective antibodies were used to identify G$\alpha_{q/11}$ and phospholipase C$_\beta$ as the active enzyme subtypes mediating agonist-induced [^{3}H]PI hydrolysis. Immunoblots indicated that the levels of G$\alpha_{q/11}$ and phospholipase C$_\beta$ were stable postmortem between 5 and 21 hours (Greenwood et al. 1995; X. Li et al. 1996). Thus, postmortem human brain retains the primary protein constituents of the phosphoinositide signal transduction system, and each constituent is activated by appropriate agents. However, this assay has several limitations in postmortem human brain, which have been discussed previously (Pacheco and Jope 1996), including the limited number of agonists that induce responses, which constrains the variety of functional receptor subtypes that can be assayed.

The availability of an assay capable of measuring phosphoinositide hydrolysis in postmortem human brain allowed us to determine whether the responses to stimuli were different in brain membranes from subjects with bipolar affective disorder and from matched control subjects. These valuable brain specimens were obtained from investigators at the Clarke Institute of Psychiatry in Toronto under the direction of Dr. Jerry Warsh, who had previously identified specific differences in G-protein subtype levels between bipolar and control subjects (Young et al. 1991).

Our investigation found that widespread alterations in stimulated [^{3}H]PI hydrolysis were not associated with bipolar affective disorder, but instead there was a selective and severe impairment (Jope et al. 1996). No differences were found between groups in the stimulation of [^{3}H]PI hydrolysis by calcium-activated phospholipase C, activation of G proteins by GTPγS or NaF, or activation of receptors by carbachol, histamine, ACPD (trans-1-aminocyclopentyl-1,3- dicarboxylic acid, a glutamatergic metabotropic receptor agonist), serotonin, or adenosine triphosphate (ATP) in membranes prepared from frontal or temporal cortices. However, in the occipital cortex, the stimulation by GTPγS of G proteins coupled to phospholipase C was 50% lower in bipolar subjects than in control subjects (Jope et al. 1996). These results showed directly in human brain that a large, selective deficit in G-protein function is associated with the phosphoinositide signal transduction system in subjects with bipolar affective disorder.

An additional intriguing observation made in this investigation was that in bipolar subjects, the brain lithium concentration was directly correlated with GTPγS-stimulated [^{3}H]PI hydrolysis in occipital cortical membranes (Jope et al. 1996). Figure 8–3 shows that [^{3}H]PI hydrolysis stimulated by 3 μM of GTPγS in seven of nine bipolar occipital cortical samples was well below responses in nonbipolar control subjects (100%), whereas two bipolar subjects had responses within the control range. Remarkably, these two bipolar subjects with responses within the normal range had the highest brain lithium concentrations, and there was a direct, significant correlation ($r = 0.725$; $P < 0.005$) between the brain lithium concentration and GTPγS-stimulated [^{3}H]PI hydrolysis. Even after omission of the two values with the highest lithium concentration and "normal" [^{3}H]PI hydrolysis in the calculation of the correlation coefficient, the relationship between lithium levels and GTPγS-stimulated [^{3}H]PI hydrolysis was significant in the remaining seven samples with depressed activity ($r = 0.60$). These findings indicate that not only is there a deficit in phosphoinositide signaling in bipolar occipital cortex, but the deficit appears to be reversed in a concentration-dependent manner by lithium. In the two cortical regions (temporal and frontal) where [^{3}H]PI hydrolysis was not impaired in bipolar subjects, there were no correlations ($r < 0.10$) between lithium levels and GTPγS-stimulated [^{3}H]PI hydrolysis, as might be expected of a biochemical process in regions not associated with the illness or with the therapeutic effect of lithium. In other words, lithium appears to influence impaired phosphoinositide signaling in bipolar subjects but not to affect unimpaired systems. Alternatively, it is possible that disease-associated deficits in the phosphoinositide system in the temporal and frontal cortices were completely reversed by lithium treatment, whereas the signaling system in the occipital cortex was only partially reversed by lithium. The latter explanation appears less likely because of the low lithium levels in many of the bipolar brain samples.

These findings provide strong corroboration of numerous previous indirect indications of aberrant signaling through the phosphoinositide signal transduction system in subjects with affective disorders, although further studies are necessary to identify more precisely the mechanism and extent of the impairment. The reduced response to GTPγS in bipolar subjects is likely caused by a deficit in G-protein function rather than in levels because we reported that $G\alpha_{q/11}$ is the primary G protein mediating [^{3}H]PI hydrolysis in human brain membranes (Jope et al. 1994b, 1994c), and $G\alpha_{q/11}$ levels were increased, not decreased, in bipolar occipital cortex (Warsh et al. 1994). Increased $G\alpha_{q/11}$ levels may be an adaptive response to the impaired function, but because little is known about the regulation of $G\alpha_{q/11}$ expression, this is purely conjecture. The mechanism causing the impaired function of $G\alpha_{q/11}$ has not been identified, although we suggested that regulation of GTP–guanosine diphosphate (GDP) exchange may be involved because activation of G proteins by NaF was not impaired to the same extent as the response to

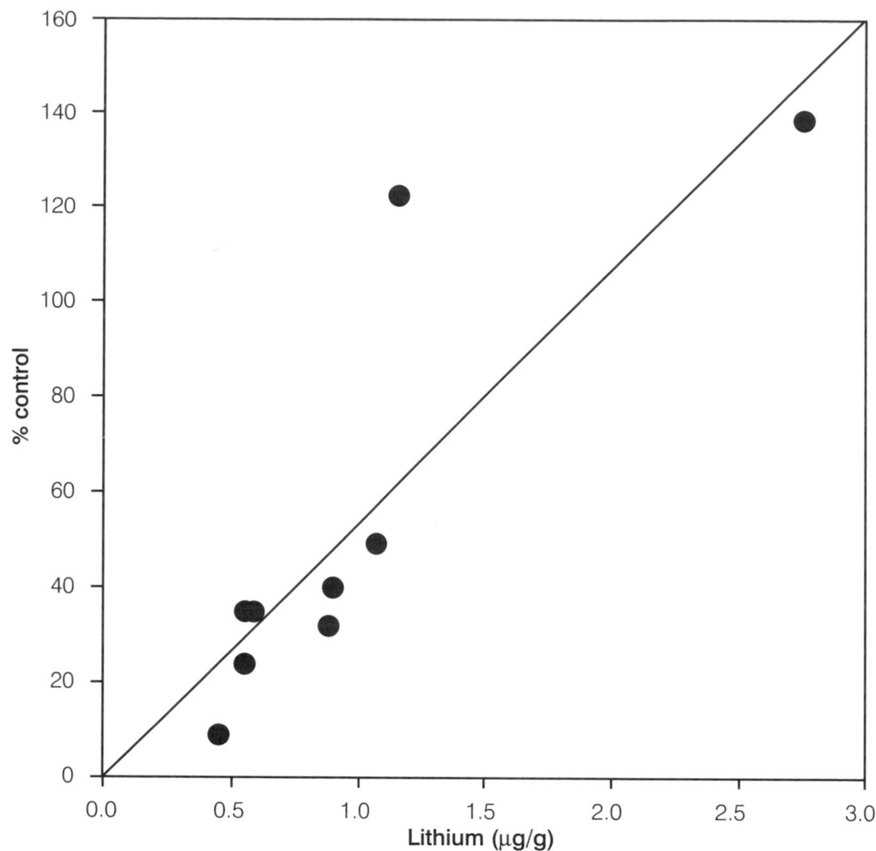

Figure 8–3. Relationship between brain lithium levels and 3 μM guanosine triphosphate (GTP)γS-stimulated [^{3}H] phosphatidylinositol (PI) hydrolysis in occipital cortex of bipolar subjects. Values for [^{3}H]PI hydrolysis in bipolar subjects are given as the percentage of responses obtained in psychiatrically healthy control subjects. The correlation coefficient ($r = 0.725$; $P < 0.005$) was obtained by linear regression analysis.
Source. Data from Jope et al. 1996.

GTPγS (Jope et al. 1996). The reason for the selective localization of the deficit in the occipital cortex is not known. It seems likely that phosphoinositide signaling in other brain regions besides the occipital cortex may be impaired in bipolar subjects and influenced by lithium treatment. The findings of impaired phosphoinositide signaling in the occipital cortex need not indicate that this region is of primary importance in the clinical manifestations of bipolar affective disorder. What the data do show is that the occipital cortex is one region (of only three examined) in which phosphoinositide signaling is impaired, and it seems likely that, rather than being unique to the occipital cortex, other brain regions that have not yet been examined are likewise affected. Thus, these findings provide data from human brain stem that in a limited number of brain regions, a deficit in phosphoinositide signaling exists in bipolar subjects. Further studies in other brain regions and in additional subjects should help to clarify the extent to which the function of the phosphoinositide system is impaired in bipolar brain.

To test if the alterations observed in phosphoinositide signaling activity in postmortem brain tissue from subjects with bipolar disorder were selectively associated with this disorder, activities were measured in tissue from subjects with other disorders. Deficits in phosphoinositide signaling in selective brain regions were also identified in postmortem brain from subjects with major depression (Pacheco et al. 1996). In contrast, brain-selective increases, rather than decreases, in phosphoinositide signaling activity were found in brain tissue from subjects with schizophrenia, whereas no alterations were found in samples from subjects with chronic alcohol dependence (Jope et al. 1998). Thus, both bipolar disorder and major depression were found to be associated with deficits in the activity of the phosphoinositide signal transduction system, although with differential brain region susceptibilities. It is interesting to speculate that this impairment in both bipolar disorder and major depression may contribute to some of the mood fluctuations common to these two disorders.

SUMMARY

Our laboratory has used various experimental strategies to identify signaling systems that are susceptible to modulation by lithium and that may contribute to the etiology of bipolar affective disorder. The findings of altered phosphoinositide signaling in human brain associated with bipolar affective disorder, taken in conjunction with the numerous animal and in vitro studies of lithium's actions, leave little doubt that this is an important component of affective disorders and of lithium's therapeutic effects. In addition, evidence continues to accumulate that lithium modulates the expression of specific genes and the levels of proteins of primary importance in signaling systems. Integration of these disparate actions of lithium into a comprehensive understanding of its mechanism of action remains a challenge. Toward this goal, evidence was recently summarized that supports the hypothesis that lithium's modulatory effects on signaling systems may be primarily directed toward stabilizing fluctuations in activities, as opposed to unidirectionally increasing or decreasing activities

(Jope 1999a). Additionally, it was proposed that current findings support the proposal that multiple, rather than individual, sites of action underlie the complex therapeutic effects of lithium (Jope 1999b). Short-term therapeutic effects of lithium may be derived from its modulatory actions on signaling systems and the associated changes in the expression of selective genes. Long-term therapeutic benefits may be derived from these actions along with neuroprotective capabilities, including downregulation of the activation of proapoptotic signaling molecules such as p53 (Lu et al. 1999) and modulation of neural plasticity through alterations of the cytoskeleton (Lesort et al. 1999; Xie et al. 1998). Thus, current evidence suggests that integration of multiple biochemical alterations is needed to achieve a greater understanding of the biochemical bases for bipolar disorder and the mechanisms of action of therapeutic agents.

REFERENCES

Arenander AT, de Vellis J, Herschman HR: Induction of c-fos and TIS genes in cultured rat astrocytes by neurotransmitters. J Neurosci Res 24:107–114, 1989

Belmaker RH, Bersudsky Y, Agam G, et al: How does lithium work on manic depression? Clinical and psychological correlates of the inositol theory. Annu Rev Med 47:47–56, 1996

Berridge MJ, Downes CP, Hanley MR: Lithium amplifies agonist-dependent phosphatidylinositol responses in brain and salivary glands. Biochem J 206:587– 595, 1982

Casebolt TL, Jope RS: Effects of chronic lithium treatment on protein kinase C and cyclic AMP-dependent protein phosphorylation. Biol Psychiatry 29:233–243, 1991

Chen G, Manji HK, Hawver DB, et al: Chronic sodium valproate selectively decreases protein kinase C α and ε in vitro. J Neurochem 63:2361–2364, 1994

Claro E, Wallace MA, Lee HM, et al: Carbachol in the presence of guanosine 5'-*O*-(3-thiotriphosphate) stimulates the breakdown of exogenous phosphatidylinositol 4,5-bisphosphate, phosphatidylinositol 4-phosphate, and phosphatidylinositol by rat brain membranes. J Biol Chem 264:18288–18295, 1989

Colin SF, Chang H-C, Mollner S, et al: Chronic lithium regulates the expression of adenylate cyclase and Gi-protein α subunit in rat cerebral cortex. Proc Natl Acad Sci U S A 88:10634–10637, 1991

Goodnight JA, Mischak H, Kolch W, et al: Immunocytochemical localization of eight protein kinase C isozymes overexpressed in NIH 3T3 fibroblasts. J Biol Chem 270:9991–10001, 1995

Greenwood AF, Powers RE, Jope RS: Phosphoinositide hydrolysis, Gαq, phospholipase C, and protein kinase C in postmortem human brain: effects of postmortem interval, subject age, and Alzheimer's disease. Neuroscience 69:125– 138, 1995

Grimes CA, Jope RS: Cholinergic stimulation of Egr-1 DNA binding activity requires protein kinase C and MEK activation and is inhibited by sodium valproate in SH-SY5Y cells. J Neurochem (in press)

Hudson CJ, Young LT, Li PP, et al: CNS signal transduction in the pathophysiology and pharmacotherapy of affective disorders and schizophrenia. Synapse 13:278–293, 1993

Jope RS: Lithium selectively potentiates cholinergic activity in rat brain. Prog Brain Res 98:317–322, 1993

Jope RS: A bimodal model for the mechanism of action of lithium. Mol Psychiatry 4:21–25, 1999a

Jope RS: Anti-bipolar therapy: mechanism of action of lithium. Mol Psychiatry 4:117–128, 1999b

Jope RS, Song L: AP-1 and NF-κB stimulated by carbachol in human neuroblastoma SH-SY5Y cells are differentially sensitive to inhibition by lithium. Mol Brain Res 50:171–180, 1997

Jope RS, Williams MB: Lithium and brain signal transduction systems. Biochem Pharmacol 47:429–441, 1994

Jope RS, Song L, Li X, et al: Impaired phosphoinositide hydrolysis in Alzheimer's disease brain. Neurobiol Aging 15:221–226, 1994a

Jope RS, Song L, Powers R: Agonist-induced, GTP-dependent, phosphoinositide hydrolysis in postmortem human brain membranes. J Neurochem 62:180–186, 1994b

Jope RS, Song L, Powers R: [^{3}H]Phosphatidylinositol hydrolysis in postmortem human brain membranes is mediated by the G-proteins Gq/11 and phospholipase C-β. Biochem J 304:655–659, 1994c

Jope RS, Song L, Li PP, et al: The phosphoinositide signal transduction system is impaired in bipolar affective disorder brain. J Neurochem 66:2402–2409, 1996

Jope RS, Song L, Grimes CA, et al: Selective increases in phosphoinositide signaling activity and G-protein levels in postmortem brain from subjects with schizophrenia or alcohol dependence. J Neurochem 70:763–771, 1998

Kalasapudi VD, Sheftel G, Divish MM, et al: Lithium augments fos protooncogene expression in PC12 pheochromocytoma cells: implications for therapeutic action of lithium. Brain Res 521:47–54, 1990

Kofman O, Belmaker RH: Biochemical, behavioral, and clinical studies of the role of inositol in lithium treatment and depression. Biol Psychiatry 34:839–852, 1993

Lenox RH, Watson DG, Patel J, et al: Chronic lithium administration alters a prominent PKC substrate in rat hippocampus. Brain Res 570:333–340, 1992

Lesort M, Jope RS, Johnson GVW: Insulin biphasically modulates tau phosphorylation: involvement of glycogen synthase kinase-3β and fyn tyrosine kinase. J Neurochem 72:576–584, 1999

Li PP, Tam Y-K, Young LT, et al: Lithium decreases Gs, Gi-1 and Gi-2 α-subunit mRNA levels in rat cortex. Eur J Pharmacol 206:165–166, 1991

Li X, Jope RS: Selective inhibition of the expression of signal transduction proteins by lithium in nerve growth factor-differentiated PC12 cells. J Neurochem 65:2500–2508, 1995

Li X, Mumby SM, Greenwood AF, et al: Pertussis toxin-sensitive G-protein α-subunits: production of monoclonal antibodies and detection of differential increases upon differentiation of PC12 and LA-N-5 cells. J Neurochem 64:1107–1117, 1995

Li X, Greenwood AF, Powers R, et al: Effects of postmortem interval, age, and Alzheimer's disease on G-proteins in human brain. Neurobiol Aging 17:115–122, 1996

Lu R, Song L, Jope RS: Lithium attenuates p53 levels in human neuroblastoma SH-SY5Y cells. NeuroReport 10:1123–1125, 1999

Manji HK: G proteins: implications for psychiatry. Am J Psychiatry 149:746–760, 1992

Manji HK, Lenox RH: Long-term action of lithium: a role for transcriptional and posttranscriptional factors regulated by protein kinase C. Synapse 16:11–28, 1994

Manji HK, Etcheberrigaray R, Chen G, et al: Lithium decreases membrane-associated protein kinase C in hippocampus: selectivity for the α isozyme. J Neurochem 61: 2303–2310, 1993

Morrisett RA, Jope RS, Snead OC: Status epilepticus is produced by administration of cholinergic agonists to lithium treated rats: comparison with kainic acid. Exp Neurol 98:594–605, 1987

Ormandy GC, Song L, Jope R: Analysis of the convulsant-potentiating effects of lithium in rats. Exp Neurol 111:356–361, 1991

Pacheco MA, Jope RS: Phosphoinositide signaling in human brain. Prog Neurobiol 50:255–273, 1996

Pacheco MA, Jope RS: Modulation of carbachol-stimulated AP-1 DNA binding activity by agents therapeutic for bipolar disorder in human neuroblastoma SH-SY5Y cells. Mol Brain Res (in press)

Pacheco MA, Stockmeier C, Meltzer HY, et al: Alterations in phosphoinositide signaling and G-protein levels in depressed suicide brain. Brain Res 723:37–45, 1996

Sherman WR, Gish BG, Honchar MP, et al: Effects of lithium on phosphoinositide metabolism in vivo. Federation Proceedings 45:2639–2646, 1986

Tricklebank MD, Singh L, Jackson A, et al: Evidence that a proconvulsant action of lithium is mediated by inhibition of myo-inositol phosphatase in mouse brain. Brain Res 558:145–148, 1991

Unlap MT, Jope RS: Lithium attenuates NGF-induced activation of AP-1 DNA binding activity in PC12 cells. Neuropsychopharmacology 17:12–17, 1997

Warsh JJ, Mathews R, Young LT, et al: Brain Gαq/11 and phospholipase C-β1 immunoreactivity in bipolar affective disorder (abstract). Can J Physiol Pharmacol 72:545, 1994

Williams MB, Jope RS: Distinctive rat brain immediate early gene responses to seizures induced by lithium plus pilocarpine. Molecular Brain Research 25:80–89, 1994a

Williams MB, Jope RS: Lithium potentiates phosphoinositide-linked 5-HT receptor stimulation in vivo. NeuroReport 5:1118–1120, 1994b

Williams MB, Jope RS: Circadian variation in rat brain AP-1 DNA binding activity after cholinergic stimulation: modulation by lithium. Psychopharmacology (Berl) 122:363–368, 1995a

Williams MB, Jope RS: Modulation by inositol of cholinergic and serotonergic-induced seizures in lithium-treated rats. Brain Res 685:169–178, 1995b

Xie H, Litersky JM, Hartigan JA, et al: The interrelationship between selective tau phosphorylation and microtubule association. Brain Res 798:173–183, 1998

Young LT, Li PP, Kish SJ, et al: Postmortem cerebral cortex $G_s\alpha$-subunit levels are elevated in bipolar affective disorder. Brain Res 553:323–326, 1991

CHAPTER 9

A MOLECULAR TARGET FOR THE LONG-TERM ACTION OF LITHIUM IN THE BRAIN

A Phosphoprotein Substrate of Protein Kinase C

Robert H. Lenox, M.D., Robert K. McNamara, Ph.D., and David G. Watson, Ph.D.

LITHIUM AND THE PATHOBIOLOGY OF BIPOLAR DISORDER

For the past several years, ongoing studies in our laboratory have been focused on identifying molecular targets for the therapeutic action of lithium in the brain in the treatment of bipolar disorder. Bipolar disorder predisposes patients to a periodic clinical manifestation of prominent changes in affective state that have been attributed to a biological vulnerability for dysregulation in critical brain regions related to the limbic system and associated cortical and subcortical areas (Goodwin and Jamison 1990; Lenox 1987). Although most

We would like to acknowledge the dedicated technical support of Ms. Rebeca Olarte and Ms. Sharlynn Sweeney. We also would like to thank Dr. Alan Aderem for providing the murine MARCKS cDNA and Mr. Nikolas Karkanias for his assistance with Figure 9–1. We would like to express our appreciation to Mrs. Angela C. Carter for her secretarial support in preparation of the manuscript. These studies were supported in part by National Institute of Mental Health Grant MH-50105.

previous drug development efforts have been aimed at the treatment of the affective states of mania or depression, the unique clinical action of lithium is its ability to prophylactically stabilize the underlying disease process by effectively reducing the frequency and severity of the profound mood cycling in in the majority of patients with classical bipolar I disorder (Lenox and Manji 1995; Manji et al. 1995). Reasonable evidence suggests that once the disease process has been triggered and clinically manifest, long-term adaptive changes in the central nervous system set the stage for predisposing an individual to more frequent and severe affective episodes over time (Post et al. 1992). It is also well recognized that the most efficacious pharmacological treatments for both mania and depression have a significant delay in their onset of action, and clinically relevant behavioral changes persist beyond treatment discontinuation (Suppes et al. 1991).

Dysregulation of transsynaptic signaling would appear to be a likely physiological process accounting for the often wild oscillations in behavioral states associated with bipolar disorder (Hudson et al. 1993; Lenox 1987); and neuroplastic events associated with neurotransmission may represent the biological mechanism for the long-term nature of the physiological changes associated with both the progression of the disease and the pharmacological properties of treatments. Thus, unlike drug treatments for depression or psychosis, a better understanding of the molecular targets for the long-term action of lithium in the brain at clinically relevant therapeutic concentrations may lead us to a better psychopharmacological approach and, in concert with molecular genetic strategies, also may bring us closer to the pathogenesis of the disorder.

LITHIUM AND PHOSPHOINOSITIDE SIGNALING

Numerous studies, including our own, over the past several years have confirmed that receptor-coupled phosphatidylinositol 4,5-bisphosphate (PIP_2) hydrolysis, which generates two second messengers (inositol 1,4,5-trisphosphate [IP_3], which mobilizes intracellular calcium, and diacylglycerol [DAG], which activates protein kinase C [PKC]), is an important site for the acute action of lithium in the brain (for reviews, see Berridge 1989; Lenox and Manji 1995; Manji and Lenox 1994; Rana and Hokin 1990). Lithium, by virtue of an interaction with one of two magnesium (Mg^{2+}) enzyme binding sites, is an uncompetitive inhibitor of inositol 1-monophosphatase (IMPase), which catalyzes the breakdown of the inositol polyphosphates and the generation of free inositol (Atack et al. 1995; Pollack et al. 1994; Figure 9–1; see also Atack, Chapter 1, in this volume). Because the brain has limited access to inositol other than that derived from recycling of the inositol polyphosphates and because the affinity of phosphatidylinositol (PI) synthase is relatively low, Berridge et al. (1989) suggested that a major physiological consequence of lithium's action is derived through a depletion of free inositol required to recombine with cytidine monophosphate (CMP)–phosphatidate to replenish the phosphoinositide signaling pool (see Manji et al., Chapter 7, and Jope et al., Chapter 8, in this volume). Thus, lithium might be expected to be most effective in systems undergoing the highest rate of receptor-mediated PIP_2 hydrolysis. As a consequence of inositol depletion in the presence of lithium, receptor-mediated accumulation of DAG or CMP-phosphatidate has been observed in several cell types and in the brain. This increase is reversed by the addition of inositol (Downes and Stone 1986; Drummond and Raeburn 1984; Godfrey 1989). Our laboratory and others have used agonist-induced accumulation of CMP-phosphatidate in both cell models and brain as a sensitive index of intracellular inositol deficiency during activation of receptor-coupled phospholipase C (PLC) pathways (Jenkinson et al. 1994; Kennedy et al. 1990; Lenox and Watson 1994; Stubbs and Agranoff 1993). We therefore hypothesized that the action of chronic lithium may stem initially from its potent effects in inhibiting the recycling of inositol through the receptor-mediated hydrolysis of PIP_2 and ultimately may be explained by its indirect action in accumulating DAG (Lenox 1987, 1988) and subsequent change in the activation of PKC (isozymes), altering the relative "constitutive phosphorylation" of key phosphoprotein substrates (Figure 9–1).

MYRISTOYLATED ALANINE-RICH C KINASE SUBSTRATE

One PKC substrate is the myristoylated alanine-rich C kinase substrate (MARCKS) (see reviews by Aderem 1992; Blackshear 1993). Genes encoding MARCKS have been cloned and sequenced from rodent (Erusalimsky et al. 1991), bovine (Stumpo et al. 1989), and human sources (Harlan et al. 1991). Sequence analysis of the protein from different species has identified two highly conserved functional domains (Blackshear 1993). The protein contains a consensus sequence for cotranslational myristoylation, which plays an important role in anchoring the protein to the membrane, and a phosphorylation site domain, which has been identified as the site of interaction with both the binding of calmodulin and the cross-linking of actin (Graff et al. 1989a; Hartwig et al. 1992). PKC-mediated phosphorylation of MARCKS in vitro appears to occur at three of the four serine residues within the lysine-rich phosphorylation site domain and is catalyzed by multiple PKC isozymes with the exception of ζ

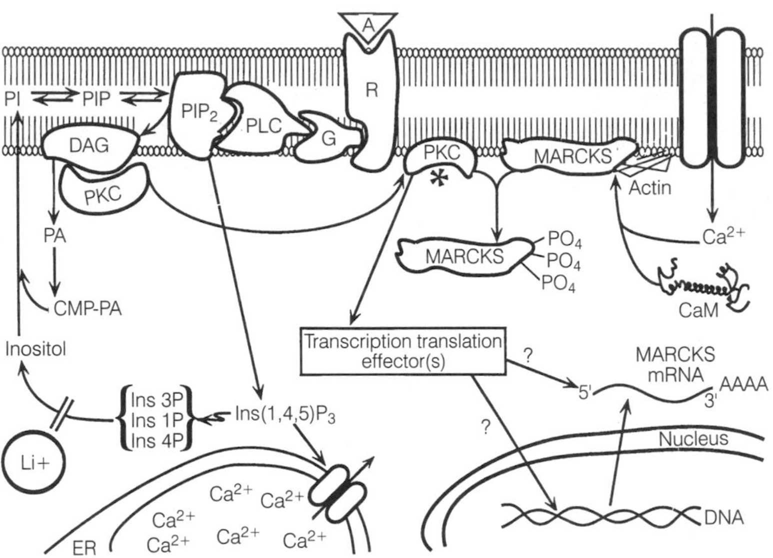

Figure 9–1. Proposed model for lithium (Li^+) regulation of myristoylated alanine-rich C kinase substrate (MARCKS). Agonist (A) occupancy of the receptor (R) binding site results in G-protein (G)–mediated coupling and activation of phospholipase C (PLC), which induces the hydrolysis of phosphatidylinositol 4,5-bisphosphate (PIP_2) and the generation of two second messengers: diacylglycerol (DAG) and *myo*-inositol 1,4,5- trisphosphate [Ins(1,4,5)P_3]. Ins(1,4,5)P_3 binds to receptors in the endoplasmic reticulum (ER) and releases intracellular calcium (Ca^{2+}). DAG is an endogenous activator of protein kinase C (PKC). Lithium inhibits the enzyme inositol 1-monophosphatase (IMPase), which prevents the recycling of inositol, resulting in an accumulation of metabolites in the DAG pathway during stimulation of receptor signaling. Activation of PKC* initiates a number of post-translational events, including translocation of PKC to the membrane, where it can phosphorylate the MARCKS protein, which then translocates to the cytosolic fraction. In the phosphorylated form, MARCKS no longer binds calmodulin (CaM) or cross-link actin, altering compartmental intracellular calcium signaling and affecting cytoskeletal restructuring. In addition, in the presence of chronic lithium and receptor activation, there is a downregulation of MARCKS protein expression, which may result from destabilization of MARCKS messenger RNA (mRNA) via phosphoprotein effector interactions, as yet unknown, with the 3′ -untranslated region (3′ -UTR). *Note.* PI = phosphoinositide; PO_4 = phosphate; Ins 3P, Ins 1P, Ins 4P = inositol phosphates; CMP-PA = cytidine monophosphorylphosphatidate; AAAA = polyadenylation.

(Fujise et al. 1994; Heemskerk et al. 1993). In addition, relative to other major PKC substrates in brain (i.e., GAP-43 and neurogranin), MARCKS is a preferred substrate for a mixed preparation of PKC isozymes α, β, and γ (Sheu et al. 1995).

MARCKS protein has been shown to be reversibly phosphorylated by several pharmacological agents and growth-promoting factors, including muscarinic agonists, vasopressin, bradykinin, endothelin, platelet-derived growth factor, and phorbol ester, all of which activate PKC through different signal transduction pathways (Blackshear et al. 1987; Erusalimsky and Rozengurt 1989; Erusalimsky et al. 1988; Herget and Rozengurt 1994; Isacke et al. 1986; Issandou and Rozengurt 1990; Rodnight and Perrett 1986; Rodriguez-Pena et al. 1986; Zachary et al. 1986). An important feature of MARCKS is its stimulation-dependent translocation between the cytoplasmic and membrane fractions, which is regulated by PKC-mediated phosphorylation (Allen and Aderem 1995; Rosen et al. 1990; Swierczynski and Blackshear 1995; Thelen et al. 1991). As a result, the subcellular distribution of the MARCKS protein has been implicated in the regulation of physiological events such as signal transduction and neurotransmitter release in the brain (Rodriguez-Pena et al. 1986; Wang et al. 1988, 1989). The calcium dependent binding of calmodulin to MARCKS is inhibited by phosphorylation, thereby making this protein potentially instrumental in coordinating PKC and calcium activation through redistribution of calmodulin for appropriate regulation of intracellular signaling (Graff et al. 1989b; Lui et al. 1994; Mangels and Gnegy 1990; McIlroy et al. 1991; Sawai et al. 1993). Furthermore, by virtue of its action in cross-linking actin filaments at the plasma membrane (Hartwig et al. 1992), MARCKS protein may play a significant role in translating extracellular signals to calcium-calmodulin–dependent and PKC-regulated intracellular events associated with actin-plasticity and actin–plasma membrane interaction.

MARCKS is enriched in neuronal growth cones and is highly expressed in brain during postnatal development (McNamara and Lenox 1998; Wees et al. 1998), and mutant mice not expressing MARCKS exhibit abnormal brain development characterized by collosal and commisural axon agenesis and cortical lamination abnormalities (Stumpo et al. 1995; Swierczynski et al. 1996). Immunohistochemical and in situ hybridization studies in adult rat brain have found MARCKS to be preferentially expressed in regions associated with a high degree of retained plasticity, including the hippocampus, amygdala, and hypothalamus, and is localized to small dendritic branches and axon terminals (McNamara and Lenox 1997; Ouimet et al. 1990). In the mature central nervous system, MARCKS expression is elevated during axonal regeneration (Schnizer et al. 1997), and adult mutant mice expressing MARCKS at 50% exhibit significant spatial learning deficits that are transgenically "rescued" (McNamara et al. 1998). Moreover, the induction of hippocampal long-term potentiation, a physiological model of activity-dependent synaptic plasticity, produces a significant elevation in MARCKS phosphorylation (Ramakers et al., in press). Collectively, these data suggest that MARCKS is an important determinant of neuronal plasticity during development as well as in the mature brain. Its reduction following the long-term administration of lithium may therefore alter neuroplastic events to stabilize aberrant neuronal activity in key brain regions.

LITHIUM, PROTEIN KINASE C, AND MARCKS

Studies in our laboratory have found that MARCKS may represent a molecular target for the action of chronic lithium in the brain (Lenox et al. 1992). In rats chronically exposed to lithium, resulting in clinically relevant therapeutic levels (1 mM) in brain, we observed a major reduction in the in vitro PKC-mediated phosphorylation of two major substrates, 83 kDa and 45 kDa, in the hippocampus. Although we found no evidence for significant changes in the total PKC activity or its subcellular distribution in hippocampal slices prepared from these animals, subsequent studies have reported a reduction in the PKCα isozyme in the hippocampus of rats exposed to chronic lithium in a similar model (Manji et al. 1993). Western blot analysis identified the 83-kDa phosphoprotein as MARCKS. In vivo levels of MARCKS in rat hippocampus were significantly reduced after chronic lithium exposure (Figure 9–2). Additionally, the reduction in MARCKS protein expression persisted in animals withdrawn from lithium for 40 hours. Under these withdrawal conditions, lithium serum levels were well below therapeutic levels. Finally, the down-regulation in MARCKS protein expression was not observed in animals after acute (2-hour) lithium chloride (LiCl) treatment. In light of the potential role of PKC substrates such as MARCKS in signal transduction and the fact that changes in the intracellular concentration of MARCKS appear to parallel the time course of the clinical action of lithium, we suggested the possible involvement of these proteins in lithium's mechanism of action in the treatment of bipolar disorder.

LITHIUM-INDUCED REGULATION OF MARCKS PROTEIN IN HN33 CELLS

To further investigate the long-term action of lithium in the brain, and to examine its role in the regulation of MARCKS, we selected a cell system that was

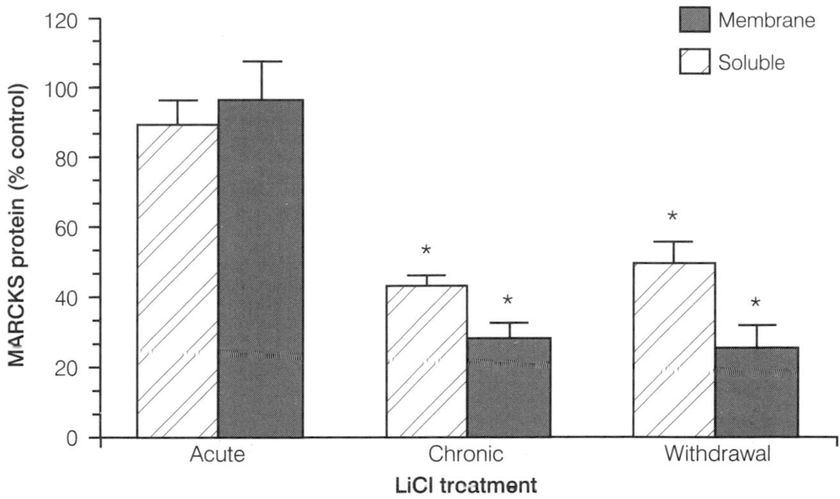

Figure 9–2. Chronic lithium–induced downregulation of myristoylated alanine-rich C kinase substrate (MARCKS) protein in rat brain hippocampus. Chronic lithium male Sprague-Dawley rats (*n* = 7) were fed Purina Lab Rat Chow containing 1.70 g/kg lithium chloride (LiCl) for 2 weeks, followed by diet containing 2.55 g/kg LiCl for an additional 2 weeks. Control animals received standard diet under parallel conditions. Withdrawal animals (*n* = 3) received the above treatment with lithium and were returned to control diet 40 hours before sacrifice. Acute lithium rats (*n* = 3) receiving an intraperitoneal injection of LiCl (5 mEq/kg body weight) were sacrificed 2 hours after injection. Following homogenization of the hippocampus, soluble and membrane fractions were prepared and MARCKS protein quantitated by Western blot analysis, as previously described (Lenox et al. 1992). Mean brain lithium levels: acute, 1.20 mM; chronic, 0.92 mM; withdrawal, 0.13 mM. Value represents mean ± SD. *Significantly different from acute group, $P < 0.001$.

devoid of the limitations of in vivo studies but that retained the potential for physiologically relevant research. For these studies, we used the HN33 immortalized hippocampal cell line derived from the somatic cell fusion of primary hippocampal neurons and N18TG2 neuroblastoma cell. These cells have morphological and cytoskeletal features that are typical of neuronal cells but that are not expressed by neuroblastoma cells. These cells also have electrophysiological features similar to those of hippocampal cells in culture (Lee et al. 1990). We identified the MARCKS protein in the HN33 cells by Western blot and found that it was located in both the soluble and the membrane fractions, with predominant (75%–80%) localization in the soluble fraction under resting conditions. Furthermore, we found that exposure of HN33 cells to phorbol esters rapidly downregulated PKC activity, leading to a PKC-dependent downregulation in MARCKS protein levels (Watson et al. 1994), similar to findings in nonneuronal cells (Brooks et al. 1991; Linder et al. 1992). The immortalized hippocampal HN33 cell line, therefore, appears to be an excellent in vitro model in which to examine the effects of chronic lithium on PKC and PKC substrate (i.e., MARCKS) regulation in the brain and to address the hypothesis that these effects are related to the known action of lithium on receptor-mediated PI hydrolysis and long-term changes in PKC regulation.

We demonstrated that chronic exposure of HN33 cells to LiCl (1–10 mM) produces a dose- and time-dependent downregulation of MARCKS protein (Table 9–1) (Watson and Lenox 1996). Maximum reduction in MARCKS protein levels was observed in cells in inositol-deficient media exposed to lithium for 7–10 days. Although a lithium-induced reduction in MARCKS protein was evident in the soluble fraction even at 1 mM under these resting conditions, significant reductions in MARCKS protein were observed in both the soluble and the membrane fractions after exposure to 5 and 10 mM of lithium. The lithium-induced reduction in MARCKS was dependent on the inositol concentration present in the medium, with as little as 0.1 mM of *myo*-inositol preventing the lithium downregulation of MARCKS protein levels. In addition, we determined that lithium-induced downregulation of MARCKS protein is reversed over a similar period of time by removing lithium from the medium or by adding high concentrations of inositol (10 mM).

Although lithium is a potent uncompetitive inhibitor of IMPase, this property is not shared by other members of the alkali metal family (sodium [Na^+], rubidium [Rb^+], cesium [Cs^+]). To demonstrate the specificity of lithium's effect on MARCKS protein downregulation, HN33 cells were exposed to rubidium chloride (RbCl) under the same conditions used with long-term

Table 9–1. Lithium-induced downregulation of MARCKS protein in HN33 cells[a]

LiCl (mM)	MARCKS protein, % controls (±SEM)[b]	
	Soluble	Membrane
1.0	63.4 (8.2)*	88.9 (4.7)
5.0	55.5 (5.0)*	76.1 (7.3)*
10.0	36.2 (5.7)*	51.0 (2.1)*

Note. MARCKS = myristoylated alanine-rich C kinase substrate. LiCl = lithium chloride.
[a]HN33 cells were grown in inositol-free Dulbecco's modified Eagle Medium (DMEM) containing 5% fetal bovine serum (FBS).
[b]MARCKS protein levels were determined by Western blot analysis following 10 days of LiCl exposure and are expressed as the percentage of MARCKS protein in cells cultured in the absence of LiCl. *$P < 0.01$, Fisher (PLSD) test (compared with controls, defined as 100%).

LiCl exposure. Following both acute- and long-term RbCl exposure, MARCKS protein levels were measured with Western blot analysis. Results of these experiments are shown in Table 9–2. Neither short- (1 day) nor long-term (3–7 days) exposure of HN33 cells to RbCl at concentrations of 1–10 mM had a significant effect on the expression of MARCKS protein. There was also no evidence for RbCl-induced alteration of MARCKS protein cellular distribution.

These data are consistent with our hypothesis that the action of chronic lithium may stem from its known acute effects of inhibiting the recycling of inositol through the receptor-mediated hydrolysis of PIP_2 and that the activation of PKC isozyme activities (via accumulation of metabolites in the DAG pathway) results in a cascade of events leading to MARCKS protein downregulation.

LITHIUM, INOSITOL, AND SPECIFICITY OF ACTION IN THE BRAIN

Our hypothesis for the mechanism of action of lithium as outlined earlier in this chapter and diagrammed in Figure 9–1 rests on several related events that have direct and indirect support: 1) lithium inhibition of IMPase, 2) activated receptor-coupled PI hydrolysis, 3) relative depletion of inositol, 4) relative in-

Table 9–2. MARCKS protein expression in HN33 cells following RbCl exposure[a]

Length of exposure (days)	RbCl (mM)	MARCKS protein, % controls[b]	
		Soluble	Membrane
1	1.0	98.7	95.9
	10.0	102.2	101.8
3	1.0	104.8	102.4
	10.0	100.6	92.3
7	1.0	93.5	98.9
	10.0	87.6	99.6

Note. MARCKS = myristoylated alanine-rich C kinase substrate. RbCl = rubidium chloride.
[a]HN33 cells were grown in inositol-free Dulbecco's modified Eagle Medium (DMEM) containing 5% fetal bovine serum (FBS).
[b]MARCKS protein levels were determined by Western blot analysis and are expressed as the percentage of MARCKS protein in cells cultured in the absence of RbCl. The data represent the mean of two separate experiments.

crease in DAG and/or CMP-phosphatidate, 5) DAG activation of PKC isozymes, and 6) phosphorylation and downregulation of MARCKS. Ample evidence indicates that lithium is an active uncompetitive inhibitor of IMPase, with an IC_{50} (0.1–0.8 mM) well within its therapeutic range, but the conditions under which one can observe relative inositol depletion in brain remain to be identified. Brain concentrations of *myo*-inositol have been estimated to be as high as 10 mM, and because PI synthase has a K_m of 0.8–1.0 mM for inositol, a relative reduction of approximately 10-fold would be required to significantly alter either PI resynthesis or DAG/CMP-phosphatidate accumulation. However, studies performed in our laboratory and others lend considerable support to our hypothesis that it is just this relative depletion of inositol in the presence of therapeutically relevant concentrations of lithium that will in part determine the specificity of lithium action to selective brain regions and neuronal cell populations.

First, as noted in an earlier section, the brain has limited access to exogenous inositol other than that derived from PI cycling. Moreover, as Gani et al. (1993) elegantly outlined, inositol homeostasis is cell specific and dependent on the presence of activated uptake mechanisms and the relative activity of inositol influx versus efflux. Furthermore, sodium-dependent inositol transport systems can be regulated by agonist stimulation, as is the case for 1321N astrocytoma cells in which receptor-PLC activation inhibits inositol uptake via calcium and/or PKC-dependent mechanisms. Second, Gray et al. (1994) observed in three different cell types differential effects of lithium on muscarinic-stimulated CMP-phosphatidate accumulation, which were critically dependent on cellular inositol homeostasis. Their findings also suggested that whereas glial cells were able to maintain intracellular concentrations considerably in excess of the medium, neuronal cells do not contain a significant reserve of free intracellular *myo*-inositol. Similar findings of differences in inositol and PI metabolism between neuronal and glial cells were reported by Glanville et al. (1989). Bevilacqua et al. (1994) used autoradiographic approaches in brain slices to show that inositol-reversible receptor-mediated accumulation of labeled CMP-phosphatidate in the presence of lithium is preferentially localized to neuronal populations as compared with glia in both hippocampus and neocortex. Thus, despite the high reported values of inositol in brain, much of the inositol may be associated with either nonneuronal or selective neuronal populations within the brain that may confer relative insensitivity for lithium-induced inositol depletion. In accordance with this premise, the receptor-stimulated accumulation of CMP-phosphatidate in brain in the presence of lithium apparently is dependent on not only the brain region under examination but also the specific receptor-coupled PI response (Heacock et al. 1993).

POTENTIATION OF LITHIUM-INDUCED MARCKS REGULATION: RECEPTOR ACTIVATION

Studies in our laboratory have confirmed the presence of populations of muscarinic receptors coupled to the PI signaling pathway in our subclone of the HN33 cells. In cells exposed to chronic lithium, stimulation of the muscarinic receptor–mediated PI hydrolysis pathway by the addition of carbachol to the medium potentiated the lithium-induced downregulation of MARCKS. Significant reductions in MARCKS protein were observed in both the soluble and the membrane fractions of these activated cells in the presence of inositol and as little as 1 mM of lithium (Figure 9–3). The MARCKS downregulation, however, was dependent on the relative concentrations of inositol present in the medium. In these experiments, the downregulation of MARCKS induced by carbachol stimulation and 1 mM of lithium was apparent even in the presence of added inositol (0.5 μM) but was prevented by the addition of 5.0 μM of inositol (Figure 9–4). These data provide evidence that downregulation of the PKC substrate MARCKS may be a consequence of lithium-induced intracellular inositol depletion in cells experiencing high and persistent activation of receptor-mediated PI hydrolysis and inositol recycling. These data lend further support to our hypothesis that the specificity of lithium's therapeutic action may lie within selective brain regions and signaling pathways unique to the pathobiology of bipolar disorder, in which the following are seen: 1) an increase in receptor activation, 2) therapeutic concentrations of lithium, 3) a relative depletion of inositol, and 4) the expression of MARCKS protein. Under these conditions, our data showed the downstream effects of chronic lithium on the regulation of MARCKS expression, which we believe is a key to the neuroplastic events associated with the long-term action of lithium in stabilization of patients with bipolar disorder.

EFFECT OF VALPROATE AND CARBAMAZEPINE ON MARCKS PROTEIN EXPRESSION

Although lithium remains the drug of choice for the treatment of classic forms of bipolar disorder, anticonvulsant drugs such as valproate (VPA) and carbamazepine (CBZ) have become popular alternative treatments in clinical practice, especially for patients with atypical or rapid-cycling bipolar illness. In

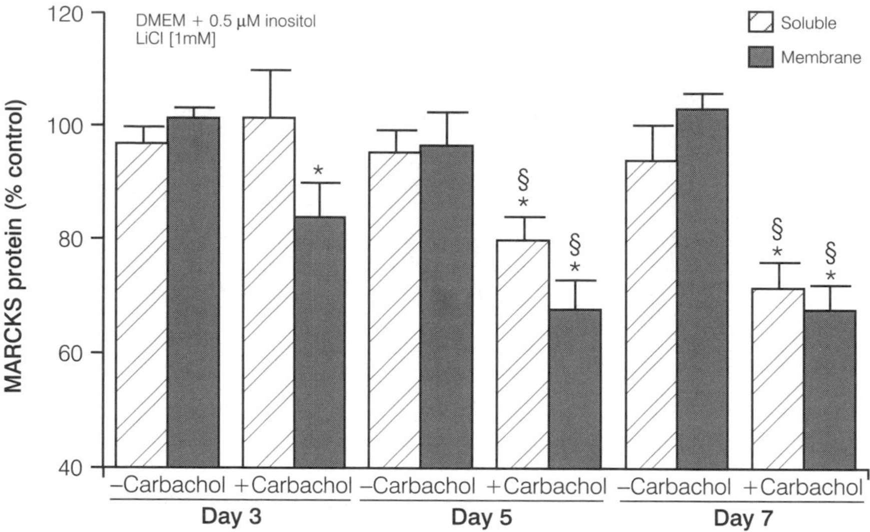

Figure 9–3. Time course of carbachol-stimulated lithium-induced down-regulation of myristoylated alanine-rich C kinase substrate (MARCKS) protein in HN33 cells. Cells were exposed to 1 mM of lithium chloride (LiCl) in Dulbecco's modified Eagle Medium (DMEM) containing 0.5 μM *myo*-inositol, with or without 1 mM carbachol. Cells were collected following 3, 5, or 7 days of exposure. Soluble and membrane fractions were prepared and MARCKS protein quantitated by Western blot analysis. Results are expressed as the percentage of MARCKS protein in cells cultured in the same medium in the absence of lithium (mean ± SD). *Significantly different from carbachol group, $P < 0.01$. §Significantly different from day 3 group, $P < 0.01$.

particular, the therapeutic efficacy of the anticonvulsant drugs such as VPA, a simple branched-chain carboxylic acid, was approved by the U.S. Food and Drug Administration (FDA) in 1995 as an effective alternative treatment of acute mania, particularly for patients not responding to lithium (Bowden et al. 1994; Calabrese and Delucchi 1989). As with lithium, the mechanisms mediating the therapeutic properties of VPA are poorly understood. Moreover, whether the therapeutic effects of VPA and lithium are mediated by a common mechanism is an intriguing question; however, definitive studies documenting its efficacy in the prophylaxis of recurrent affective episodes in patients with bipolar disorder remain to be carried out. Indeed, both lithium and VPA have a delayed onset as well as residual activity after treatment discontinuation, suggesting that both drugs might exert their effects via long-term neuroplastic events in the brain. In light of our data related to lithium, the MARCKS protein is a candidate target that also may be affected by VPA.

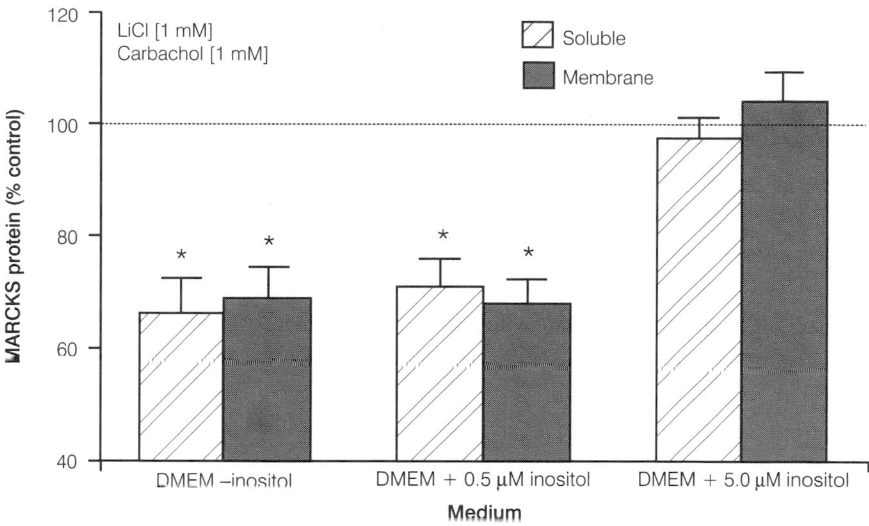

Figure 9–4. Effect of carbachol and *myo*-inositol on the lithium-induced downregulation of myristoylated alanine-rich C kinase substrate (MARCKS) protein in HN33 cells. Cells were exposed to 1 mM of lithium chloride (LiCl) in Dulbecco's modified Eagle Medium (DMEM) lacking inositol or in medium containing 0.5 or 5.0 μM of *myo*-inositol and 1 mM of carbachol. Following 7 days of exposure, soluble and membrane fractions were prepared and MARCKS protein quantitated by Western blot analysis. Results are expressed as the percentage of MARCKS protein in cells cultured in the same medium in the absence of lithium (mean ± SD). *Significantly different from 5.0 μM inositol group, $P < 0.01$.

To examine the effects of VPA or CBZ on MARCKS protein expression, HN33 cells were grown in inositol-free Dulbecco's modified Eagle Medium (DMEM) supplemented with 5% fetal bovine serum and exposed to 0.5, 1.0, or 1.5 mM of VPA or 10, 25, or 100 μM of CBZ for up to 7 days. Recommended therapeutic plasma concentrations for VPA are in the range of 0.8 mM and for CBZ are in the range of 50 μM. Following VPA or CBZ exposure, soluble and membrane fractions were prepared by centrifugation at 100,000 × *g*. MARCKS protein levels were measured with Western blot analysis by using a rabbit polyclonal MARCKS antiserum and quantitated by scanning laser densitometric analysis. Chronic (3–7 days), but not acute (1 day), exposure to VPA resulted in the downregulation of MARCKS protein levels in both the soluble and the membrane fractions of HN33 cells (Table 9–3). In comparison, there was no evidence for CBZ-induced alterations in MARCKS protein expression or intracellular distribution. Additional studies have subsequently demonstrated that this property of regulation of MARCKS expression is not

Table 9–3. MARCKS protein levels in HN33 cells following exposure to valproate or carbamazepine[a]

Drug and amount	Exposure (days)	MARCKS protein, % controls[b]	
Valproate (mM)		Soluble	Membrane
0.5	1	102.1	98.3
1.0	1	95.4	94.9
0.5	3	90.5	44.5
1.0	3	76.8	62.0
1.5	3	60.2	20.2
0.5	7	66.8	71.4
1.0	7	54.3	60.0
Carbamazepine (μM)			
10.0	3	103.8	94.5
25.0	3	94.2	96.1
100.0	3	109.0	89.2
10.0	7	103.6	94.0
25.0	7	99.8	91.1
100.0	7	104.3	88.5

Note. MARCKS = myristoylated alanine-rich C kinase substrate.

[a]HN33 cells were grown in inositol-free Dulbecco's modified Eagle Medium (DMEM) containing 5% fetal bovine serum (FBS).

[b]MARCKS protein levels were determined by Western blot analysis and are expressed as the percentage of MARCKS protein in cells cultured in the absence of drug. The data represent the mean of two separate experiments.

shared by a number of drugs in other classes of psychotropic agents, including opiates, benzodiazepines, and neuroleptics (Watson et al. 1998).

The effects of VPA we observed on MARCKS protein levels in the HN33 hippocampal cell are similar to preliminary findings in the C6 glioma cell line (Chen et al. 1994; G. Chen, personal communication, 1995). In their study, 3- to 7-day exposure to therapeutic concentrations of VPA produced a decrease in total PKC activity, a selective reduction in the immunolabeling of PKCα and PKCε, and a decrease in the immunolabeling of MARCKS protein in both the membrane and the soluble fractions. The observed effects on MARCKS protein were not found after 1-day exposure. These data suggest that VPA and lithium may share a common site of action, via a PKC-dependent regulation of MARCKS protein expression in brain. However, because little evidence supports an action of VPA on phosphoinositide signaling, the precise mechanism of the PKC interaction for these two drugs likely differs.

LOCALIZATION OF MARCKS MESSENGER RNA IN RAT BRAIN HIPPOCAMPUS BY IN SITU HYBRIDIZATION

As noted earlier in this chapter (see section, "Lithium, Protein Kinase C, and MARCKS"), our laboratory demonstrated that chronic, but not acute, in vivo lithium treatment resulted in a dramatic reduction in hippocampal MARCKS protein levels in rats (Lenox et al. 1992). These findings are of particular interest in that the hippocampal formation has been implicated as a region that may contribute to bipolar symptoms. For example, manic patients show a significant reduction in the volume of the right hippocampus (Swayze et al. 1992) and reduced blood flow to the basal region of the right temporal lobe, which houses the hippocampal formation (Migliorelli et al. 1993). Because MARCKS has been implicated in neuroplastic events, including cytoskeletal restructuring, transmembrane signaling, and neurotransmitter release (Blackshear 1993), its reduction in the hippocampus after chronic lithium treatment would be predicted to reduce hippocampal plasticity and function; indeed, a major side effect of lithium treatment associated with noncompliance is a disturbance of cognitive processes, including memory (Lenox and Manji 1995). Whether this effect of lithium on hippocampal plasticity also contributes to its therapeutic efficacy in the treatment of bipolar illness remains to be determined.

Studies conducted in our laboratory have characterized the constitutive distribution of MARCKS messenger RNA (mRNA) in the adult rat hippocampus with in situ hybridization histochemistry. Antisense hybridization indicates that MARCKS mRNA is not uniformly expressed in the adult rat hippocampus: MARCKS hybridization is highest in granule cells, moderate in CA1 pyramidal cells, and low to absent in CA2 and CA3 pyramidal cells and in hilar neurons (Figure 9–5). The distribution of MARCKS mRNA in the hippocampus agrees with the known distribution of MARCKS protein (Ouimet et al. 1990). For example, MARCKS immunoreactivity is high in the hilus, which is the terminal field for numerous granule cell axons and axon collaterals (Claiborne et al. 1986), but absent from the granule cell layer or the molecular layer (granule cell dendrites), indicating localization of the protein to granule cell axons.

Previous reports indicated that MARCKS message levels can be regulated at the posttranscriptional level via PKC-mediated processes. Specifically, activation of PKC with phorbol esters appears to lead to a reduction in the MARCKS mRNA half-life (Brooks et al. 1992; Linder et al. 1992), a finding that is consistent with our report of reduced MARCKS protein expression in

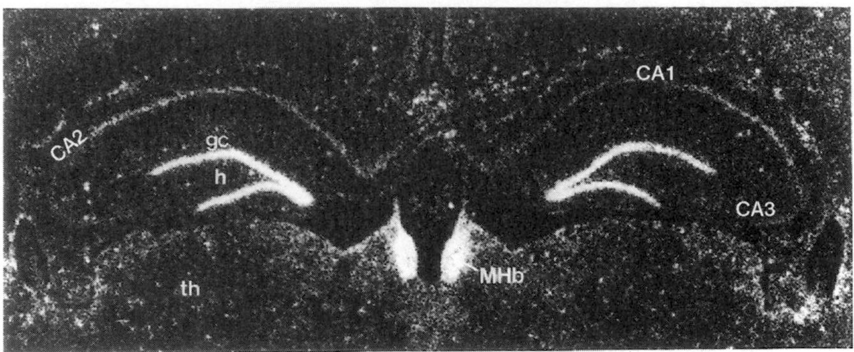

Figure 9–5. Localization of myristoylated alanine-rich C kinase substrate (MARCKS) gene expression in the dorsal hippocampus of the adult rat by in situ hybridization histochemistry. gc = granule cell layer; h = hilus; mHb = medial habenula nucleus; th = thalamus.

immortalized hippocampal neurons after phorbol ester treatment (Watson et al. 1994). If PKC activity regulates MARCKS message levels in vivo, then the constitutive distribution pattern observed in the hippocampal formation could be reflective of regional PKC activity and/or regional localization of specific PKC isozymes. That is, the high expression of MARCKS message in granule cells would indicate either a low level of constitutive PKC activity or the absence of a specific PKC isozyme that selectively interacts with MARCKS message. Conversely, the low level of message expression in CA2 and CA3 pyramidal cells may indicate a high level of constitutive PKC activity or the expression of a specific PKC isozyme. It is noteworthy that the distribution of MARCKS message in the hippocampus is the inverse to the distribution of a second major PKC substrate, GAP-43 (F1, B-50, pp46, P57, neuromodulin), which is also regulated posttranscriptionally by PKC, but its half-life is instead increased by phorbol ester–induced PKC activity (Perrone-Bizzozero et al. 1993). As would be predicted, then, GAP-43 message is highly expressed in CA3 pyramidal cells but is at low to absent levels in granule cells (Meberg and Routtenberg 1991). Determining which PKC isozymes are involved in the regulation of MARCKS message levels in the hippocampus will therefore be of great interest.

CONCLUSION

Our discovery of the lithium-induced regulation of MARCKS offers us a window through which we can begin to understand the downstream molecular effect of long-term lithium on neuroplastic events modulating signaling pathways in critical regions of the brain that may be associated with its therapeutic efficacy in bipolar disorder. The regulation of both the intracellular localization of the MARCKS protein and its expression has become a focus of investigation in several cell systems outside of the brain. Studies using site-directed mutagenesis have highlighted the importance of MARCKS phosphorylation site domain in regulating its membrane/cytosol translocation and have just begun to examine the specificity of the action of PKC isozymes in this event (Swierczynski and Blackshear 1995). As noted in this chapter, studies of fibroblasts indicated that transcription and translation are both required for the phorbol ester–induced downregulation of the MARCKS protein, which may be mediated through a posttranscriptional mechanism involving a destabilization of mRNA. A similar series of studies are under way to examine precisely the mechanism by which chronic lithium induces such a PKC-mediated regulation of the expression of the MARCKS protein in neuronal cell populations and the brain.

REFERENCES

Aderem A: The MARCKS brothers: a family of protein kinase C substrates. Cell 71:713–716, 1992

Allen LH, Aderem A: Protein kinase C regulates MARCKS cycling between the plasma membrane and lysosomes in fibroblasts. EMBO J 14:1109–1121, 1995

Atack JR, Broughton HB, Pollack SJ, et al: Inositol monophosphatase—a putative target for Li^+ in the treatment of bipolar disorder. Trends Neurosci 18:343–349, 1995

Berridge MJ: Inositol triphosphate, calcium, lithium, and cell signaling. JAMA 262:1834–1841, 1989

Berridge MJ, Downes CP, Hanley MR. Neural and developmental actions of lithium: a unifying hypothesis. Cell 59:411–419, 1989

Bevilacqua JA, Downes CP, Lowenstein PR: Visualization of agonist-stimulated inositol phospholipid turnover in individual neurons of the rat cerebral cortex and hippocampus. Neuroscience 60:945–958, 1994

Blackshear PJ: The MARCKS family of cellular protein kinase C substrates. J Biol Chem 268:1501–1504, 1993

Blackshear PJ, Stumpo DJ, Huang J, et al: Protein kinase C-dependent and -independent pathways of proto-oncogene induction in human astrocytoma cells. J Biol Chem 262:7774–7781, 1987

Bowden CL, Brugger AM, Swann AC, et al: Efficacy of divalproex vs. lithium and placebo in the treatment of mania. JAMA 271:918–924, 1994

Brooks SF, Herget T, Erusalimsky JD, et al: Protein kinase C activation potently down-regulates the expression of its major substrate, 80K, in Swiss 3T3 cells. EMBO J 10:2497–2505, 1991

Brooks SF, Herget T, Broad S, et al: The expression of 80K/MARCKS, a major substrate of protein kinase C (PKC), is down-regulated through PKC-dependent and -independent pathways. J Biol Chem 267:14212–14218, 1992

Calabrese JR, Delucchi GA: Phenomenology of rapid cycling manic-depression and its treatment with VPA. J Clin Psychiatry 50:30–34, 1989

Chen G, Manji HK, Hawver DB, et al: Chronic sodium valproate selectively decreases protein kinase C α and ε in vitro. J Neurochem 63:2361–2364, 1994

Claiborne BJ, Amaral DG, Cowan WM: A light and electron microscopic analysis of the mossy fibers of the rat dentate gyrus. J Comp Neurol 246:435–458, 1986

Downes CP, Stone MA: Lithium-induced reduction in intracellular inositol supply in cholinergically stimulated parotid gland. Biochem J 234:199–204, 1986

Drummond AH, Raeburn CA: The interaction of lithium with thyrotropin releasing hormone-stimulated lipid metabolism in GH3 pituitary tumor cells. Biochem J 224:129–136, 1984

Erusalimsky JD, Rozengurt E: Vasopressin rapidly stimulates protein kinase C in digitonin-permeabilized Swiss 3T3 cells: involvement of a pertussis toxin-sensitive guanine nucleotide binding protein. J Cell Physiol 141:253–261, 1989

Erusalimsky JD, Friedberg I, Rozengurt E: Bombesin diacylglycerols, and phorbol esters rapidly stimulate the phosphorylation of an M_r = 80,000 protein kinase C substrate in permeabilized 3T3 cells: effect of guanine nucleotides. J Biol Chem 263:19188–19194, 1988

Erusalimsky JD, Brooks SF, Herget T, et al: Molecular cloning and characterization of the acidic 80-kDa protein kinase C substrate from rat brain. J Biol Chem 266:7073–7080, 1991

Fujise A, Mizuno K, Udea Y, et al: Specificity of the high affinity interaction of protein kinase C with a physiological substrate, myristoylated alanine-rich protein kinase C substrate. J Biol Chem 269:31642–31648, 1994

Gani D, Downes CP, Batty IH, et al: Lithium and *myo*-inositol homeostasis. Biochimica et Biophysica ACTA 1177:253–269, 1993

Glanville NT, Byers DM, Cook HW, et al: Differences in the metabolism of inositol and phosphoinositides by cultured cells of neuronal and glial origin. Biochimica et Biophysica ACTA 1004:169–179, 1989

Godfrey PP: Potentiation by lithium of CMP-phosphatidate formation in carbachol-stimulated rat cerebral-cortical slices and its reversal by *myo*-inositol. Biochem J 258:621–624 1989

Goodwin FK, Jamison KR: Manic-Depressive Illness. New York, Oxford University Press, 1990

Graff JM, Gordon JI, Blackshear PJ: Myristoylated and nonmyristoylated forms of a protein are phosphorylated by protein kinase C. Science 246:503–506, 1989a

Graff JM, Young TM, Johnson JD, et al: Phosphorylation-regulated calmodulin binding to a prominent cellular substrate for protein kinase C. J Biol Chem 264:21818–21823, 1989b

Gray DW, Challiss RAJ, Nahorski SR: Differential effects of lithium on muscarinic cholinoceptor-stimulated CMP-phosphatidate accumulation in cerebellar granule cells, CHO-M3 cells, and SH-SY5Y neuroblastoma cells. J Neurochem 63: 1354–1360, 1994

Harlan DM, Graff JM, Stumpo DJ, et al: The human myristoylated alanine-rich C kinase substrate (MARCKS) gene (MACS). J Biol Chem 266:14399–14405, 1991

Hartwig JH, Thelen M, Rosen A, et al: MARCKS is an actin filament crosslinking protein regulated by protein kinase C and calcium-calmodulin. Nature 356:618–622, 1992

Heacock AM, Seguin EB, Agranoff BW: Measurement of receptor-activated phosphoinositide turnover in rat brain: nonequivalence of inositol phosphate and CDP-diacylglycerol formation. J Neurosci 60:1087–1092, 1993

Heemskerk FM, Chen HC, Huang FL. Protein kinase C phosphorylates Ser^{152}, Ser^{156} and Ser^{163} but not Ser^{160} of MARCKS in rat brain. Biochem Biophys Res Commun 190:236–241, 1993

Herget T, Rozengurt E: Bombesin, endothelin and platelet-derived growth factor induce rapid translocation of the myristoylated alanine-rich C kinase substrate in Swiss 3T3 cells. Eur J Biochem 2254:539–548, 1994

Hudson CJ, Young LT, Li PP, et al: CNS signal transduction in the pathophysiology and pharmacotherapy of affective disorders and schizophrenia. Synapse 13:278–293, 1993

Isacke CM, Meisenhelder J, Brown KD, et al: Early phosphorylation events following the treatment of Swiss 3T3 cells with bombesin and the mammalian bombesin-related peptide, gastrin-releasing peptide. EMBO J 5:2889–2898, 1986

Issandou M, Rozengurt E: Bradykinin transiently activates protein kinase C in Swiss 3T3 cells: distinction from activation by bombesin and vasopressin. J Biol Chem 265:11890–11896, 1990

Jenkinson S, Nahorski SR, Challiss RAJ: Disruption by lithium of phosphatidylinositol-4,5-bisphosphate supply and inositol-1,4,5-trisphosphate generation in chinese hamster ovary cells expressing human recombinant m_1 muscarinic receptors. Mol Pharmacol 46:1138–1148 1994

Kennedy ED, Challiss RAJ, Ragan CI, et al: Reduced inositol polyphosphate accumulation and inositol supply induced by lithium in stimulated cerebral cortex slices. Biochem J 267:781–786, 1990

Lee HJ, Hammond DN, Large TH, et al: Neuronal properties and trophic activities of immortalized hippocampal cells from embryonic and young adult mice. J Neurosci 10:1779–1787, 1990

Lenox RH: Role of receptor coupling to phosphoinositide metabolism in the therapeutic action of lithium. Adv Exp Med Biol 221:515–530, 1987

Lenox RH: Lithium interaction with the phosphoinositide system and protein kinase C in the nervous system, in Progress in Catecholamine Research, Vol 42C. Edited by Belmaker RH, Sandler M, Dahlstrom A. New York, Alan R Liss, 1988, pp 327–335

Lenox RH, Manji HK: Lithium, in The American Psychiatric Press Textbook of Psychopharmacology. Edited by Schatzberg AF, Nemeroff CB. Washington, DC, American Psychiatric Press, 1995, pp 303–349

Lenox RH, Watson DG: Lithium and the brain: a psychopharmacological strategy to a molecular basis for manic-depressive illness. Clin Chem 40:309–314, 1994

Lenox RH, Watson DG, Patel J, et al: Chronic lithium administration alters a prominent PKC substrate in rat hippocampus. Brain Res 570:333–340, 1992

Linder D, Gschwendt M, Marks F: Phorbol ester-induced down-regulation of the 80-kDa myristoylated alanine-rich C-kinase substrate-related protein in Swiss 3T3 fibroblasts. J Biol Chem 267:24–26, 1992

Lui JP, Engler D, Funder JW, et al: Arginine vasopressin (AVP) causes the reversible phosphorylation of the myristoylated alanine-rich C kinase substrate (MARCKS) protein in the ovine anterior pituitary: evidence that MARCKS phosphorylation is associated with adrenocorticotropin (ACTH) secretion. Mol Cell Endocrinol 1055:217–226, 1994

Mangels LA, Gnegy ME: Muscarinic receptor-mediated translocation of calmodulin in SK-N-SH human neuroblastoma cells. Mol Pharmacol 37:820–826, 1990

Manji HK, Lenox RH: Long term action of lithium: a role for transcriptional and post-transcriptional factors regulated by protein kinase C. Synapse 16:11–28, 1994

Manji HK, Etcheberrigaray R, Chen G, et al: Lithium decreases membrane-associated protein kinase C in hippocampus: selectivity for the α-isozyme. J Neurochem 61:2303–2310, 1993

Manji HK, Potter WZ, Lenox RH: Signal transduction pathways; molecular targets for lithium's action. Arch Gen Psychiatry 52:531–543, 1995

McIlroy BK, Walters JD, Blackshear PJ, et al: Phosphorylation-dependent binding of a synthetic MARCKS peptide to calmodulin. J Biol Chem 266:4959–4966, 1991

McNamara RK, Lenox RH: Comparative distribution of myristoylated alanine-rich C kinase substrate (MARCKS) and F1/GAP-43 gene expression in the adult rat brain. J Comp Neurol 379:48–71, 1997

McNamara RK, Lenox RH: Distribution of protein kinase C substrates MARCKS and MRP in the postnatal developing rat brain. J Comp Neurol 397:337–356, 1998

McNamara RK, Stumpo DJ, Morel LM, et al: Effects of reduced myristoylated alanine rich C-kinase substrate expression on spatial learning in mutant mice: transgenic rescue and interaction with gene background. Proc Natl Acad Sci U S A 95:14517–14522, 1998

Meberg PJ, Routtenberg A: Selective expression of protein F1 (GAP-43) mRNA in pyramidal but not granule cells of the hippocampus. Neuroscience 45:721–733, 1991

Migliorelli R, Starkstein SE, Teson A, et al: SPECT findings in patients with primary mania. J Neuropsychiatry Clin Neurosci 5:379–383, 1993

Ouimet CC, Wang JKT, Walaas SI, et al: Localization of the MARCKS (87 kDa) protein, a major specific substrate for the protein kinase C, in rat brain. J Neurosci 10:1683–1698, 1990

Perrone-Bizzozero NI, Cansino VV, Kohn DT: Post-translational regulation of GAP-43 gene expression in PC12 cells through protein kinase C-dependent stabilization of the mRNA. J Cell Biol 120:1263–1270, 1993

Pollack SJ, Atack JR, Knowles MR, et al: Mechanism of inositol monophosphatase, the putative target of lithium therapy. Proc Natl Acad Sci U S A 91:5766–5770, 1994

Post RM, Leverich GS, Altshuler L, et al: Lithium-discontinuation-induced refractoriness: preliminary observations. Am J Psychiatry 149:1727–1729, 1992

Ramakers GMJ, McNamara RK, Lenox RH, et al: Differential changes in the phosphorylation of the protein kinase C substrates MARCKS and GAP-43/B-50 following schaffer collateral long-term potentiation and long-term depression. J Neurochem (in press)

Rana RS, Hokin LE: Role of phosphoinositides in transmembrane signaling. Physiol Rev 70:115–164, 1990

Rodnight R, Perrett C: Protein phosphorylation and synaptic transmission: receptor mediated modulation of protein kinase C in a rat brain fraction enriched in synaptosomes. J Physiol 81:340–348, 1986

Rodriguez-Pena A, Zachary I, Rozengurt E: Rapid dephosphorylation of a M_r 80000 protein, a specific substrate of protein kinase C upon removal of phorbol esters, bombesin and vasopressin. Biochem Biophys Res Commun 140:379–385, 1986

Rosen A, Keenan KF, Thelen M, et al: Activation of protein kinase C results in the displacement of its myristoylated, alanine-rich substrate from punctate structures in macrophage filopodia. J Exp Med 172:1211–1215, 1990

Sawai T, Negishi M, Nishigaki N, et al: Enhancement by protein kinase C of prostacyclin receptor-mediated activation of adenylate cyclase through a calmodulin/myristoylated alanine-rich C kinase substrate (MARCKS) system in IC2 mast cells. J Biol Chem 268:1995–2000, 1993

Schnizer RA, McNamara RK, Streit WJ, et al: Differential expression of MARCKS, MRP & GAP-43 mRNA in the facial nucleus during neuronal regeneration and degeneration. Society for Neuroscience Abstracts 23:612, 1997

Sheu FS, Huang FL, Huang KP: Differential responses of protein kinase C substrates (MARCKS, neuromodulin, and neurogranin) phosphorylation to calmodulin and S100. Arch Biochem Biophys 316:335–342, 1995

Stubbs EB, Agranoff BW: Lithium enhances muscarinic receptor-stimulated CDP-diacylglycerol formation in inositol-depleted SK-N-SH neuroblastoma cells. J Neurochem 60:1292–1299, 1993

Stumpo DJ, Graff JM, Albert KA, et al: Molecular cloning, characterization, and expression of a cDNA encoding the "80- to 87-kDa" myristoylated alanine-rich C kinase substrate: a major cellular substrate for protein kinase C. Proc Natl Acad Sci U S A 86:4012–4016, 1989

Stumpo DJ, Bock CB, Tuttle JS, et al: MARCKS deficiency in mice leads to abnormal brain development and perinatal death. Proc Natl Acad Sci U S A 92:944–948, 1995

Suppes T, Baldessarini RJ, Faedda GI, et al: Risk of recurrence following discontinuation of lithium treatment in bipolar disorder. Arch Gen Psychiatry 48:1082–1088, 1991

Swayze VW, Andreasen NC, Alliger RJ, et al: Subcortical and temporal structures in affective disorder and schizophrenia: a magnetic resonance imaging study. Biol Psychiatry 31:221–240, 1992

Swierczynski SL, Blackshear PJ: Membrane association of the myristoylated alanine-rich C kinase substrate (MARCKS) protein: mutational analysis provides evidence for complex interactions. J Biol Chem 270:13436–13445, 1995

Swierczynski SL, Siddhanti SR, Tuttle JS, et al: Nonmyristoylated MARCKS complements some but not all of the developmental defects associated with MARCKS deficiency in mice. Dev Biol 179:135–147, 1996

Thelen M, Rosen A, Nairn AC, et al: Regulation by phosphorylation of reversible association of a myristoylated protein kinase C substrate with the plasma membrane. Nature 351:320–322, 1991

Wang JKT, Walaas SI, Greengard P: Protein phosphorylation in nerve terminals: comparison of calcium/calmodulin-dependent and calcium/diacylglycerol-dependent systems. J Neurosci 8:281–288, 1988

Wang JKT, Walaas SI, Sihra TS, et al: Phosphorylation and associated translocation of the 87-kDa protein, a major protein kinase C substrate, in isolated nerve terminals. Proc Natl Acad Sci U S A 86:2253–2256, 1989

Watson DG, Lenox RH: Chronic lithium-induced down-regulation of MARCKS in immortalized hippocampal cells: potentiation by muscarinic receptor activation. J Neurochem 67:767–777, 1996

Watson DG, Wainer BH, Lenox RH: Phorbol ester- and retinoic acid-induced regulation of the protein kinase C substrate MARCKS in immortalized hippocampal cells. J Neurochem 63:1666–1674, 1994

Watson DG, Watterson JM, Lenox RH: Sodium valproate down-regulates the myristoylated alanine-rich C kinase substrate (MARCKS) in immortalized hippocampal cells: a property unique to PKC-mediated mood stabilization J Pharmacol Exp Ther 285:307–316, 1998

Wees EA, McNamara RK, Meberg PJ, et al: The PKC substrate MARCKS is enriched in neuronal growth cones and developmentally regulated in the rat hippocampus. Society for Neuroscience Abstracts 24:537, 1998

Zachary I, Sinnett-Smith JW, Rozengurt E: Early events elicited by bombesin and structurally related peptides in quiescent Swiss 3T3 cells, I: activation of protein kinase C and inhibition of epidermal growth factor binding. J Cell Biol 102:2211–2222, 1986

CHAPTER 10

LITHIUM, CARBAMAZEPINE, AND VALPROATE IN AFFECTIVE ILLNESS

Biochemical and Neurobiological Mechanisms

Robert M. Post, M.D., Susan R. B. Weiss, Ph.D.,
Mike Clark, Ph.D., De-Maw Chuang, Ph.D.,
Christopher Hough, Ph.D., and He Li, Ph.D.

LITHIUM

Lithium has been the paradigmatic treatment for bipolar illness, effective in both the acute treatment of mania and the long-term prophylaxis of manic and depressive episodes. Although its efficacy as a treatment for depression in monotherapy is controversial, overwhelming data support its role as an augmentation treatment in conjunction with virtually every known antidepressant (Kramlinger and Post 1989b). Interestingly, this therapeutic effect in augmentation treatment may have a faster onset than in monotherapy and suggests differential mechanisms of action (de Montigny et al. 1981; Post and Chuang 1991).

CARBAMAZEPINE

Over the last 20 years, recognition has been increasing that carbamazepine, widely used in the treatment of seizure disorders and paroxysmal pain syndromes such as trigeminal neuralgia, also has a spectrum of efficacy in bipolar illness (Okuma 1993; Post 1990; Post et al. 1996a, 1996b). Nineteen controlled studies using various designs support its efficacy in acute mania, in most instances with a time course and effect magnitude comparable to that of neuroleptics (123 of 203 [61%] improved response) (Post et al., in press).

Carbamazepine's acute antidepressant properties are less well delineated than its antimanic properties, but the data are highly suggestive that in some treatment-refractory depressed patients, it has both acute and prophylactic efficacy (Post et al. 1996a, 1996b). Sixteen of 17 partially controlled trials support the prophylactic efficacy of carbamazepine for both manic and depressive recurrences in bipolar illness (Post et al., in press). Fifteen studies compared carbamazepine with lithium in a randomized design, 1 compared carbamazepine with placebo, and 1 used a double-blind, off-on-off-on (BABA) design. The overall improved response rate was 62% (217 of 350) in controlled studies and 62% (390 of 629) in open studies. In addition, several studies supported the efficacy of carbamazepine in conjunction with lithium in the treatment of acute episodes (Kramlinger and Post 1989a, 1989b) and rapid cycling, in which the combination is more effective than either drug used alone (Denicoff et al. 1997; Di Costanzo and Schifano 1991; Okuma 1993).

VALPROATE

Valproate or its congener valpromide was initially reported (in open studies) to be effective acutely and in long-term prophylaxis of bipolar disorder (Lambert 1984; Lambert et al. 1975). These studies were followed up with double-blind, on-off-on (ABA) studies by Emrich and associates (1985) that reported efficacy in acute mania and in long-term prophylaxis. Double-blind studies comparing valproate with lithium and placebo have now been completed in several centers (Bowden et al. 1994; Freeman et al. 1992; Pope et al. 1991), the data of which supported the recent U.S. Food and Drug Administration (FDA) approval in 1996 of valproate in the treatment of acute mania. Valproate's efficacy in acute depression has not been systematically tested, but considerable open trial evidence is suggestive of its effectiveness in long-term prophylaxis, particularly in some rapid-cycling patients inadequately responsive to lithium, carbamazepine, or the combination (Calabrese and Delucchi 1989, 1990; Keck et al. 1992;

Schaff et al. 1993; Sharma et al. 1993). Some studies suggest that the combination of lithium and valproate may be required for patients who discontinue lithium after the addition of valproate and subsequently have breakthrough episodes (Emrich et al. 1985).

Valproate is widely recognized for its broad-spectrum anticonvulsant properties, including efficacy in the treatment of absence seizures, which carbamazepine can often exacerbate. Additionally, studies have reported valproate utility in migraine syndromes (Balfour and Bryson 1994) and anxiety disorders (Keck et al. 1993).

CLINICAL OVERVIEW—DIFFERENTIAL AND OVERLAPPING RESPONSE

Lithium and the two mood-stabilizing anticonvulsants carbamazepine and valproate appear to share certain commonalities in the treatment of bipolar illness. Their efficacy in acute mania is more robust or better demonstrated than in acute depression, and all three drugs appear to have utility in long-term prophylaxis, either alone or in combination with one another (Post et al. 1996a). Given this spectrum of common clinical targets, with differences in other aspects of their profiles, one is tempted to look for common mechanisms of action that could account for efficacy in affective illness.

This approach, however, has limitations, particularly given the preliminary view alluded to previously that differential clinical response may occur among different subtypes of bipolar illness. Moreover, excellent evidence indicates that response to one mood stabilizer does not necessarily predict response to another (Denicoff et al. 1997; Post 1990; Post et al. 1996a, 1996b), suggesting that patients with different pathophysiologies may be responsive to some mood stabilizers but not others.

Given this perspective, and considering the extensive use of mood stabilizers in combination, it is highly likely that differences in action among the mood stabilizers will account for the differential responses in monotherapy and additive responses in combination therapy (Post and Chuang 1991; Post et al. 1992, 1994). With the advent of lithium, it was hoped that discerning lithium's mechanism of action would rapidly lead to a better understanding of illness pathophysiology and the development of additional treatments specifically targeting more focused mechanisms. This has not been the case; in fact, it can be argued that the opposite has occurred. Lithium has a panoply of effects on a variety of neurotransmitter, receptor, second-messenger, and intracellular systems, most of which have been hypothesized to play a role in its clinical profile of efficacy and to be disordered in the affective illnesses (Post and Chuang 1991). Within the caveats noted above, however, it may be possible to balance lithium's effects against the other agents and to assess both common and differential effects on putative systems thought to be implicated in affective illness.

We organize the following neurobiological review and discussion on the sequential mechanistic themes ranging from extracellular to intracellular and presynaptic to postsynaptic. This discussion progresses from considering effects on neurotransmitters, receptors, and second-messenger mechanisms to ion channels, gene transcription, and neuropeptide regulation as putative candidates for the psychotropic action of the mood stabilizers. This progression also approximately follows the historical developments of affective illness theories and the putative mechanisms of action of these mood-stabilizing agents but does not necessarily sequentially relate to the most likely candidate systems involved in the agents' psychotropic effects. As newer treatment developments (briefly alluded to) and more targeted therapies become available, there should be an increasingly rapid link of mechanisms of action to therapeutic effect and, ultimately, better prediction of pharmacological response.

CLASSICAL NEUROTRANSMITTER-RECEPTOR SYSTEMS

Norepinephrine

Lithium exerts a variety of effects on noradrenergic mechanisms, including increased synaptosomal reuptake and downregulation of noradrenergic responsivity at a level of both receptor binding and blocking of β-receptor activation of adenylate cyclase (Belmaker et al. 1991; Post et al. 1984). Carbamazepine's effects on noradrenergic metabolism are complex, including decreases in norepinephrine turnover (Maitre et al. 1984), weak reuptake blockade (Purdy et al. 1977), and contrary to the actions of most other putative antidepressant substances, upregulation rather than downregulation of β-receptors following chronic administration (G. Chen et al. 1992). Parenthetically, this effect could account for carbamazepine's atypical antidepressant properties in some patients, including those who are unresponsive to more traditional tricyclic and related compounds. Few data putatively link valproate's effects on noradrenergic metabolism with its clinical mechanism of action.

Carbamazepine's effects on noradrenergic metabolism, nonetheless, are instructive from several perspectives; which actions of carbamazepine are important to its antimanic effects, including its ability to decrease stimulated-induced release of norepinephrine and to inhibit norepinephrine turnover, remains an open issue (Post et al. 1985). It is of considerable interest that noradrenergic tone is necessary for carbamazepine's anticonvulsant effects in some models (Crunelli et al. 1981; Quattrone and Samanin 1977; Quattrone et al. 1978) but is unnecessary in others (Quattrone et al. 1981). The α_2-agonist clonidine blocks the anticonvulsant effects of carbamazepine against electroconvulsive shock (Crunelli et al. 1981; Fischer and Muller 1988), whereas the α_2-agonist yohimbine blocks carbamazepine's effects on amygdala-kindled seizures (Post et al. 1993b). Thus, it is clear that even when a putative biochemical effect of the drug is linked to its mechanism of action in one type of seizure or psychiatric syndrome, this may not be the case for all of the subcategories and subtypes of that syndrome.

Dopamine

Lithium appears to exert many indirect effects on dopamine release and receptors (Bunney and Garland-Bunney 1987), as does carbamazepine (Post et al. 1980). Lithium and carbamazepine do not appear to be easily classifiable as either direct or indirect agonists or antagonists, although lithium has been reported to block aspects of cocaine-related sensitization and receptor supersensitivity. Maitre et al. (1984) reviewed evidence that carbamazepine and the other mood stabilizers decrease dopamine turnover via mechanisms that are as yet unknown. Most recently, Baptista et al. (1993) indicated that carbamazepine blocks cocaine-induced increases in dopamine overflow in the nucleus accumbens as measured by in vivo dialysis. This effect could account for the observation of Aigner and colleagues (1990) that carbamazepine inhibits cocaine intake in self-administration in the rhesus monkey, a process thought to be mediated by accumbens dopaminergic mechanisms. The extent to which all of the mood stabilizers share some ability to indirectly block dopaminergic tone leaves dopamine a candidate system for the actions of these drugs in mania and clearly differentiates the mood stabilizers from the neuroleptics (which directly block dopamine receptors).

Serotonin

The serotonergic actions of the mood stabilizers are of considerable interest in relation to the hypothesized deficits of serotonin in relation to depression and cycling (Curzon 1988; Price et al. 1989; Van Praag 1984). In contrast to many antidepressants, none of the mood stabilizers appear to strongly block serotonin reuptake. However, lithium enhances tryptophan uptake and has various other indirect effects on serotonin metabolism (de Montigny et al. 1983; Price et al. 1989, 1990). Carbamazepine enhances serotonin levels in the hippocampus in epilepsy-prone rats (Dailey et al. 1995; Yan et al. 1992), with a magnitude and time course suggesting a significance to its anticonvulsant effects. Moreover, depletion of serotonin inhibits carbamazepine's actions in these animals (Dailey et al. 1995), although the mechanism of this effect is unknown. As reviewed by Calabrese et al. (1994) and Keck et al. (1994), valproate has interesting serotonergic properties (Khaitan et al. 1994), also suggesting that this system could be a putative common target system for the effects of all three mood stabilizers.

GABAergic Mechanisms

In the γ-aminobutyric acid (GABA) system, all three mood stabilizers exert important effects, decreasing GABA turnover in the frontal cortex (Bernasconi 1982). In addition, all three mood stabilizers are reported to increase $GABA_B$ receptors in the hippocampus after chronic, but not acute, administration (Motohashi 1990; Motohashi et al. 1989). These findings are interesting given that the $GABA_B$ agonist baclofen appeared to exacerbate depression in a small group of patients, and its discontinuation was associated with improvement in mood and behavior (Post et al. 1991). The data suggest the possibility that $GABA_B$ antagonists rather than agonists could have a useful antidepressant effect and that the effect of mood stabilizers on GABAergic tone could, indeed, be related to some of their psychotropic properties.

Valproate increases GABA levels by a variety of mechanisms, which is interesting in relation to the putative mood-stabilizing properties of the inhibitor of the GABA transporter gabapentin. The $GABA_B$ effects of carbamazepine are likely relevant to its effects on trigeminal neuralgia (Terrence et al. 1983). Valproate also has been reported to be effective in trigeminal neuralgia (Balfour and Bryson 1994), but lithium has not, presenting another interesting clinical point for study.

Acetylcholine

All three drugs appear to have differential effects on cholinergic metabolism: lithium augments cholinergic effects and impairs cholinergic supersensitivity adaptations (Bunney and Garland-Bunney 1987), carbamazepine increases choline levels in the striatum (Consolo et al. 1976), and valproate has unspecified effects. However, each of these substances lacks anticholinergic side effects that are typical of the tricyclic antidepressants. In light of recent data suggesting the utility of choline supplementation in some treatment-refractory disorders (Stoll et al. 1996), one could question whether carbamazepine's action on this system, or lithium's indirect effects, could be important to their mood-stabilizing properties.

Adenosine

Carbamazepine has relatively selective effects on adenosine A_1 receptors (Clark and Post 1989; Daval et al. 1989; Elphick et al. 1990; Marangos et al. 1983). This is of considerable interest because during chronic administration, electroconvulsive therapy (ECT) upregulates adenosine A_1 receptors. Biber et al. (1999) believe that carbamazepine could modulate the phosphatidylinositol (PI) system via its inhibition of the adenosine A_1 receptor because adenosine synergistically potentiates the actions of acetylcholine, norepinephrine, and histamine on PI. The effects of valproate on this system are unknown.

Glutamatergic Effects

Many indirect effects of carbamazepine on glutamate systems have been hypothesized. Lampe and Bigalke (1990) reported that carbamazepine, but not phenytoin, inhibited current induced by *N*-methyl-D-aspartate (NMDA) in spinal cord neurons, although Olpe (1991) did not replicate these findings. The observations of Lancaster and Davies (1992) that carbamazepine inhibited NMDA-induced depolarization in cortical wedges prepared from epilepsy-prone mice and the observations of Gao and Chuang (1992) that carbamazepine, in supratherapeutic doses, induced slow neurotoxicity in cultured cerebellar granule cells by an NMDA-reversible mechanism are congruous with a possible site of action of carbamazepine on NMDA receptors. Suggestive of yet another area of convergence between carbamazepine and valproate, Zeise et al. (1991) reported that valproate, in a dose-related fashion, suppressed transient depolarization induced by NMDA applied iontophoretically to neocortical pyramidal cells.

Carbamazepine displaces $[^3H]$-MK-801 binding and inhibits NMDA-induced phosphoinositide turnover in cerebellar granule cells (Gao and Chuang 1992). Preliminary evidence from Hough and colleagues (1996) showed that carbamazepine attenuates NMDA receptor-gated calcium influx in these neurons. Chronic treatment of these cells leads to appropriate changes consistent with an acute inhibitory effect on glutamate receptors. Cerebellar granule cells may be differentially or more sensitive to these effects than those in the hippocampus, which could account for the prominent effects of carbamazepine on ataxia and nystagmus in toxic overdose clinical situations.

Interestingly, carbamazepine and lamotrigine decrease release of excitatory amino acids, whereas lithium increases release of glutamate in primate cerebral cortex slices (Dixon et al. 1994).

Benzodiazepine Receptors: Peripheral- Versus Central-Type

Carbamazepine is a relatively potent antagonist at peripheral-type (p-type) benzodiazepine receptors (Marangos et al. 1990; Weiss and Post 1991; Weiss et al. 1986), otherwise called the mitochondrial benzodiazepine receptors. These receptors are thought to modulate calcium influx (Le Fur et al. 1985; Mestre et al. 1985) and neurosteroid biosynthesis (Krueger 1995).

To the extent that neurosteroids are modulated by p-type receptors, this would provide a conceptual basis for how a p-type benzodiazepine ligand such as carbamazepine could also influence GABA systems because several of the neurosteroids are active at GABA and glutamate receptors (Morrow et al. 1990; Purdy et al. 1977).

In contrast, valproate appears to be active, at least in part, through its multiple effects on GABAergic mechanisms and thus could indirectly influence central-type benzodiazepine receptors. These effects are also of interest in relation to the preliminary suggestions of the mood-stabilizing effects of gabapentin, which acts on a GABA transporter (Beydoun et al. 1995). Lithium does not appear to be directly active at either central- or p-type benzodiazepine receptors, but it also could affect this complex via indirect GABAergic mechanisms noted above. In contrast to these three mood-stabilizing drugs, clonazepam is a selective central-type benzodiazepine ligand; clonazepam and diazepam do not show cross-tolerance to carbamazepine in the amygdala-kindled seizure model (Weiss et al. 1985).

EFFECTS ON SECOND-MESSENGER SYSTEMS

G Proteins and Adenylate Cyclase

Effects on second-messenger signal transduction mechanisms are a particularly intriguing potential mechanism of action of the mood stabilizers, in light of the postulated excesses in behavioral and affective responsivity that occur in bipolar illness. We and others have postulated that one of the ways around the conundrum of how a single drug such as lithium carbonate can be effective in both manic and depressive phases of the illness is to consider that mania and depression are representative of excessive activity in neural systems mediating excitation or inhibition (Post and Chuang 1991; Post et al. 1992). To the extent that such overexcursions of primary or secondary compensatory mechanisms (Post and Weiss 1992) are ultimately found to be involved in the pathophysiology of bipolar illness, the ability to dampen these overexcursions at the level of guanine nucleotide binding proteins (G proteins) and signal transduction coupling mechanisms could provide a conceptual basis for the biphasic effects on mood.

This concept is even more promising in light of recent evidence that G-protein dysfunction can be found in the blood elements and, in some instances, in autopsy specimens of bipolar patients compared with control subjects. These data are more extensively reviewed elsewhere (Avissar and Schreiber 1992b; Avissar et al. 1996, 1997; Manji 1992; Schreiber et al. 1991; Young et al. 1994) and are even more intriguing from the perspective that other putative mood-stabilizing agents also exert important effects on second messengers.

Belmaker and associates (1991) reviewed evidence that lithium's ability to inhibit adenylate cyclase activity could be linked to its mechanism of action. More recently, Manji et al. (1995) and Avissar and Schreiber (1992a) postulated direct effects of lithium on G-protein function. Although not all investigators have replicated these findings, a variety of data support some effect on either G-protein levels or G-protein function. In addition, the work of Avissar and Schreiber (1992a) suggested that lithium, carbamazepine, valproate, and possibly ECT (Avissar et al. 1990) share some common effects on G proteins. Note that data summarized earlier (Post et al. 1982) indicated that carbamazepine, like lithium, was able to inhibit various stimulated adenylate cyclase activities (i.e., by norepinephrine, adenosine, potassium chloride, ouabain, and veratridine).

In addition, carbamazepine is reported to block nitroprusside stimulation of cyclic guanosine monophosphate (cGMP) (Schubert et al. 1991), a finding of considerable interest in relation to the recent linkage of this transduction mechanism to nitric oxide and nitric oxide synthase pathways. The direct and indirect effects of the mood stabilizers and nitric oxide synthase remain to be more directly and comparatively assessed.

Several studies indicated that lithium and the mood-stabilizing anticonvulsants differentially affect G-protein levels and functions (Colin et al. 1991; Lesch et al. 1991; Li et al. 1991; Manji et al. 1995). Whether these are ultimately related to their mechanisms of action remains an exciting area of investigation.

Phosphoinositol Turnover and Protein Kinase C

Other intracellular messengers, including protein kinase C (PKC) and various elements in the phosphoinositide turnover transduction mechanism, appear to be the target for lithium and the mood-stabilizing anticonvulsants (Manji et al. 1995). Chronic (5-week), but not subchronic (1-week), lithium treatment resulted in a selective decrease in the level of PKC isozyme α in the CA1 region of rat hippocampus (Manji et al. 1993). Interestingly, valproate, another antimanic drug, also induced a selective loss of PKC isozyme α and PKCε in C6 glioma cells after treatment for 6–7 days (G. Chen et al. 1994). These observations suggest that PKC isozyme downregulation could be a common mechanism underlying the therapeutic effect of these two drugs. These data led Bebchuk et al. (in press) to assess the possible efficacy of the PKC inhibitor tamoxifen in acute mania, with initial studies showing positive results.

Lithium is clearly known to inhibit phosphoinositol turnover at several steps, with a particularly marked inhibition on the inositol monophosphatase converting inositol monophosphate, for free inositol. Several other phosphatases—inositol 1,3,4-trisphosphate (IP_3) and inositol 1,4-bisphosphate (IP_2)—are more weakly inhibited by lithium. Most interestingly, lithium, carbamazepine, and valproate have been shown to have differential effects on this phosphatase activity: lithium decreases inositol monophosphatase, carbamazepine increases inositol monophosphatase, and valproate has no effect (Vadnal and Parthasarathy 1995).

To the extent that carbamazepine and valproate are effective in either a different subgroup of patients or patients in a different phase of illness progression, such differential second-messenger effects become very interesting. If one is postulating excesses in initial effects, adaptations, or counterregulatory effects, it becomes possible to see how inhibition of the phosphatase enzyme and subsequent decreases in PI turnover might be of use in some instances, whereas other instances would require a carbamazepine-like stimulation. The effects of these agents during chronic administration (i.e., a situation more likely related to psychotropic effects) remain to be determined, however.

The noncompetitive inhibition of lithium makes its effects on the PI cycle "use dependent," (i.e., it has effects on systems that are activated or overactivated) (Atack et al. 1993). This is an interesting partial parallel to carbamazepine, which exerts use-dependent effects on other overactive systems (i.e., both in blocking sodium channels and in calcium influx through the NMDA receptor) as discussed.

Interpretation of the lithium data is further confounded by the fact that inositol replacement can overcome lithium side effects in some instances and by recent data that inositol alone, in the absence of lithium, is effective in some patients with refractory depression and anxiety disorders (Benjamin et al. 1995; Levine et al. 1995). Because phosphatase inhibition by lithium should, theoretically, impair inositol recycling, it becomes an interesting problem to consider how inositol itself (in the absence of lithium) could be of therapeutic value. Some side effects (polyuria and polydipsia) may be related to inositol depletion; carbamazepine, which has an opposing side-effect profile, might be even further potentiated by inositol.

ION CHANNELS

Calcium Influx and Ion Channel Effects

Intracellular calcium is a major cellular transduction mechanism that plays a key role in neurotransmission, second-messenger effects, and cellular homeostasis at many levels. Considerable data support a role for calcium in the affective disorders, ranging from the original findings of a high incidence of mood disorders in hyper- and hypoparathyroidism to evidence of calcium dysregulation in the affective disorders (Carman et al. 1984). Most recently, a noteworthy series of studies reported increased intracellular calcium in the blood elements of patients with unipolar and bipolar depressive illness (Dubovsky et al. 1994). This increase is present in some studies in the basal condition and in many others in the stimulated condition, with either serotonin, thrombin, or platelet-activating factor (see review in Post et al., in press). Could these peripheral intracellular markers parallel a similar phenomenon occurring intracerebrally? What is the molecular mechanism or pathophysiology of this increased intracellular accumulation, and could it be used to better target therapeutic interventions? These types of questions remain to be answered with appropriate clinical and preclinical studies.

It is noteworthy that the recent psychopharmacology of affective illness supports a role for this ion. There is a rich literature of the efficacy of the L-type calcium channel blocker verapamil in manic patients in a series of small but controlled, double-blind studies (Dubovsky 1993). Antidepressant effects were disappointing, however (Hoschl and Kozeny 1989). This led us to explore other subtypes of L-type calcium channel blockers of the dihydropyridine class, such as nimodipine, isradipine, and amlodipine.

Preliminary data support the efficacy of nimodipine in some patients with rapid- and ultradian-cycling bipolar illness and in patients with recurrent brief depressions, as documented in BABA double-blind designs (McDermut et al. 1995; Pazzaglia et al. 1993, 1998). These data raise the possibility that inhibition of calcium influx by L-type calcium channels may, in fact, contribute to the antimanic and antidepressant effects observed. In this regard, it is noteworthy that various animal models suggest that calcium channel blockers are active and positive in these tests of antidepressant efficacy. Responders to nimodipine showed cross-responsivity to the dihydropyridine L-type calcium channel blocker isradipine but not to the phenylalkylamine verapamil (Pazzaglia et al. 1998).

Carbamazepine is not active at L-type calcium channels. However, it does block calcium-related influx via the glutamate NMDA receptor (Hough et al. 1996). The properties of carbamazepine in this regard are most significant in that carbamazepine is a better calcium channel blocker under high-frequency and use-dependent conditions than it is in the resting state. This property, like that of type 2 sodium channels for carbamazepine and phenytoin (McLean and MacDonald 1986a; Willow et al. 1984), suggests a mechanism that could make carbamazepine particularly helpful in pathological states without impairing normal functioning.

We observed that a subgroup of patients who had a partial but definite response to the L-type calcium channel blockers had a more sustained response to the addition of carbamazepine. This suggests that the blockade of two different points of calcium entry by two different mechanisms (i.e., L-type vs. NMDA) may, in some instances, be more effective than either alone, although this must be confirmed with the appropriate clinical studies (Post et al., in press).

Moreover, we have not ruled out whether the addition of agents other than carbamazepine (not active at the NMDA receptor) would be as efficacious in augmenting nimodipine. For example, Manna (1991) reported that the combination of lithium and nimodipine is more effective than either agent alone. Lithium has numerous effects on calcium mechanics, as reviewed by Meltzer (1990), and these could also be additive or potentiative. Similarly, valproate has various effects on calcium channels, particularly on T-type calcium channels, similar to that of ethosuximide, and this action has been linked to efficacy in absence (petit mal) seizures. Complex effects of both carbamazepine and valproate have been reported on calcium spikes or currents (Elliott 1990; Gasser et al. 1988; Zona and Avoli 1990; Zona et al. 1990).

Sodium Channel Effects

Both carbamazepine and phenytoin are active at batrachotoxin type 2 sodium channels in a frequency- and membrane-depolarization–dependent fashion (Willow et al. 1984). These use-dependent properties have made sodium channels a prime candidate system for some components of the antiepileptic properties of these drugs. However, local anesthetics also bind these channels in a use-dependent manner and can produce kindled seizures that are blocked by chronic, but not acute or intermittent, carbamazepine treatment (Weiss et al. 1989). Thus, the mechanisms by which these various drugs affect and/or modulate sodium channel function require further study. Moreover, carbamazepine appears to have psychotropic effects not shared by phenytoin, but they are both equally potent on the type 2 sodium channels. Valproate also affects type 2 sodium channels but in a slightly different fashion (McLean and MacDonald 1986b), whereas lithium's ionic properties are most similar to those of sodium; how these relate to its psychotropic actions is not well defined.

Potassium Channel Effects

Carbamazepine also increases potassium conductance and provides a new candidate system for its anticonvulsant effects (Olpe et al. 1991; Zona et al. 1990). This is significant because valproate also has been reported to enhance potassium conductance (Slater and Johnston 1978; Walden et al. 1993; but see Zona and Avoli 1990), suggesting another potential common mechanism for carbamazepine and valproate.

EFFECTS ON GENE EXPRESSION

Studies by Divish et al. (1991) and Leslie et al. (1993) have reported that lithium carbonate increases *c-fos* expression. Chronic lithium markedly potentiates *fos* induction in the piriform cortex in rats treated with a serotonin type 2 receptor agonist (Leslie et al. 1993). In contrast, carbamazepine inhibits *c-fos* expression produced by kindling and other seizure inductions (Gunn et al. 1990). These findings are of considerable interest in relation to the ability of lithium to affect gene expression and neurophysiology of cerebellar granule cells. For example, lithium increases transcription factor binding to activator protein 1 (AP-1) and cyclic adenosine monophosphate (cAMP) response element binding protein (CRE) (Ozaki and Chuang 1997) and enhances the expression of M_3 muscarinic receptors but decreases M_2 muscarinic receptor levels (Gao et al. 1993). Moreover, long-term lithium treatment upregulates neuroprotective bcl-2 but downregulates proapoptotic Bax and p53 in these neurons (R. W. Chen and Chuang 1999). Additionally, lithium activates the cell-surviving PI 3-kinase/Akt signaling (Chalecka-Franaszek and Chuang 1999). These aspects of lithium's actions are likely to contribute to its neuroprotective effects against glutamate excitotoxicity (Nonaka et al. 1998a) and carbamazepine-induced apoptosis (Nonaka et al. 1998b). These findings also could be related to differential actions on white blood cell count, with carbamazepine decreasing and lithium increasing white blood cell count, possibly at the level of the colony-stimulating factor. Chronic lithium treatment has been shown to reduce brain infarct volume and suppress neurological deficits in an animal model of focal ischemia (Nonaka and Chuang 1998). This neuroprotective action also could be related to lithium's ability to induce bcl-2 in the cerebral cortex of rats (G. Chen et al. 1999b).

Valproate's effects on gene expression need to be more systematically explored, although effects on the AP-1 binding complex have been described (G. Chen et al. 1999a). This is a site of action for *c-fos* and thus also could be influenced by lithium and carbamazepine. Valproate appears to be the most teratogenic of the three mood stabilizers, with a 1%–2% incidence of spina bifida, exceeding that of carbamazepine (Lindhout et al. 1992). Lithium's teratogenicity may have been initially overestimated; it now appears to be the least teratogenic of the three mood stabilizers. Its ability to induce Ebstein's anomaly and other general cardiac malformations is only slightly greater than that in the general population (Jacobson et al. 1992).

How such effects on immediate-early gene expression come to modulate putative late-effector genes and other cellular and adaptive mechanisms during chronic administration is not yet well delineated. However, several longer-term adaptations following chronic drug administration with the mood stabilizers have been identified. These delayed changes are more likely to be associated with acute antimanic and antidepressant effects, which take time to develop, even with loading strategies (Post 1988). These effects could be related to adaptive changes at the level of modulation of neurotransmitter biosynthesis, release, reuptake, receptor, second-messenger, or neurotropic and neuropeptide systems.

The mechanism by which all three mood stabilizers upregulate $GABA_B$ receptors in the hippocampus after chronic, but not acute, administration (Motohashi 1990; Motohashi et al. 1989) has not been elucidated. However, the time course of such an effect suggests effects on gene expression, with chronic administration being required to induce such a long-term regulatory response. This concept also could be relevant to the slow onset of antimanic and (even slower onset of) antidepressant effects, despite maximum dose titration. In this manner, not until the appropriate effects on gene expression are induced with chronic administration would these agents exert their putative mechanism of action. For example, chronic lithium increases glucocorticoid type II messenger RNA (mRNA) (Pfeiffer et al. 1991) and prodynorphin and preprotachykinin mRNA in rat striatum, in addition to other peptide changes noted below (Sivam et al. 1988, 1989).

As these putative late-effector gene substrates become better understood, it might be possible to circumvent this time-dependent neuroregulatory mechanism and target the late-effector genes directly. Alternatively, an acute manipulation of sufficient potency to exert a therapeutic action long enough could be sought and used until the more chronic onset of action of the traditional mood stabilizers is achieved. Such a mechanism has been used with sleep deprivation, wherein the acute transient effects of this manipulation have been enhanced by cotreatment with lithium to prevent relapse after a night's recovery sleep and to sustain a longer antidepressant response (Baxter 1985).

Thus, elucidating the critical molecular targets and mechanisms of action of the mood stabilizers may not only allow further development of more potent and specific agents but also identify agents that ultimately have the potential for more rapid onset of action. With the ability of physostigmine to immediately produce acute antimanic effects (Janowsky et al. 1973), and sleep deprivation to acutely induce antidepressive effects (Post et al. 1987), it becomes clear that acute manic and depressive syndromes are not, inherently, unresponsive within an acute time frame, but only that the current therapeutic agents are unable to achieve this acute response.

PEPTIDES

Vasopressin

Carbamazepine and lithium have essentially opposing effects on vasopressinergic tone. Lithium inhibits vasopressin's effects at the level of adenylate cyclase, whereas carbamazepine appears to have some direct receptor-related activity (Gold et al. 1984). Thus, carbamazepine is unable to reverse lithium-induced diabetes insipidus, although, used alone, it is a useful alternative mood stabilizer for the patient with severe lithium-induced diabetes insipidus. Conversely, carbamazepine can cause hyponatremia (Joffe et al. 1986; Uhde and Post 1983; Yassa et al. 1988) and water intoxication, in part mediated through its vasopressinergic effects. Not only demeclocycline but also lithium is able to block or reverse these effects (Brewerton and Jackson 1994; Ringel and Brick 1986; Vieweg et al. 1986). Valproate's effects on vasopressin are not well delineated, and whether this system relates to the differential psychotropic or side-effect profiles of lithium or carbamazepine remains to be determined.

Substance P

Lithium and carbamazepine, on chronic administration, share the ability to upregulate substance P in the striatum of the rat brain, a finding that could preliminarily account for antidepressant effects (Hong et al. 1983; Le Douarin et al. 1983; Mitsushio et al. 1988). To our knowledge, valproate's effects on substance P have not been explored. These data are of particular interest in light of the recent reports of the antidepressant effects of substance P antagonists (Kramer et al. 1998).

Somatostatin

Interestingly, carbamazepine decreases somatostatin in the cerebrospinal fluid (CSF) of affectively ill patients (Rubinow et al. 1985), whereas nimodipine significantly increases somatostatin (Pazzaglia et al. 1995). Patients with low baseline CSF somatostatin responded better to nimodipine than did those with normal or high levels (M. A. Frye, P. J. Pazzaglia, D. Luckenbaugh, T. A. Kimbrell, J. T. Little, R. T. Dunn, M. S. George, T. Huggins, L. Vanderham, G. S. Leverich, C. Davis, D. R. Rubinow, and R. M. Post, unpublished data, May 1997). The effects of lithium and valproate on somatostatin in clinical or animal studies require further exploration.

To the extent that decreases in somatostatin are associated with cognitive impairment in Alzheimer's disease and in animal model systems of deficient learning and memory, the opposing effects of carbamazepine and nimodipine become of particular interest in relation to their pattern of psychotropic and cognitive pretargeted effects. In this regard, it is interesting that preliminary data support an effect of nimodipine in late Alzheimer's disease, although apparently not of a sufficient magnitude to be clinically relevant at this late phase of deterioration (S. Dubovsky et al., personal communication, January 1993).

Ketter et al. (1996) described a different baseline profile—an abnormal brain metabolism measured by positron-emission tomography (PET) in nimodipine compared with carbamazepine responders. The former showed the typical depressive pattern of baseline frontotemporal hypometabolism, whereas the latter showed a pattern of frontotemporal hypermetabolism, even though both were equally depressed at baseline. Differential peptidergic effects could account for these differences in response characteristics, based on presumed differential pathophysiologies.

Thyrotropin-Releasing Hormone

Chronic carbamazepine administration may be associated with increased thyrotropin-releasing hormone (TRH) levels in the CSF of patients with affective illness (Marangell et al. 1994). Whether this effect is reliable and shared by any of the other mood stabilizers remains to be further studied. The ability of an agent to increase TRH is, nonetheless, interesting in relation to recent data suggesting that some effects on gene expression in the amygdala kindling model are part of the primary pathophysiological process of seizure development (or kindled memory trace), whereas others are secondary, compensatory, and adaptive (Weiss et al. 1995). These latter effects may represent endogenous anticonvulsant mechanisms and putatively include inhibitory systems, such as $GABA_A$ and benzodiazepine receptors, that increase after seizures and increases in peptides with known anticonvulsant properties, such as TRH and cholecystokinin.

Following the view that TRH could thus be an endogenous positive adaptation in the seizure model, we explored whether it also could be acting in such a compensatory adaptive fashion in primary affective illness. Some evidence suggests TRH hypersecretion in depressed patients based on CSF studies (Banki et al. 1988; Kirkegaard et al. 1979) and in a subgroup of patients with blunted thyroid-stimulating hormone (TSH) response to TRH. If TRH were compensatory and adaptive, administering it to patients would more likely be associated with a positive antidepressant effect rather than an exacerbation of the illness if it were part of the primary pathophysiology.

Marangell and associates (1997) found, with TRH administered intrathecally and, in some instances, parenterally (Callahan et al. 1997), that subacute antidepressant effects were often observed even in refractory depressed patients. However, the positive effects of parenteral TRH could not be sustained longer than approximately 6 weeks with repeated administration in two patients in whom this was systematically explored (Callahan et al. 1997). Nonetheless, because TRH has a relatively rapid onset of action, such a manipulation raises the possibility that an appropriately delivered and targeted peptide could provide a bridging action until more chronic and sustained effects could be achieved with other manipulations.

RATIO OF PRIMARY PATHOLOGICAL TO SECONDARY COMPENSATORY MECHANISMS

Elsewhere, we have discussed in more detail how the ratio of the primary pathophysiological mechanisms balanced by endogenous compensatory mechanisms (and as supplemented by exogenous medications) could be associated with the cyclic recurrence of illness (Post and Weiss 1996). To the extent that this is shown to be the case in affective illness, it would suggest that cyclicity emerges directly out of illness-related variables (i.e., the changing ratios of the relative balance of primary pathological vs. secondary adaptive mechanisms). In this manner, one would not have to postulate the unparsimonious notion that the illness has two defects, one related to its pathophysiology and a separate defect in a "clock" mechanism. Under this rubric, all of the observed patterns of illness variation, cyclicity, and recurrence could be subsumed in one inherent process rather than specific rhythmic patterns of illness being associated with specific circadian defects, as in the case of the *per* and *timeless* mutants.

Encompassed in the perspective of effects on gene expression mediating pathological versus compensatory mechanisms, one could understand the importance of targeting different mechanisms for treatment. Thus, some agents might dampen pathological mechanisms, and others might enhance apparent illness-related abnormalities, but these latter changes, to the extent that they reflect endogenous positive adaptation, could prove useful in pursuit of optimal therapeutics. Such a view would also explain the general observations that agents effective in acute depression are often effective in long-term prophylaxis of unipolar disorders as well. The mood stabilizers also appear to share this quality that acute response may be linked to longer-term prophylactic response.

We are suggesting that the mechanisms inherent in episode termination, to the extent that they represent bimodal or mood-stabilizing properties, also might be effective in prevention. In contrast, the unimodal antidepressants such as the tricyclics could be conceptualized as potentially exacerbating cyclicity; although they have potent antidepressant properties, they cannot act as antimanic agents. Thus, unimodal antidepressants would augment changes in a depressive episode, leading to episode termination, but they might simultaneously be part of the physiology driving the illness toward the next mania.

Such a perspective also could account for the observation of the emergence of loss of efficacy via tolerance to the major mood-stabilizing agents lithium, carbamazepine, and valproate (Post et al. 1990, 1993a; Weiss et al. 1995). In these instances, one would postulate an increasing predominance of pathological processes that are finally unable to be compensated by endogenous mechanisms (such as TRH) as supplemented by exogenous medications (such as the mood stabilizers), resulting in an episode breakthrough. With the occurrence of such a breakthrough episode, a new set of transient endogenous compensatory changes may be induced, sufficient to reenable the therapeutic effects of the drug, at least temporarily. With the putative dissipation of these endogenous adaptations, and an equal or progressive engendering illness drive of the primary pathological mechanisms, breakthrough episodes may again reoccur, and so on, leading to complete loss of drug efficacy.

Given this rubric and the overall trend for increasing emergence of episode severity and/or cyclicity over the course of untreated illness (Post and Weiss 1996), or during the breakthrough of progressively more frequent and severe episodes in the face of loss of prophylactic drug efficacy via tolerance, one would postulate various clinical principles derived from this model that could be tested directly. The basic tenet is that one should treat early and aggressively enough with the most effective agents, alone or in combination, to completely suppress episodes, so that the appearance of minor episodes does not lead to more major ones and result in progressively more frequent breakthrough episodes. This view of minor "flurries" predicting more major episodes is very consistent with the data of Keller et al. (1992) from the collaborative study, as well as with the life-chart mapping in our studies (Post et al. 1993a), about how episodes can begin to reemerge in the face of loss of efficacy to the mood stabilizers lithium, carbamazepine, and valproate in patients who develop tolerance.

This theoretical perspective thus complements the empirical view that early treatment with lithium carbonate, before too many episodes occur, is much more likely to be effective than later treatment after many episodes have occurred (Denicoff et al. 1997; Gelenberg et al. 1989; O'Connell et al. 1991; Sarantidis and Waters 1981). Thus, an adequate elucidation of the mechanisms of action of the mood stabilizers in bipolar illness should include not only their acute actions, emphasized in the major portion of this chapter, but also their long-term effects on the illness and its underlying mechanisms (Weiss et al. 1995) and the appropriate means of maximizing them in order to provide the best opportunity for long-term and sustained remission in what can otherwise be a potentially lethal mood disorder.

REFERENCES

Aigner T, Weiss SRB, Post RM: Carbamazepine attenuates i.v. cocaine self-administration in rhesus monkeys (abstract). ACNP Abstracts:181, 1990

Atack JR, Prior AM, Griffith D, et al: Characterization of the effects of lithium on phosphatidylinositol (PI) cycle activity in human muscarinic m1 receptor-transfected CHO cells. Br J Pharmacol 110:809–815, 1993

Avissar S, Schreiber G: Interaction of antibipolar and antidepressant treatments with receptor-coupled G proteins. Pharmacopsychiatry 25:44–50, 1992a

Avissar S, Schreiber G: The involvement of G proteins in the pathogenesis and treatment of affective disorders. Biol Psychiatry 3:435–459, 1992b

Avissar S, Schreiber G, Aulakh CS, et al: Carbamazepine and electroconvulsive shock attenuate beta-adrenoceptor and muscarinic cholinoceptor coupling to G proteins in rat cortex. Eur J Pharmacol 189:99–103, 1990

Avissar S, Barki-Harrington L, Nechamkin Y, et al: Reduced beta-adrenergic receptor-coupled Gs protein function and Gs alpha immunoreactivity in mononuclear leukocytes of patients with depression. Biol Psychiatry 39:755–760, 1996

Avissar S, Nechamkin Y, Barki-Harrington L, et al: Differential G protein measures in mononuclear leukocytes of patients with bipolar mood disorder are state dependent. J Affect Disord. 43:85–93, 1997

Balfour JA, Bryson HM: Valproic acid: a review of its pharmacology and therapeutic potential in indications other than epilepsy. CNS Drugs 2:144–173, 1994

Banki CM, Bissette G, Arato M, et al: Elevation of immunoreactive CSF TRH in depressed patients. Am J Psychiatry 145:1526–1531, 1988

Baptista T, Weiss SRB, Post RM: Carbamazepine attenuates cocaine-induced increases in dopamine in the nucleus accumbens: an in vivo dialysis study. Eur J Pharmacol 236:39–42, 1993

Baxter LR: Can lithium carbonate prolong the antidepressant effect of sleep deprivation? (letter) Arch Gen Psychiatry 42:635, 1985

Bebchuk JM, Arfken CL, Dolan-Manji S, et al: A preliminary investigation of a protein kinase C inhibitor (tamoxifen) in the treatment of acute mania. Arch Gen Psychiatry (in press)

Belmaker RH, Avissar S, Schreiber G: Effect of lithium on human neurotransmitter receptor systems and G proteins, in Lithium and the Cell: Pharmacology and Biochemistry. Edited by Birch NJ. London, Academic Press, 1991, pp 113–119

Benjamin J, Levine J, Fux M, et al: Double-blind, placebo-controlled, crossover trial of inositol treatment for panic disorder. Am J Psychiatry 152:1084–1086, 1995

Bernasconi R: The GABA hypothesis of affective illness: influence of clinically effective antimanic drugs on GABA turnover, in Basic Mechanisms in the Action of Lithium. Proceedings of symposium held at Schloss Ringberg, F.R.G., Bavaria, October 4–6, 1981. Amsterdam, Excerpta Medica, 1982, pp 183–192

Beydoun A, Uthman BM, Sackellares JC: Gabapentin: pharmacokinetics, efficacy, and safety. Clin Neuropharmacol 18:469–481, 1995

Biber K, Fiebich BL, Gebicke-Harter P, et al: Carbamazepine-induced upregulation of adenosine A1-receptors in astrocyte cultures affects coupling to the phosphoinositol signaling pathway. Neuropsychopharmacology 20:271–278, 1999

Bowden CL, Brugger AM, Swann AC, et al: Efficacy of divalproex vs lithium and placebo in the treatment of mania. JAMA 271:918–924, 1994

Brewerton TD, Jackson CW: Prophylaxis of carbamazepine-induced hyponatremia by demeclocycline in six patients. J Clin Psychiatry 55:249–251, 1994

Bunney WE Jr, Garland-Bunney BL: Mechanisms of action of lithium in affective illness: basic and clinical implications, in Psychopharmacology: The Third Generation of Progress. Edited by Meltzer HY. New York, Raven, 1987, pp 553–565

Calabrese JR, Delucchi GA: Phenomenology of rapid cycling manic depression and its treatment with valproate. J Clin Psychiatry 50:30–34, 1989

Calabrese JR, Delucchi GA: Spectrum of efficacy of valproate in 55 patients with rapid-cycling bipolar disorder. Am J Psychiatry 147:431–434, 1990

Calabrese JR, Woyshville MJ, Rapport RT: Clinical efficacy of valproate, in Anticonvulsants in Mood Disorders. Edited by Joffe RT, Calabrese JR. New York, Marcel Dekker, 1994, pp 131–146

Callahan AM, Frye MA, Marangell LB, et al: Comparative antidepressant effects of intravenous and intrathecal thyrotropin releasing hormone: confounding effects of tolerance and implications for therapeutics. Biol Psychiatry 41:264–272, 1997

Carman JS, Wyatt ES, Smith W, et al: Calcium and calcitonin in bipolar illness, in Neurobiology of Mood Disorders. Edited by Post RM, Ballenger JC. Baltimore, MD, Williams & Wilkins, 1984, pp 340–355

Chalecka-Franaszek E, Chuang DM: Lithium activates the serine/threonine kinase Akt-1 and suppresses glutamate-induced inhibition of Akt-1 activity in neurons. Proc Natl Acad Sci U S A 96:8745–8750

Chen G, Hough C, Manji HK, et al: Desipramine and carbamazepine modulare β-adrenergic receptors βARs and βAR mRNA in vitro. Clin Pharmacol Ther 51:190, 1992

Chen G, Manji HK, Hawver DB, et al: Chronic sodium valproate selectively decreases protein kinase C alpha and epsilon in vitro. J Neurochem 63:2361–2364, 1994

Chen G, Yuan PX, Jiang YM, et al: Valproate robustly enhances AP-1 mediated gene expression. Brain Res.Mol.Brain Res 64:52–58, 1999a

Chen G, Zeng WZ, Yuan PX, et al: The mood-stabilizing agents lithium and valproate robustly increase the levels of the neuroprotective protein bcl-2 in the CNS. J Neurochem 72:879–882, 1999b

Chen RW, Chuang DM: Long term lithium treatment suppresses p53 and Bax expression but increases Bcl-2 expression: a prominent role in neuroprotection against excitotoxicity. J Biol Chem (Communication) 274:6039–6042, 1999

Clark M, Post RM: Carbamazepine, but not caffeine, is highly selective for adenosine A_1 binding sites. Eur J Pharmacol 164:399–401, 1989

Colin SF, Chang H-C, Mollner S, et al: Chronic lithium regulates the expression of adenylate cyclase and G_I-protein alpha subunit in rat cerebral cortex. Proc Natl Acad Sci U S A 88:10634–10637, 1991

Consolo S, Bianchi S, Ladinsky H: Effects of carbamazepine on cholinergic parameters in rat brain areas. Neuropharmacology 15:653–657, 1976

Crunelli V, Cervo L, Samanin R: Evidence for a preferential role of central noradrenergic neurons in electrically induced convulsions and activity of various anticonvulsants in the rat, in Neurotransmitters, Seizures and Epilepsy. Edited by Morselli PL, Lloyd KG, Loscher W. New York, Raven, 1981, pp 195–202

Curzon G: Serotonergic mechanisms of depression. Clin Neuropharmacol 11 (suppl 2):S11–S20, 1988

Dailey JW, Yan QS, Adams-Curtis LE, et al: Neurochemical correlates of antiepileptic drugs in the genetically epilepsy-prone rat (GEPR). Life Sci 58:259–266, 1995

Daval JL, Deckert J, Weiss SRB, et al: Upregulation of adenosine A_1 receptors and forskolin binding sites following chronic treatment with caffeine or carbamazepine: a quantitative autoradiographic study. Epilepsia 30:26–33, 1989

De Montigny C, Grunberg F, Mayer A, et al: Lithium induces rapid relief of depression in tricyclic antidepressant drug non-responders. Br J Psychiatry 138:252–256, 1981

De Montigny C, Cournoyer G, Morissette R: Lithium carbonate addition in tricyclic antidepressant-resistant unipolar depression: correlations with the neurobiologic actions of tricyclic antidepressant drugs and lithium ion on the serotonin system. Arch Gen Psychiatry 40:1327–1334, 1983

Denicoff KD, Smith-Jackson EE, Disney ER, et al: Comparative prophylactic efficacy of lithium, carbamazepine, and the combination in bipolar disorder. J Clin Psychiatry 58:470–478, 1997

Di Costanzo E, Schifano F: Lithium alone or in combination with carbamazepine for the treatment of rapid-cycling bipolar affective disorder. Acta Psychiatr Scand 83:456–459, 1991

Divish MM, Sheftel G, Boyle A, et al: Differential effect of lithium on fos protooncogene expression mediated by receptor and postreceptor activators of protein kinase C and cyclic adenosine monophosphate: model for its antimanic action. J Neurosci Res 28:40–48, 1991

Dixon J, Los G, Hokin L: Lithium stimulates glutamate "release" and inositol 1,4,5-trisphosphate accumulation via activation of the N-methyl-D-aspartate receptor in monkey and mouse cerebral cortex slices. Proc Natl Acad Sci U S A 91:8358–8362, 1994

Dubovsky SL: Calcium antagonists for manic-depressive illness. Neuropsychobiology 27:184–192, 1993

Dubovsky SL, Thomas M, Hijazi A, et al: Intracellular calcium signalling in peripheral cells of patients with bipolar affective disorder. Eur Arch Psychiatry Clin Neurosci 243:229–234, 1994

Elliott P: Action of antiepileptic and anaesthetic drugs on Na-and Ca-spikes in mammalian non-myelinated axons. Eur J Pharmacol 175:155–163, 1990

Elphick M, Taghavi Z, Powell T, et al: Chronic carbamazepine down-regulates adenosine A_2 receptors: studies with the putative selective adenosine antagonists PD115,199 and PD116,948. Psychopharmacology (Berl) 100:522–529, 1990

Emrich HM, Dose M, Von Zerssen D: The use of sodium valproate, carbamazepine and oxcarbazepine in patients with affective disorders. J Affect Disord 8:243–250, 1985

Fischer W, Muller M: Pharmacological modulation of central monoaminergic systems and influence on the anticonvulsant effectiveness of standard antiepileptics in maximal electroshock seizure. Biomedica Biochimica Acta 47:631–645, 1988

Freeman TW, Clothier JL, Pazzaglia P, et al: A double-blind comparison of valproate and lithium in the treatment of acute mania. Am J Psychiatry 149:108–111, 1992

Gao XM, Chuang DM: Carbamazepine-induced neurotoxicity and its prevention by NMDA in cultured cerebellar granule cells. Neurosci Lett 135:159–162, 1992

Gao X-M, Fukamauchi F, Chuang D-M: Long-term biphasic effects of lithium treatment on phospholipase C-coupled M_3-muscarinic acetylcholine receptors in cultured cerebellar granule cells. Neurochem Int 22:395–403, 1993

Gasser T, Reddington M, Schubert P: Effect of carbamazepine on stimulus-evoked Ca2+ fluxes in rat hippocampal slices and its interaction with A1-adenosine receptors. Neurosci Lett 91:189–193, 1988

Gelenberg AJ, Kane JM, Keller MB, et al: Comparison of standard and low serum levels of lithium for maintenance treatment of bipolar disorder. N Engl J Med 321: 1489–1493, 1989

Gold PW, Ballenger JC, Robertson GL, et al: Vasopressin in affective illness: direct measurement, clinical trials and response to hypertonic saline, in Neurobiology of Mood Disorders. Edited by Post RM, Ballenger JC. Baltimore, MD, Williams & Wilkins, 1984, pp 323–339

Gunn AJ, Dragunow M, Faull RL, et al: Effects of hypoxia-ischemia and seizures on neuronal and glial-like c-fos protein levels in the infant rat. Brain Res 531:105–116, 1990

Hong JS, Tilson HA, Yoshikawa K: Effects of lithium and haloperidol administration on the rat brain levels of substance P. J Pharmacol Exp Ther 224:590–593, 1983

Hoschl C, Kozeny J: Verapamil in affective disorders: a controlled, double-blind study. Biol Psychiatry 25:128–140, 1989

Hough CJ, Irwin RP, Gao X-M, et al: Carbamazepine inhibition of N-methyl-D-aspartate-evoked calcium influx in rat cerebellar granule cells. J Pharmacol Exp Ther 276:143–149, 1996

Jacobson SJ, Jones K, Johnson K, et al: Prospective multicentre study of pregnancy outcome after lithium exposure during first trimester. Lancet 339:530–533, 1992

Janowsky DS, El-Yousef MK, Davis JM: Parasympathetic suppression of manic symptoms by physostigmine. Arch Gen Psychiatry 28:542–547, 1973

Joffe RT, Post RM, Uhde TW: Effects of carbamazepine on serum electrolytes in affectively ill patients. Psychol Med 16:331–335, 1986

Keck PE Jr, McElroy SL, Vuckovic A, et al: Combined valproate and carbamazepine treatment of bipolar disorder. J Neuropsychiatry Clin Neurosci 4:319–322, 1992

Keck PE, McElroy SL, Tugrul KC, et al: Antiepileptic drugs for the treatment of panic disorder. Neuropsychobiology 27:150–153, 1993

Keck PE, McElroy SL, Bennett JA: Pharmacology and pharmacokinetics of valproic acid, in Anticonvulsants in Mood Disorders. Edited by Joffe RT, Calabrese JR. New York, Marcel Dekker, 1994, pp 27–42

Keller MB, Lavori PW, Kane JM, et al: Subsyndromal symptoms in bipolar disorder: a comparison of standard and low serum levels of lithium. Arch Gen Psychiatry 49:371–376, 1992

Ketter TA, Kimbrell TA, George MS, et al: Baseline hypermetabolism may predict carbamazepine response, and hypometabolism nimodipine response in mood disorders (abstract). XXth annual meeting of the Collegium Internationale Neuropsychologicum Congress, Melbourne, Australia, June 1996

Khaitan L, Calabrese JR, Stockmeier CA: Effects of chronic treatment with valproate on serotonin-1A receptor binding and function. Psychopharmacology (Berl) 113: 539–542, 1994

Kirkegaard C, Faber J, Hummer L, et al: Increased levels of TRH in cerebrospinal fluid from patients with endogenous depression. Psychoneuroendocrinology 4:227–235, 1979

Kramer MS, Cutler N, Feighner J, et al: Distinct mechanism for antidepressant activity by blockade of central substance P receptors. Science 281:1640–1645, 1998

Kramlinger KG, Post RM: Adding lithium carbonate to carbamazepine: antimanic efficacy in treatment resistant mania. Acta Psychiatr Scand 79:378–385, 1989a

Kramlinger KG, Post RM: The addition of lithium carbonate to carbamazepine: antidepressant efficacy in treatment-resistant depression. Arch Gen Psychiatry 46: 794–800, 1989b

Krueger KE: Molecular and functional properties of mitochondrial benzodiazepine receptors. Biochim Biophys Acta 1241:453–470, 1995

Lambert PA: Acute and prophylactic therapies of patients with affective disorders using valpromide (dipropylacetamide), in Anticonvulsants in Affective Disorders. Edited by Emrich HM, Okuma T, Muller AA. Amsterdam, Excerpta Medica, 1984, pp 33–44

Lambert PA, Carraz G, Borselli S: Le dipropylacetamide dans le traitement de la psychose maniaco-depressive. Encephale 1:25–31, 1975

Lampe H, Bigalke H: Carbamazepine blocks NMDA-activated currents in cultured spinal cord neurons. Neuroreport 1:26–28, 1990

Lancaster JM, Davies JA: Carbamazepine inhibits NMDA-induced depolarizations in cortical wedges prepared from DBA/2 mice. Experientia 48:751–753, 1992

Le Douarin C, Oblin A, Fage D, et al: Influence of lithium on biochemical manifestations of striatal dopamine target cell supersensitivity induced by prolonged haloperidol treatment. Eur J Pharmacol 93:55–62, 1983

Le Fur G, Mestre M, Carriot T, et al: Pharmacology of peripheral type benzodiazepine receptors in the heart. Prog Clin Biol Res 192:175–186, 1985

Lesch KP, Aulakh CS, Tolliver TJ, et al: Differential effects of long-term lithium and carbamazepine administration on Gsa and Gia protein in rat brain. Eur J Pharmacol (Mol Pharmacol) 20:355–359, 1991

Leslie RA, Moorman JM, Grahame-Smith DG: Lithium enhances 5-HT2A receptor-mediated c-fos expression in rat cerebral cortex. Neuroreport 5:241–244, 1993

Levine J, Barak Y, Gonzalves M, et al: Double-blind, controlled trial of inositol treatment of depression. Am J Psychiatry 152:792–794, 1995

Li PP, Tam Y, Young LT, et al: Lithium decreases Gs, Gi-1 and Gi-2 a subunit mRNA levels in rat cortex. Eur J Pharmacol 206:165–166, 1991

Lindhout D, Omtzigt JG, Cornel MC: Spectrum of neural-tube defects in 34 infants prenatally exposed to antiepileptic drugs. Neurology 42:111–118, 1992

Maitre L, Baltzer V, Mondadori C: Psychopharmacological and behavioural effects of anti-epileptic drugs in animals, in Anticonvulsants in Affective Disorders. Edited by Emrich HM, Okuma T, Muller AA. Amsterdam, Excerpta Medica, 1984, pp 3–13

Manji HK: G proteins: implications for psychiatry. Am J Psychiatry 149:746–760, 1992

Manji HK, Etcheberrigaray R, Chen G, et al: Lithium decreases membrane-associated protein kinase C in hippocampus: selectivity for the α isozyme. J Neurochem 61:2303–2310, 1993

Manji HK, Potter WZ, Lenox RH: Signal transduction pathways: molecular targets for lithium's actions. Arch Gen Psychiatry 52:531–543, 1995

Manna V: [Bipolar affective disorders and role of intraneuronal calcium: therapeutic effects of the treatment with lithium salts and/or calcium antagonist in patients with rapid polar inversion]. Minerva Medica 82:757–763, 1991

Marangell L, George MS, Bissette G, et al: Carbamazepine increases CSF thyrotropin-releasing hormone in affectively ill patients. Arch Gen Psychiatry 51:625–628, 1994

Marangell LB, George MS, Callahan AM, et al: Effects of intrathecal thyrotropin-releasing hormone (protirelin) in refractory depressed patients. Arch Gen Psychiatry 54:214–222, 1997

Marangos P, Post RM, Patel J, et al: Specific and potent interactions between carbamazepine and brain adenosine receptors. Eur J Pharmacol 93:175–182, 1983

Marangos PJ, Daval JL, Weiss SRB, et al: Carbamazepine and brain adenosine receptors, in Neonatal Seizures. Edited by Wasterlain CG, Vert P. New York, Raven, 1990, pp 203–209

McDermut W, Pazzaglia PJ, Huggins T, et al: Use of single case analyses in off-on-off-on trials in affective illness: a demonstration of the efficacy of nimodipine. Depression 2:259–271, 1995

McLean MJ, MacDonald RL: Carbamazepine and 10,11-epoxycarbamazepine produce use- and voltage-dependent limitation of rapidly firing action potentials of mouse central neurons in cell culture. J Pharmacol Exp Ther 238:727–738, 1986a

McLean MH, MacDonald RL: Sodium valproate, but not ethosuximide, produces use- and voltage-dependent limitation of high frequency repetitive firing of action potentials of mouse central neurons in cell culture. J Pharmacol Exp Ther 237:1001–1010, 1986b

Meltzer HL: Mode of action of lithium in affective disorders: an influence on intracellular calcium functions. Pharmacol Toxicol 66:84–99, 1990

Mestre M, Carriot T, Belin C, et al: Electrophysiological and pharmacological evidence that peripheral type benzodiazepine receptors are coupled to calcium channels in the heart. Life Sci 36:391–400, 1985

Mitsushio H, Takashima M, Mataga N, et al: Effects of chronic treatment with trihexyphenidyl and carbamazepine alone or in combination with haloperidol on substance P content in rat brain: a possible implication of substance P in affective disorders. J Pharmacol Exp Ther 245:982–989, 1988

Morrow AL, Pace JR, Purdy RH, et al: Characterization of steroid interactions with gamma-aminobutyric acid receptor-gated chloride ion channels: evidence for multiple steroid recognition sites. Mol Pharmacol 37:263–270, 1990

Motohashi N: GABA receptor alterations after chronic lithium—in comparison with carbamazepine and sodium valproate. Clin Neuropharmacol 13:207–208, 1990

Motohashi N, Ikawa K, Kariya T: $GABA_B$ receptors are up-regulated by chronic treatment with lithium or carbamazepine: GABA hypothesis of affective disorders. Eur J Pharmacol 166:95–99, 1989

Nonaka S, Chuang DM: Neuroprotective effects of chronic lithium on focal cerebral ischemia in rats. Neuroreport. 9:2081–2084, 1998

Nonaka S, Hough CJ, Chuang DM: Chronic lithium treatment robustly protects neurons in the central nervous system against excitotoxicity by inhibiting N-methyl-D-aspartate receptor-mediated calcium influx. Proc.Natl.Acad.Sci U S A 95:2642–2647, 1998a

Nonaka S, Katsube N, Chuang DM: Lithium protects rat cerebellar granule cells against apoptosis induced by anticonvulsants, phenytoin and carbamazepine. J Pharmacol.Exp Ther 286:539–547, 1998b

O'Connell RA, Mayo JA, Flatow L, et al: Outcome of bipolar disorder on long-term treatment with lithium. Br J Psychiatry 159:123–129, 1991

Okuma T: Effects of carbamazepine and lithium on affective disorders. Neuropsychobiology 27:138–145, 1993

Olpe HR: Mechanism of action of antiepileptic drugs with special reference to carbamazepine (abstract). Abstracts, World Congress of Biological Psychiatry, Florence, Italy, June 1991, p 185

Olpe H, Kolb CN, Hausdorf A, et al: 4-Aminopyridine and barium chloride attenuate the anti-epileptic effect of carbamazepine in hippocampal slices. Experientia 47:254–257, 1991

Ozaki N, Chuang DM: Lithium increases transcription factor binding to AP-1 and cyclic AMP-responsive element in cultured neurons and rat brain. J Neurochem 69:2336–2344, 1997

Pazzaglia PJ, Post RM, Ketter TA, et al: Preliminary controlled trial of nimodipine in ultra-rapid cycling affective dysregulation. Psychiatry Res 49:257–272, 1993

Pazzaglia PJ, George MS, Post RM, et al: Nimodipine increases CSF somatostatin in affectively ill patients. Neuropsychopharmacology 13:75–83, 1995

Pazzaglia PJ, Post RM, Ketter TA, et al: Nimodipine monotherapy and carbamazepine augmentation in patients with refractory recurrent affective illness. J Clin Psychopharmacol 18:404–413, 1998

Pfeiffer A, Veilleux S, Barden N: Antidepressant and other centrally acting drugs regulate glucorticoid receptor messenger RNA levels in rat brain. Psychoneuroendocrinology 16:505–515, 1991

Pope HG, McElroy SL, Keck PE Jr, et al: Valproate in the treatment of acute mania. Arch Gen Psychiatry 48:62–68, 1991

Post RM: Time course of clinical effects of carbamazepine: implications for mechanisms of action. J Clin Psychiatry 49:35–46, 1988

Post RM: Prophylaxis of bipolar affective disorders. International Review of Psychiatry 2:277–320, 1990

Post RM, Chuang D-M: Mechanism of action of lithium: comparison and contrast with carbamazepine, in Lithium and the Cell: Pharmacology and Biochemistry. Edited by Birch NJ. London, Academic Press, 1991, pp 199–241

Post RM, Weiss SRB: Endogenous biochemical abnormalities in affective illness: therapeutic vs. pathogenic. Biol Psychiatry 32:469–484, 1992

Post RM, Weiss SRB: A speculative model of affective illness cyclicity based on patterns of drug tolerance observed in amygdala-kindled seizures. Mol Neurobiol 13:33–60, 1996

Post RM, Jimerson DC, Bunney WE Jr, et al: Dopamine and mania: behavioral and biochemical effects of the dopamine receptor blocker pimozide. Psychopharmacology 67:297–305, 1980

Post RM, Ballenger JC, Uhde TW, et al: Effect of carbamazepine on cyclic nucleotides in CSF of patients with affective illness. Biol Psychiatry 17:1037–1045, 1982

Post RM, Jimerson DC, Ballenger JC, et al: Cerebrospinal fluid norepinephrine and its metabolites in manic-depressive illness, in Neurobiology of Mood Disorders. Edited by Post RM, Ballenger JC. Baltimore, MD, Williams & Wilkins, 1984, pp 539–553

Post RM, Rubinow DR, Uhde TW, et al: Effects of carbamazepine on noradrenergic mechanisms in affectively ill patients. Psychopharmacology 87:59–63, 1985

Post RM, Uhde TW, Rubinow DR, et al: Differential time course of antidepressant effects following sleep deprivation, ECT, and carbamazepine: clinical and theoretical implications. Psychiatry Res 22:11–19, 1987

Post RM, Leverich GS, Rosoff AS, et al: Carbamazepine prophylaxis in refractory affective disorders: a focus on long-term follow-up. J Clin Psychopharmacol 10:318–327, 1990

Post RM, Ketter TA, Joffe RT, et al: Lack of beneficial effects of l-baclofen in affective disorders. Int Clin Psychopharmacol 6:197–207, 1991

Post RM, Weiss SRB, Chuang D-M: Mechanisms of action of anticonvulsants in affective disorders: comparisons with lithium. J Clin Psychopharmacol 12:23S–35S, 1992

Post RM, Ketter TA, Denicoff K, et al: Assessment of anticonvulsant drugs in patients with bipolar affective illness, in Human Psychopharmacology: Methods and Measures. Edited by Hindmarch I, Stonier PD. Chichester, England, John Wiley & Sons, 1993a, pp 211–245

Post RM, Weiss SRB, Aigner TG: Carbamazepine in the treatment of cocaine abuse, in Biological Basis of Substance Abuse. Edited by Korenman SG, Barchas JD. New York, Oxford University Press, 1993b, pp 443–462

Post RM, Weiss SRB, Chuang D, et al: Mechanisms of action of carbamazepine in seizure and affective disorders, in Anticonvulsants in Mood Disorders. Edited by Joffe RT, Calabrese JR. New York, Marcel Dekker, 1994, pp 43–92

Post RM, Ketter TA, Pazzaglia PJ, et al: Rational polypharmacy in the bipolar affective disorders. Epilepsy Res 11 (suppl):153–180, 1996a

Post RM, Ketter TA, Denicoff K, et al: The place of anticonvulsant therapy in bipolar illness. Psychopharmacology (Berl) 128:115–129, 1996b

Post RM, Pazzaglia PJ, Ketter TA, et al: Carbamazepine and nimodipine in refractory bipolar illness: efficacy and mechanisms, in Pharmacotherapy for Mood, Anxiety, and Cognitive Disorders. Edited by Halbreich U, Montgomery S. Washington, DC, American Psychiatric Press (in press)

Price LH, Charney DS, Delgado PL, et al: Lithium treatment and serotoninergic function: neuroendocrine and behavioral responses to intravenous tryptophan in affective disorder. Arch Gen Psychiatry 46:13–19, 1989

Price LH, Charney DS, Delgado PL, et al: Lithium and serotonin function: implications for the serotonin hypothesis of depression. Psychopharmacology (Berl) 100:3–12, 1990

Purdy RE, Julien RM, Fairhurst AS: Effect of carbamazepine on the in vitro uptake and release of norepinephrine in adrenergic nerves of rabbit aorta and in whole brain synaptosomes. Epilepsia 18:251–257, 1977

Quattrone A, Samanin R: Decreased anticonvulsant activity of carbamazepine in 6-hydroxydopamine-treated rats. Eur J Pharmacol 41:333–336, 1977

Quattrone A, Crunelli V, Samanin R: Seizure susceptibility and anticonvulsant activity of carbamazepine, diphenylhydantoin and phenobarbitol in rats with selective depletions of brain monoamines. Neuropharmacology 17:643–647, 1978

Quattrone A, Annunziato L, Aguglia V, et al: Carbamazepine, phenytoin and phenobarbital do not influence brain catecholamine uptake, in vivo, in male rats. Archives Internationales de Pharmacodynamic et de Therapie 252:180–185, 1981

Ringel RA, Brick JF: Perspective on carbamazepine-induced water intoxication: reversal by demeclocycline. Neurology 36:1506–1507, 1986

Rubinow DR, Post RM, Gold PW, et al: Effects of carbamazepine on cerebrospinal fluid somatostatin. Psychopharmacology 85:210–213, 1985

Sarantidis D, Waters B: Predictors of lithium prophylaxis effectiveness. Prog Neuropsychopharmacol 5:507–510, 1981

Schaff MR, Fawcett J, Zajecka JM: Divalproex sodium in the treatment of refractory affective disorders. J Clin Psychiatry 54:380–384, 1993

Schreiber G, Avissar S, Danon A, et al: Hyperfunctional G proteins in mononuclear leukocytes of patients with mania. Biol Psychiatry 29:273–280, 1991

Schubert T, Stoll L, Muller WE: Therapeutic concentrations of lithium and carbamazepine inhibit cGMP accumulation in human lymphocytes. Psychopharmacology (Berl) 104:43–50, 1991

Sharma V, Persad E, Mazmanian D, et al: Treatment of rapid cycling bipolar disorder with combination therapy of valproate and lithium. Can J Psychiatry 38:137–139, 1993

Sivam SP, Takeuchi K, Li S, et al: Lithium increases dynorphin A(1-8) and prodynorphin mRNA levels in the basal ganglia of rats. Molecular Brain Research 3:155–164, 1988

Sivam SP, Krause JE, Takeuchi K, et al: Lithium increases rat striatal beta- and gamma-preprotachykinin messenger RNAs. J Pharmacol Exp Ther 248:1297–1301, 1989

Slater GE, Johnston D: Sodium valproate increases potassium conductance in aplysia neurones. Epilepsia 19:379–384, 1978

Stoll AL, Sachs GS, Cohen BM, et al: Choline in the treatment of rapid-cycling bipolar disorder: clinical and neurochemical findings in lithium-treated patients. Biol Psychiatry 40:382–388, 1996

Terrence CF, Sax M, Fromm GH, et al: Effect of baclofen enantiomorphs on the spinal trigeminal nucleus and steric similarities of carbamazepine. Pharmacology 27:85–94, 1983

Uhde TW, Post RM: Effects of carbamazepine on serum electrolytes: clinical and theoretical implications. J Clin Psychopharmacol 3:103–106, 1983

Vadnal R, Parthasarathy R: Myo-inositol monophosphatase: diverse effects of lithium, carbamazepine, and valproate. Neuropsychopharmacology 12:277–285, 1995

Van Praag HM: Depression, suicide, and serotonin metabolism in the brain, in Neurobiology of Mood Disorders. Edited by Post RM, Ballenger JC. Baltimore, MD, Williams & Wilkins, 1984, pp 601–618

Vieweg WV, Yank GR, Rowe WT, et al: Increase in white blood cell count and serum sodium level following the addition of lithium to carbamazepine treatment among three chronically psychotic male patients with disturbed affective states. Psychiatr Q 58:213–217, 1986

Walden J, Altrup U, Reith H, et al: Effects of valproate on early and late potassium currents of single neurons. Eur Neuropsychopharmacol 3:137–141, 1993

Weiss SRB, Post RM: Contingent tolerance to carbamazepine: a peripheral-type benzodiazepine mechanism. Eur J Pharmacol 193:159–163, 1991

Weiss SRB, Post RM, Patel J, et al: Differential mediation of the anticonvulsant effects of carbamazepine and diazepam. Life Sci 36:2413–2419, 1985

Weiss SRB, Post RM, Marangos PJ, et al: Peripheral-type benzodiazepines: behavioral effects and interactions with the anticonvulsant effects of carbamazepine, in Kindling III. Edited by Wada JA. New York, Raven, 1986, pp 375–389

Weiss SRB, Post RM, Szele F, et al: Chronic carbamazepine inhibits the development of local anesthetic seizures kindled by cocaine and lidocaine. Brain Res 497:72–79, 1989

Weiss SRB, Clark M, Rosen JB, et al: Contingent tolerance to the anticonvulsant effects of carbamazepine: relationship to loss of endogenous adaptive mechanisms. Brain Res Rev 20:305–325, 1995

Willow M, Kuenzel EA, Catterall WA: Inhibition of voltage-sensitive sodium channels in neuroblastoma cells and synaptosomes by the anticonvulsant drugs diphenylhydantoin and carbamazepine. Mol Pharmacol 25:228–234, 1984

Yan QS, Mishra PK, Burger RL, et al: Evidence that carbamazepine and antiepilepsirine may produce a component of their anticonvulsant effects by activating serotonergic neurons in genetically epilepsy-prone rats. J Pharmacol Exp Ther 261:652–659, 1992

Yassa R, Iskandar H, Nastase C, et al: Carbamazepine and hyponatremia in patients with affective disorder. Am J Psychiatry 145:339–342, 1988

Young LT, Warsh JJ, Kish SJ, et al: Reduced brain 5-HT and elevated NE turnover and metabolites in bipolar affective disorder. Biol Psychiatry 35:121–127, 1994

Zeise ML, Kasparow S, Zieglgansberger W: Valproate suppresses N-methyl-D-aspartate-evoked, transient depolarizations in the rat neocortex in vitro. Brain Res 544:345–348, 1991

Zona C, Avoli M: Effects induced by the antiepileptic drug valproic acid upon the ionic currents recorded in rat neocortical neurons in cell culture. Exp Brain Res 81: 313–317, 1990

Zona C, Tancredi V, Palma E, et al: Potassium currents in rat cortical neurons in culture are enhanced by the antiepileptic drug carbamazepine. Can J Physiol Pharmacol 68:545–547, 1990

CHAPTER 11

POTENTIATION OF IMMEDIATE-EARLY GENE *c-fos* EXPRESSION IN CEREBRAL CORTEX BY CHRONIC LITHIUM TREATMENT AFTER 5-HT_{2A} RECEPTOR ACTIVATION

R. A. Leslie, Ph.D., and
J. M. Moorman, Ph.D.

Despite the highly successful use of lithium for the treatment of bipolar disorder (Prien et al. 1984), its mechanism of action is still poorly understood. One suggestion that has received much attention has been termed the *inositol depletion hypothesis* (Berridge and Irvine 1989; Berridge et al. 1982), which states that the inhibition of phosphoinositide turnover in especially active neurons by lithium may explain its therapeutic effects. This hypothesis developed from the fact that lithium administration, both in vitro and in vivo, can result in depletion of intracellular inositol, an action assumed to be caused by its inhibition of the enzyme inositol monophosphatase (Hallcher and Sherman 1980).

The inositol depletion hypothesis remains controversial, and several lines

We wish to thank Drs. Mike Clark and Guy Kennett for comments on the manuscript and Professor David Grahame-Smith for his constant support and invaluable discussions throughout the studies reported here.

of evidence are not entirely consistent with it. Some basic and clinical studies have used administrations of several isomers of inositol, including the biologically active isomer *myo*-inositol, which is implicated in phosphatidylinositol (PI) turnover, in order to investigate the hypothesis. Behavioral and other studies have shown reversal of effects of lithium on the administration of large amounts of inositol, which are consistent with the effects of lithium in attenuating PI turnover via its inhibition of inositol monophosphatase (Belmaker et al. 1995; Wood and Goodwin 1987). In contrast, some recent trials with psychiatric patients have found successful results of treatment with oral *myo*-inositol, such that symptoms of depression and other affective disorders have been ameliorated (Belmaker et al. 1995). These authors suggested that entirely different neurobiological mechanisms (perhaps involving separate neurotransmitters or second-messenger systems) might be affected by inositol in the different experimental paradigms. Thus, alleviation of depression by exogenous inositol may not be inconsistent with the inositol depletion hypothesis, which implies that the usefulness of lithium in bipolar affective disorder is the result of its ability to attenuate inositol levels. In any case, a direct link between the inhibitory effect of lithium on the PI cycle and its therapeutic efficacy has yet to be identified. In addition, the inositol depletion hypothesis does not adequately explain the long lag phase that commonly occurs between lithium's initial administration and the onset of several of its therapeutic benefits. Lithium has many effects on central nervous system (CNS) neurons, both on neurotransmitter-receptor interactions and on aspects of intracellular signaling that are not necessarily associated with PI metabolism, and one or more of these other effects may be important for its therapeutic effectiveness.

Many studies have shown that lithium affects the synthesis, turnover, release, and uptake of the amine neurotransmitter 5-hydroxytryptamine (serotonin; 5-HT) (Wood and Goodwin 1987). Furthermore, it enhances the effects of serotonergic antidepressant drugs, particularly in cases of tricyclic-resistant depression (Heninger et al. 1983). Although the number (B_{max}) and function of 5-HT_{2A} receptors are modulated by several antidepressant therapies, lithium's effect on this serotonin receptor subtype is not straightforward. The 5-HT_2 family of serotonin receptors is of particular interest because it activates, through a guanine nucleotide binding protein (G protein) linkage, the hydrolysis of phospholipase C (PLC), which activates the diacylglycerol (DAG) and inositol 1,4,5-trisphosphate (IP_3) second-messenger systems. Lithium's involvement in modulating 5-HT_{2A} receptor function is probably not a simple matter of it altering receptor number or affinity, because many investigations have failed to show a consistent effect (Goodwin et al. 1986; Hotta et al. 1986; Maggi and Enna 1980; Treiser et al. 1981). The functional consequences of lithium on 5-HT_{2A} receptor activity, as measured by behavioral responses, are equally ambiguous (Friedman et al. 1979; Goodwin et al. 1986; Harrison-Read 1979; Kofman and Levin 1995).

We used immunocytochemistry to investigate the expression of the protein product (Fos) of the immediate-early gene (IEG) *c-fos* as a tool to explore the interactions of lithium and serotonin.

ENHANCEMENT BY CHRONIC LITHIUM OF 5-HT_{2A}, BUT NOT 5-HT_{1A}, RECEPTOR–ACTIVATED *c-fos* EXPRESSION IN RAT CEREBRAL CORTEX

The effect of chronic lithium administration on the expression of *c-fos*, following the activation of 5-HT_{1A} or 5-$HT_{2A/2C}$ receptors, was used to monitor the distribution of Fos in adult rat brain. Previously, we showed (Leslie et al. 1993a) that administration of the 5-$HT_{2A/2C}$ receptor agonist 2,5-dimethoxy-4-iodophenylisopropylamine (DOI) resulted in a distinct pattern of Fos immunoreactivity in rat brain, which correlated well with the distribution of 5-HT_{2A} receptor binding sites (Appel et al. 1990). Similarly, challenge of animals with the selective 5-HT_{1A} receptor agonist 8-hydroxy-2-(di-*n*-propylamino) tetralin (8-OH-DPAT) resulted in a characteristic but distinct pattern of Fos-like immunoreactivity (FLI) in rat forebrain (Leslie et al. 1993b).

Male Sprague-Dawley rats (250–300 g) were used in these studies. Animals were housed with a 12-hour light-dark cycle and fed ad libitum. Animals were handled daily for at least a week before any assessment of *c-fos* activity in the brain to ensure that effects of stress on Fos expression were minimized. At least four animals per group were used, and the groups consisted of rats challenged with intraperitoneal DOI–hydrogen chloride (HCl; 8 mg/kg), 8-OH-DPAT (2 mg/kg), or saline vehicle, with or without lithium pretreatment. Rats were treated with either acute intraperitoneal injection of 3 mEq/kg of lithium chloride (LiCl) in distilled water or chronic administration (1–3 weeks) of rat chow containing lithium carbonate (0.1% weight/weight). Rats from both control and lithium dietary groups had free access to tap water and 0.9% normal saline. Following injection with the serotonin receptor agonist, animals were perfused for immunocytochemical examination of brain tissue. Prior to perfusion, blood samples were taken from all animals for analysis of lithium plasma levels by atomic absorption spectroscopy. Dietary lithium resulted in lithium plasma levels in the range of 0.4–0.6 mEq/L. All control animals had lithium plasma levels of less than 0.01 mEq/L.

For immunocytochemistry, animals were anesthetized and perfused transcardially with 100 mL of normal saline followed by 100 mL of 4% paraformaldehyde in 0.1 M sodium phosphate buffer. Brains were postfixed in the same fixative for at least another 24 hours, and 100-μm Vibratome sections were cut and collected in sodium phosphate buffer. Sections were preincubated for 30 minutes in 1% H_2O_2 and then incubated for 3 days in a polyclonal primary antiserum raised against residues 2–16 of the N-terminal region of the Fos molecule (Cambridge Research Chemicals, UK). After routine treatment for immunocytochemistry with the avidin-biotin complex procedure followed by a chromogen reaction in 0.05% 3,3′ -diaminobenzidine, sections were mounted on glass slides, air dried, and examined microscopically. In cells showing FLI, numbers of immunoreactive cell nuclei in a standard tissue area in each section (approximately 0.03 mm^2) were counted. Counts were made over the appropriate brain nucleus in sections taken from four separate experiments in each case, and means ± standard error of the mean (SEM) were calculated. Results were analyzed by unpaired Student's t test and were considered significant at $P < 0.05$.

Time course experiments revealed that Fos protein began to be detectable 30 minutes after treatment with DOI, reached a maximum level (i.e., most dense reaction product within cell nuclei was evident) at 3 hours, and then declined to background or near background levels during subsequent examinations (Figure 11–1). For example, at 24 and 48 hours postinjection with DOI, very little FLI was detectable anywhere in the brain. For all subsequent experiments, a time of 3 hours after the final drug challenge was chosen for preparation of tissues for immunocytochemistry.

Effects of 5-$HT_{2A/2C}$ Receptor Activation on Fos Expression

Examination of rat brain sections from animals that had received saline vehicle injections, acute lithium injections, or chronic lithium treatment followed by saline vehicle challenge showed very low levels of FLI, similar in most cases to those seen in completely drug-naive animals (i.e., resembling basal Fos activity).

Administration of DOI alone to experimental rats resulted in a characteristic pattern of FLI in certain cortical and subcortical areas of the brain (Leslie et al. 1993a; Moorman and Leslie 1998). FLI was elevated over baseline in various regions of the cerebral cortex and the mamillary bodies, bed nucleus of the stria terminalis, amygdala, and corpus striatum (Table 11–1). The amounts of FLI varied considerably in different cortical regions; for example, in the somatosensory cortex, FLI was characteristically high in a single layer

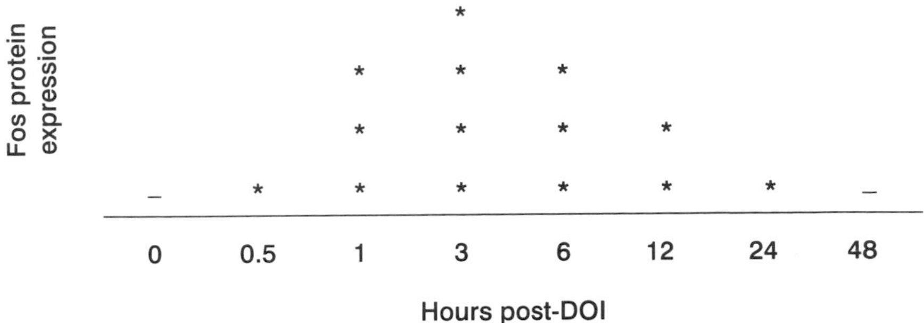

Figure 11–1. Time course of Fos protein expression as monitored by immunocytochemistry in rat cerebral cortex following systemic challenge with 2,5-dimethoxy-4-iodophenylisopropylamine (DOI) (see text). Symbols:
– = background levels of expression;
* = just detectable above background;
** = light expression above background;
*** = moderate expression above background;
**** = strong expression above background.

(layer Va; Figure 11–2), whereas levels were only moderate anywhere in the piriform cortex (Figure 11–3). Very little or no FLI was detectable in some brain regions known to contain 5-HT_{2A} receptor ligand binding sites—for example, in the ventral dentate gyrus of the hippocampus (Pazos et al. 1985).

Pretreatment with the 5-HT_{2A} receptor antagonist spiperone (Kennett and Curzon 1991) attenuated FLI caused by DOI treatment in several cortical and subcortical brain regions (Table 11–1). In areas in which no such attenuation occurred, such as the caudate nucleus, olfactory tubercle, and nucleus accumbens, treatment with spiperone alone followed by a control saline injection resulted in FLI in these same brain regions, suggesting that this drug itself was involved in the positive Fos response in these regions. This elevation of *c-fos* expression is most likely the result of the action of spiperone in these brain regions as a dopamine D_2 receptor antagonist as well as a potent and selective (among 5-HT_2 receptors) 5-HT_{2A} receptor antagonist (Dragunow et al. 1990; Leslie et al. 1993a). In contrast, pretreatment with the 5-$HT_{2A/2C}$ receptor antagonist ritanserin significantly attenuated the DOI-induced FLI in most regions in which it was expressed (Table 11–1). Control animals given ritanserin followed by a saline injection and animals injected with only saline vehicle showed very little FLI in all brain regions (Table 11–1). The results suggest that at least the cortical FLI observed in these studies was largely caused by activation of 5-HT_{2A} receptors by DOI (Leslie et al. 1993a; Moorman and Leslie 1998).

Table 11–1. Fos protein expression in rat forebrain following DOI administration

	Sal	DOI	DOI + spiperone	DOI + ritanserin	Spiperone	Ritanserin
Medial amygdala	0	28.8 ±3.4	13.5 ±2.5*	2.3 ±1.2*	0	0
Mamillary nucleus	0	25.5 ±2.1	18.5 ±3.5	3.0 ±2.5*	1.0 ±0.4	4.0 ±2.3
Bed nucleus of the stria terminalis	0	14.0 ±3.6	19.7 ±7.7	2.3 ±0.3*	3.0 ±2.4	1.0 ±1.0
Caudate nucleus	0	17.4 ±2.0	20.7 ±2.6	2.0 ±2.0*	10.0 ±0.8	0
Piriform cortex	1	10.0 ±0.8	7.7 ±0.8	4.0 ±2.0	3.0 ±0.8	3.0 ±0.6
Cingulate cortex	0	17.4 ±2.5	9.7 ±1.2*	1.7 ±1.7*	1.0 ±0.8	0
Parietal (somatosensory region, layer Va) cortex	0	21.6 ±2.5	8.0 ±0.6*	0.7 ±0.7*	0	0

Note. Values indicate numbers of immunoreactive cells in specific brain nuclei counted in tissue sections within an area of 0.03 mm^2. Numbers are means ± SEM. Abbreviations and conditions: Sal = saline vehicle controls; DOI = 8 mg/kg DOI (2,5-dimethoxy-4-iodophenylisopropylamine); DOI + spiperone = 1 mg/kg spiperone followed by 8 mg/kg DOI; DOI + ritanserin = 0.4 mg/kg ritanserin followed by DOI; spiperone = 1 mg/kg spiperone followed by saline vehicle; ritanserin = 0.4 mg/kg ritanserin followed by saline vehicle. All drugs were given intraperitoneally.

*$P < 0.05$ (unpaired Student's *t* test) compared with DOI alone.

Source. Adapted from Leslie RA, Moorman JM, Coulson A, et al.: "Serotonin$_{2/1c}$ Receptor Activation Causes a Localized Expression of the Immediate-Early Gene c-fos in Rat Brain: Evidence for Involvement of Dorsal Raphe Nucleus Projection Fibres." *Neuroscience* 53:457–463,1993. Copyright 1993, with kind permission from Elsevier Science Ltd., The Boulevard, Langford Lane, Kidlington, UK.

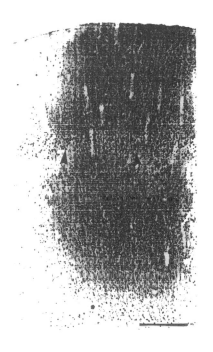

Figure 11–2. Transverse section through somatosensory (SI) cortex of a rat treated with 8 mg/kg 2,5-dimethoxy-4-iodophenylisopropylamine (DOI). Fos-like immunoreactivity (FLI) is concentrated in the nuclei of cells in layer Va in this region of cortex (arrowheads). Scale bar = 350 μm.
Source. Adapted from Leslie RA, Moorman JM, Coulson A, et al.: "Serotonin$_{2/1C}$ Receptor Activation Causes a Localized Expression of the Immediate-Early Gene c-fos in Rat Brain: Evidence for Involvement of Dorsal Raphe Nucleus Projection Fibres." *Neuroscience* 53:457–463, 1993. Copyright 1993, with kind permission from Elsevier Science Ltd., The Boulevard, Langford Lane, Kidlington, UK.

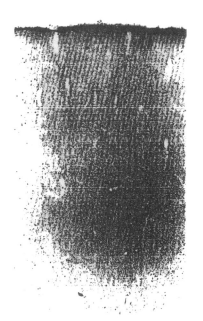

Figure 11–3. Transverse section through a similar region of somatosensory cortex as shown in Figure 11–2, but taken from a rat treated with 2 mg/kg 8-hydroxy-2-(di-*n*-propylamino) tetralin (8-OH-DPAT). A small amount of Fos-like immunoreactivity (FLI) was induced throughout the layers of the cortex. (Magnification as in Figure 11–2.)
Source. Adapted from Leslie RA, Moorman JM, Grahame-Smith DG: "Lithium Enhances 5-HT$_{2A}$ Receptor-Mediated c-fos Expression in Rat Cerebral Cortex." *Neuroreport* 5:241–244, 1993. Used with permission from Rapid Science Ltd.

Some sections were double-immunostained for the Fos protein and for neuron-specific enolase (NSE) or for glial fibrillary acidic protein (GFAP); separate and optically distinct chromogen reactions were used to differentiate the results. Cortical areas contained cells that were clearly stained for both Fos and NSE (Leslie et al. 1993a). Most neurons and most Fos-positive cells appeared to be immunostained for NSE. In contrast, many NSE-positive cells throughout the brain showed no FLI. Cells in sections incubated in separate antisera recognizing Fos protein and GFAP did not contain double-labeled cells (Leslie et al. 1993a).

Effects of 5-HT$_{1A}$ Receptor Activation on Fos Expression

Administration of the 5-HT$_{1A}$ receptor agonist 8-OH-DPAT resulted in FLI in a relatively homogeneous distribution throughout the various layers of the cerebral cortex in the rat, a pattern very different from that observed in animals that had been treated with DOI. This was most noticeable in somatosensory and cingulate cortices, which exhibited a layered pattern of FLI after DOI but no such layering after 8-OH-DPAT (Figure 11–4). The caudal piriform cortex was also much more heavily stained after 8-OH-DPAT than after DOI administration (compare Figure 11–5 with Figure 11–4).

Effects of Lithium on DOI-Induced Fos Expression

Preliminary experiments with acute lithium injections (3 mEq/kg of LiCl intraperitoneally) resulted in variable effects on DOI-induced FLI, which appeared to be dependent on the lithium plasma level. For example, animals that received lithium 5 hours before DOI challenge generally had lithium levels of between 0.6 and 0.8 mEq/L. DOI-induced behavior and FLI in such animals were indistinguishable from those in animals that had not received lithium. However, the lithium plasma level of one animal in this group was 1.1 mEq/L. This animal experienced convulsions, and dense FLI was observed in its caudal piriform cortex. Similarly, animals that received an injection of lithium 7 hours before DOI challenge had convulsions, and FLI was seen in their piriform cortices. Animals in this group had lithium plasma levels of 0.9–1.0 mEq/L. In contrast, one animal that received lithium 16 hours before DOI (resulting in a lithium plasma level of 0.14 mEq/L) had no convulsions, and DOI-induced FLI was similar to that in control animals. Thus, it appears that acute lithium

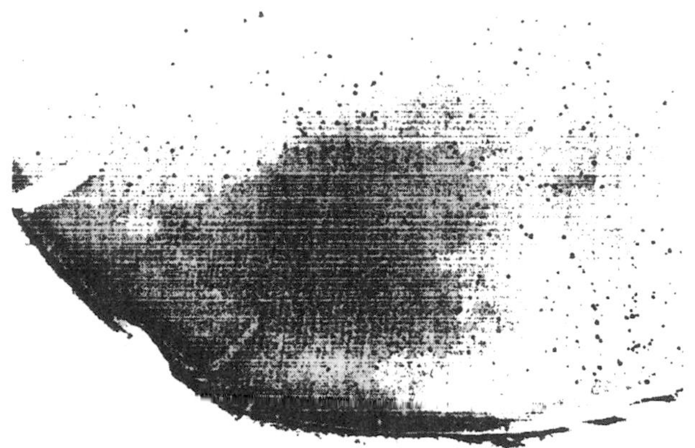

Figure 11–4. Transverse section through the caudal piriform cortex of a rat that had been treated with 2 mg/kg 8-hydroxy-2-(di-*n*-propylamino) tetralin (8-OH-DPAT). Note the relatively dense distribution (compare with Figure 11–5) of Fos-like immunoreactivity (FLI). (Magnification as in Figure 11–2.)
Source. Adapted from Leslie RA, Moorman JM, Grahame-Smith DG: "Lithium Enhances 5-HT_{2A} Receptor-Mediated c-fos Expression in Rat Cerebral Cortex." *Neuroreport* 5:241–244, 1993. Used with permission from Rapid Science Ltd.

administration modulates DOI-induced behavior and Fos expression only when the levels of lithium in plasma exceed 0.9 mEq/L.

Pretreatment of animals with dietary lithium for at least 1 week before DOI challenge (resulting in lithium plasma levels of 0.4–0.6 mEq/L) had consistent and profound effects on the induction of Fos expression (Leslie et al. 1993b; Moorman and Leslie 1998). For example, such treatment resulted in the expression of Fos in the nuclei of many neurons throughout the cortical layers of the cingulate, frontal, and somatosensory cortices after DOI treatment, especially in the superficial layers, such that the previous layered appearance of immunostained cells in these cortical areas was no longer evident. Notably, this effect of lithium was a result of an increase in FLI in cortical layers that previously had low FLI rather than a decrease in the number of Fos-positive nuclei in layer Va (Table 11–2). In the claustrum, lithium pretreatment also resulted in a significant increase in the number of Fos-positive cells after DOI treatment. The most dramatic effect of chronic lithium administration on DOI-induced FLI, however, was seen in the caudal piriform cortex. Whereas this region of cortex expressed little Fos above baseline levels in animals that had received a control diet before DOI treatment, a dense band of Fos-positive nuclei was seen in the pyramidal cell layer of this region of piriform cortex in lithium-treated rats (compare Figure 11–6 with Figure 11–3; see Table 11–2).

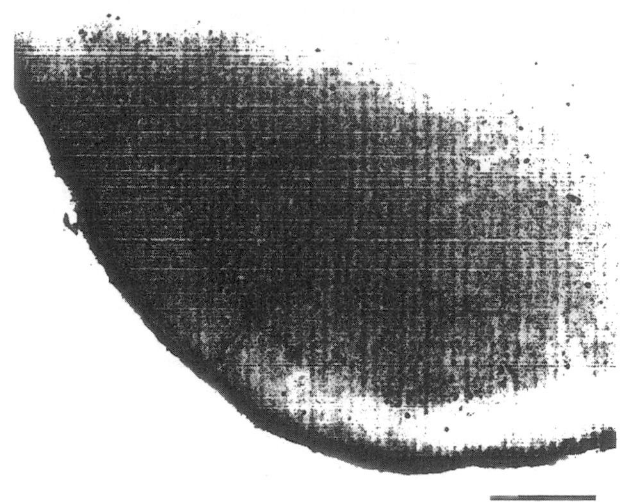

Figure 11–5. Section from rat indicated in Figure 11–2, but taken through the caudal piriform cortex. Note the relative lack of Fos-like immunoreactivity (FLI) in this region of cortex after 2,5-dimethoxy-4-iodophenylisopropylamine (DOI) treatment. Scale bar = 350 μm.
Source. Adapted from Leslie RA, Moorman JM, Grahame-Smith DG: "Lithium Enhances 5-HT_{2A} Receptor-Mediated c-fos Expression in Rat Cerebral Cortex." *Neuroreport* 5:241–244, 1993. Used with permission from Rapid Science Ltd.

In a small percentage (<20%) of cases, lithium-treated rats challenged with DOI had convulsions (severe partial tonic-clonic seizures involving only the upper body, often referred to as *limbic seizures*) that were sometimes fatal. When the brains of such animals were examined for FLI, a very robust Fos response was seen in the dentate gyrus of the hippocampus. No FLI above basal levels was ever seen in the hippocampi of any of our animals that had not experienced such convulsions.

COMPLEX EFFECTS OF CHRONIC LITHIUM ADMINISTRATION ON SEROTONIN RECEPTOR-ACTIVATED BEHAVIOR

To compare the effects of lithium on IEG expression in the brain with another functional measure of serotonin receptor activation, we performed some be-

Table 11–2. Distribution of Fos immunoreactivity following lithium pretreatment

	Li/DOI	Cont/DOI	Li/DPAT	Cont/DPAT	Li/ saline
Piriform cortex	>50*	3.3 ±0.3	7.0 ±2.5	3.0 ±0.5	0.5 ±0.4
Somatosensory cortex (I)	20.2 ±5.7	3.2 ±1.0	2.3 ±0.5	1.3 ±0.5	0
Somatosensory cortex (Va)	21.3 ±2.0	22.3 ±2.3	1.7 ±0.2	0.3 ±0.3	0
Somatosensory cortex (Vb)	7.5 ±0.9*	3.5 ±0.2	0.5 ±0.2	0.5 ±0.2	0
Somatosensory cortex (VI)	7.2 ±1.8	3.8 ±1.0	0.8 ±0.1	0.3 ±0.3	0
Claustrum	19.0 ±2.5*	9.7 ±0.1	6.3 ±0.3	6.5 ±0.6	2.2 ±0.9
Preoptic area	17.0 ±1.7	14.5 ±1.8	6.7 ±0.7	10.0 ±1.1	1.8 ±1.1
Putamen	9.8 ±0.6	12.0 ±0.4	2.0 ±0.5	0	0.3 ±0.3

Note. Values indicate numbers of immunoreactive cells in specific brain nuclei counted in tissue sections within an area of 0.03 mm^2. Numbers are means ±SEM.

*$P < 0.05$ (unpaired Student's t test) compared with cont/DOI. Li = lithium; Cont = saline vehicle control; DOI = 2,5-dimethoxy-4-iodophenylisopropylamine; DPAT = 8-hydroxy-2-(di-*n*-propylamino) tetralin (8-OH-DPAT).

Source. Adapted from Leslie RA, Moorman JM, Grahame-Smith DG: "Lithium Enhances 5-HT_{2A} Receptor-Mediated c-fos Expression in Rat Cerebral Cortex." *Neuroreport* 5:241–244, 1993. Used with permission from Rapid Science Ltd.

havioral experiments that examined the effects of the 5-HT_{2A} receptor agonist DOI on rat motor function. Two groups of animals were tested. Prior to drug challenge, one group received a lithium-containing diet and the other group received normal rat chow for 3 weeks. On test days, animals were habituated in separate cages for at least 60 minutes before an intraperitoneal injection of 8 mg/kg of DOI. Locomotor activity was then monitored by a computerized Opto-Varimex II activity monitor (Columbus Instruments, Columbus, OH), and the number of head shakes was counted manually, each for a period of 30 minutes immediately after DOI injection. Three hours after injection, animals were perfused for immunocytochemical examination of brain tissue. Blood samples were taken from all animals for plasma lithium analysis to ensure that plasma levels remained within desired levels (0.4–0.6 mEq/L).

DOI administration to rats resulted in behavior that has been shown to be mediated by 5-$HT_{2A/2C}$ receptor activation (Pranzatelli 1990). Such behavior involved characteristic head shakes, rearing, and back-muscle twitches. Pretreatment of animals with chronic dietary lithium for 3 weeks resulted in a

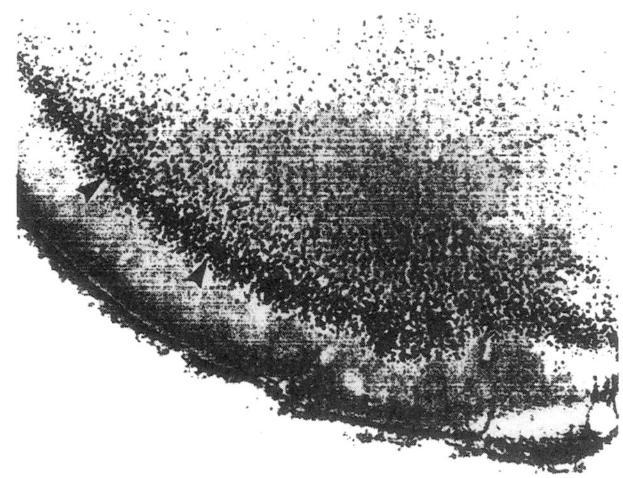

Figure 11–6. Transverse section through caudal piriform cortex of a rat that had been treated with 8 mg/kg 2,5-dimethoxy-4-iodophenylisopropylamine (DOI) following chronic pretreatment with dietary lithium. Note the very dense distribution of fos-like immunoreactivity (FLI) in layer II (arrowheads). (Magnification as in Figure 11–3.)
Source. Adapted from Leslie RA, Moorman JM, Grahame-Smith DG: "Lithium Enhances 5-HT_{2A} Receptor-Mediated c-fos Expression in Rat Cerebral Cortex." *Neuroreport* 5:241–244, 1993. Used with permission from Rapid Science Ltd.

slight, nonsignificant reduction in the mean number of head shakes and in a significant enhancement of locomotor activity counted in a 30-minute period immediately after DOI administration (Figures 11–7 and 11–8).

FUNCTIONAL IMPLICATIONS OF THE CHRONIC LITHIUM-INDUCED ENHANCEMENT OF FOS EXPRESSION FOLLOWING DOI CHALLENGE

Chronic lithium treatment in rats resulted in a remarkable potentiation of Fos expression in several regions of the cerebral cortex following challenge with the 5-$HT_{2A/2C}$ receptor agonist DOI. In particular, pyramidal cells of the caudal piriform cortex, which are almost devoid of any FLI in control animals or in those given DOI alone, showed very dense labeling after chronic lithium

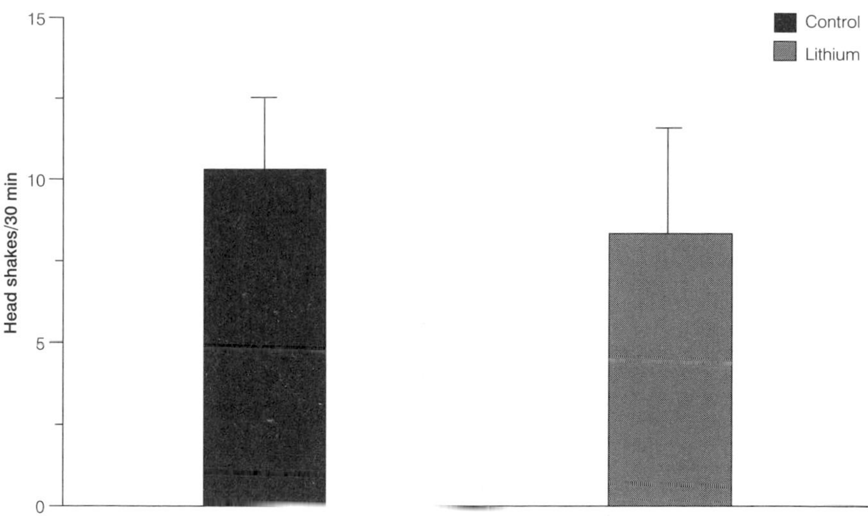

Figure 11–7. Mean numbers of head shakes (± SEM) counted in rats during a period of 30 minutes immediately after an injection of 2,5-dimethoxy-4-iodophenylisopropylamine (DOI) (8 mg/kg, ip), with or without previous chronic treatment with dietary lithium ($n = 6$).

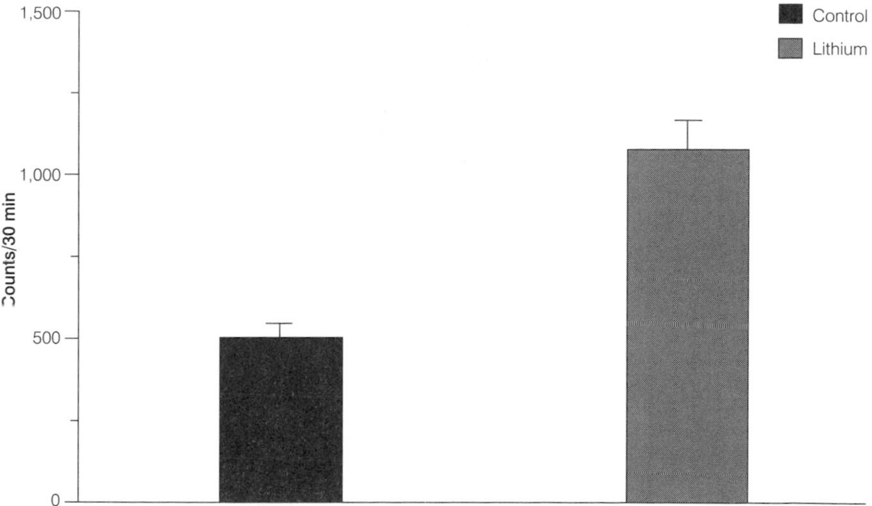

Figure 11–8. Total locomotor activity (i.e., numbers of light beam crossings ±SEM) counted during a 30-minute period immediately after administration of 2,5-dimethoxy-4-iodophenylisopropylamine (DOI) ($n = 6$). Comparison of lithium-free rats with those pretreated with chronic dietary lithium. *$P < 0.05$ (unpaired Student's t test).

treatment. Other cortical regions also showed a similar, if less spectacular, enhancement. Although the number of Fos-positive cells increased in the cerebral cortex (and the claustrum) after lithium pretreatment, no other brain region (even those showing FLI after DOI challenge alone) had such an enhancement. Chronic lithium treatment in animals had no effect on basal Fos expression, seen as a response to saline vehicle injection.

The results described in this chapter may appear to be difficult to reconcile with reported effects of lithium on the density of 5-HT_{2A} receptors. Although the results of such studies are somewhat conflicting, they have indicated that lithium treatment results in either no change or a reduction in the density of these sites. For example, Hotta et al. (1986) reported that chronic lithium pretreatment in rats reduced the number of 5-HT_{2A} receptor binding sites in both the hippocampus and the cortex. In contrast, Maggi and Enna (1980) and Treiser et al. (1981) found that such treatment decreased the number of 5-HT_{2A} receptor ligand binding sites in the rat hippocampus but not in the cortex. Goodwin et al. (1986) found that chronic lithium treatment had no effect on the density of cortical 5-HT_{2A} receptor binding sites in mice, whereas Wajda et al. (1986) detected a decrease in the number of these sites in this brain area in rats. The *c-fos* results reported here, however, showed that the induction of 5-$HT_{2A/2C}$ receptor–mediated Fos is increased after chronic lithium treatment, which might suggest a corresponding increase in the numbers of this receptor subtype after such treatment. However, such an increase in the density of this receptor subtype after long-term lithium administration has not been reported. Thus, an alternative explanation for the enhancement of DOI-induced Fos expression after chronic lithium administration must be sought.

Little is known about the precise neuronal distribution and function of 5-HT_{2A} receptors in cortical neuronal networks, so it is difficult to determine the functional implications of our results. In our studies, most cells in the caudal piriform cortex, which expressed FLI after lithium pretreatment and DOI challenge, had the morphological appearance of pyramidal projection neurons. It is possible, however, that a subpopulation of Fos-positive cells in our studies were γ-aminobutyric acid (GABA)–ergic interneurons. Reports in the literature have suggested that both projection neurons and interneurons in the cortex may bear 5-HT_{2A} receptors. Some studies have suggested that 5-HT_{2A} receptors occur on GABAergic cells in the cortex (Burnet et al. 1995; Morilak et al. 1993; Sheldon and Aghajanian 1991) and/or on pyramidal cells (Arenada and Andrade 1991; Burnet et al. 1995; Davies et al. 1987). Most electrophysiological studies reported that activation of 5-HT_{2A} receptors in the brain resulted in depolarizing (excitatory) responses in the postsynaptic cells (i.e., postsynaptic to serotonergic input neurons) that bear them (North and

Uchimura 1991). This may not be universally true, however, because in vitro studies of this receptor subtype have shown that cells bearing 5-HT_{2A} receptors can have hyperpolarizing responses following their activation (Elliott et al. 1995).

Another factor that must be taken into account regarding the function of the agonist DOI is the potential presence of another subtype of 5-HT_2 receptors in the brain. The 5-HT_{2B} receptor, which has an affinity for DOI similar to that of both the 5-HT_{2A} and the 5-HT_{2C} receptor (Baxter et al. 1995), may be present in the rat brain at the messenger RNA (mRNA) level (Flanigan et al. 1995) and as expressed protein (Duxon et al. 1995). Selective ligands for this receptor generally are not yet available, so it is impossible to determine whether some of the effects we report here are the result of 5-HT_{2B} receptor activation as opposed to 5-HT_{2A} receptor effects of DOI administration. When such ligands become available, it will be interesting to study this question.

IMPLICATIONS OF THE INOSITOL DEPLETION HYPOTHESIS

A well-documented effect of lithium is its modulatory action on the PI cycle via its inhibition of a number of phosphatases, principally inositol monophosphatase (Hallcher and Sherman 1980). Interestingly, this action of lithium implies a *reduction* of PI-mediated neuronal responses, and, indeed, chronic lithium treatment in rats results in an inhibition of serotonin- stimulated PI hydrolysis (Godfrey et al. 1989b; Kendall and Nahorski 1987). This effect might be predicted to reduce DOI-induced *c-fos* expression after chronic lithium treatment, but the opposite effect was observed in the present study. One explanation for this may be that although lithium results in a depletion of certain components of the PI cycle, such as inositol and IP_3, other metabolites may be enhanced

For example, DAG, phosphatidic acid, and cytidine monophosphate phosphatidate have been shown to be elevated in the presence of lithium in some tissues, including brain (Godfrey et al. 1989a). This effect was predictable, however, because cytidine monophosphate phosphatidate requires inositol to resynthesize inositol phosphates for the regeneration of phosphatidylinositol 4,5-bisphosphate (PIP_2). Consequently, if inositol is not available, cytidine monophosphate phosphatidate, phosphatidic acid, and DAG are likely to accumulate. Because DAG activates protein kinase C (PKC), one consequence of an increase in the levels of DAG within cells is likely to be an enhancement in the activation, or persistent activation, of this enzyme. Activation of PKC has been linked to the induction of several IEGs, including *c-fos* (Sheng and Greenberg 1990); thus, an increase in the activity of PKC as a result of lithium treatment may, in part, explain the enhanced 5-HT_{2A} receptor–mediated Fos expression following such treatment in our studies.

In support of the above-mentioned hypothesis, studies with PC12 pheochromocytoma cells have shown that lithium specifically enhanced PKC-mediated *c-fos* mRNA expression but had no effect on receptor or postreceptor activation of adenylate cyclase (Kalasapudi et al. 1990). In addition, Weiner et al. (1991) found that acute and chronic lithium treatment augmented PKC-linked *c-fos* expression after muscarinic M_1 receptor activation, but such treatment had no effect on cyclic adenosine monophosphate (cAMP)–linked expression of this IEG. Considering that activation of the 5-HT_{2A} receptor, like the muscarinic M_1 receptor, is linked to hydrolysis of PI, it appears that lithium may exert an enhancing effect only on *c-fos* expression via PI-linked mechanisms but not via receptors linked to adenylate cyclase, even though a cAMP response element regulates the expression of *c-fos*.

COMPARISON OF LITHIUM-INDUCED INCREASES IN *c-fos* EXPRESSION WITH BEHAVIORAL EFFECTS OF LITHIUM

Chronic lithium treatment before DOI challenge resulted in a small, nonsignificant reduction in the number of head shakes in a 30-minute period after injection. Previous studies reported that long-term lithium administration to rats (Hotta et al. 1986) or mice (Goodwin et al. 1986) resulted in a significant reduction in the number of presumed 5-HT_{2A} receptor–mediated head shakes or wet dog shakes (Kofman and Levin 1995). Any discrepancies between our results and those of the earlier studies may relate to the different drugs used. We used the selective 5-$HT_{2A/2C}$ receptor agonist DOI in our experiments, whereas other investigators used relatively nonselective serotonin receptor activators (5-hydroxytryptophan: Hotta et al. 1986; and 5-methoxydimethyltryptamine: Goodwin et al. 1986; Kofman and Levin 1995).

Although chronic lithium treatment slightly reduced DOI-induced head shakes, it significantly *enhanced* locomotor activity monitored during the same interval. Furthermore, this increase in locomotor activity occasionally culminated in severe limbic seizures that were sometimes fatal. Such effects were never seen in rats fed lithium-free food, even at higher (up to 32 mg/kg) doses of DOI. Recent studies (Williams and Jope 1994, 1995) showed that lithium induced a marked increase in electroencephalogram (EEG) activity in the rat cortex following challenge with DOI, which is consistent with the increased locomotor activity we report here.

Thus, lithium has opposite effects on two different behavioral effects of DOI. Complex anatomical distributions of the receptors involved may help to explain this apparent paradox. Although cortical activity is certainly involved in the 5-HT_{2A} receptor–mediated locomotor behavior that was enhanced by chronic lithium (and note that it was in the cerebral cortex where lithium dramatically potentiated the induction of Fos), the nuclei directing head shake behavior appear to be located within the caudal brain stem and spinal cord (Bedard and Pycock 1977; Handley and Singh 1986) and not in the forebrain. Perhaps the most parsimonious explanation for these differences in effects of lithium could relate to the involvement of different neurotransmitter and/or second-messenger systems in these two behaviors.

IMPORTANCE OF SEIZURE ACTIVITY IN THE *c-fos* RESPONSE

The DOI-induced behavioral activation seen after lithium treatment in the present study usually involved only movements of the forelimbs and facial muscles of the rats and also included rearing and falling. These limbic motor seizures are thought to be analogous to complex partial seizures in humans (Olney et al. 1986). Limbic motor seizures can be evoked in the rat by infusion of the GABA_A receptor antagonist bicuculline into an epileptogenic site within the endopiriform nucleus, known as the *area tempestas* (Piredda and Gale 1985), an area where we found enhanced DOI-induced Fos expression after lithium pretreatment. Other researchers have shown that applications of bicuculline into the area tempestas resulted in the expression of *c-fos* mRNA in other limbic areas, including the piriform cortex, olfactory bulb, and hippocampus (Maggio et al. 1993). Moreover, the piriform cortex has been shown to express dense *c-fos* mRNA and Fos protein in various seizure models (Popovici et al. 1990; Simonato et al. 1991). Such studies also have reported more moderate inductions of this IEG in other regions of the cerebral cortex, such as the somatosensory cortex, after seizure activity. Thus, those brain areas in which $5\text{-HT}_{2A/2C}$ receptor–mediated Fos expression increased after lithium pretreatment—specifically, the piriform and somatosensory cortices and claustrum—have been shown to express Fos in several seizure paradigms. These data suggest that such an increase in the number of Fos-positive nuclei seen after lithium treatment may result from the involvement of these areas in seizure activity (Williams and Jope 1994, 1995).

Lithium has a proconvulsant effect on the muscarinic cholinergic system and in the rat lowers the seizure threshold to the muscarinic agonist pilocarpine by a factor of at least 13 (Ormandy et al. 1991). Such an effect of lithium appeared to be specific to cholinergic agonists because lithium had no effect on the responses to a number of other convulsants such as pentylenetetrazol or kainate (Ormandy et al. 1991). Weiner et al. (1991) showed that acute and chronic lithium treatment in rats before pilocarpine challenge also enhanced the expression of *c-fos* mRNA in the brain and that this effect was mediated by M_1 receptors linked to PI hydrolysis. Such results, coupled with the findings with DOI detailed earlier in this chapter, imply that lithium may have proconvulsant effects only on responses mediated by agonists acting at receptors coupled to PI hydrolysis (Leslie et al. 1993b; Moorman and Leslie 1998; Williams and Jope 1995).

CONCLUSION

The results of the experiments reported in this chapter indicate that lithium alters IEG expression in the brain in an anatomically and pharmacologically specific manner that appears to be consistent with a proconvulsant action of lithium on 5-$HT_{2A/2C}$ receptor–mediated activity. Although convulsions sometimes occur in humans following lithium toxicity, such effects are usually seen only at very high plasma concentrations (2.5 mEq/L and higher; Price and Heninger 1994), yet the effects of lithium on the *c-fos* response in the rat occurred at much lower levels (within the therapeutic range for humans). The cellular mechanisms behind the effects of lithium on IEG expression reported here are not clear. However, seizures, certainly those propagated in the area tempestas, are thought to be caused by a disturbance in the balance between neuronal inhibition (e.g., by GABAergic cells) and excitation. Because lithium has effects on numerous neurotransmitter systems, an action on glutamatergic or GABAergic transmission may explain some of these effects. Certainly, lithium can affect G-protein function in complex ways (see Manji et al, Chapter 7, in this volume), and such interactions may well be involved. Other possible explanations may involve the action of lithium on the turnover of inositol phosphates in PI-linked receptor systems, and the apparent selectivity for lithium potentiation of PI-linked receptors of the serotonin and acetylcholine families strongly suggests that such mechanisms are important. In keeping with this idea, lithium administration to rats increases the levels of the PI-linked second-messenger DAG, which may result in the overactivation of neurons.

The therapeutic relevance of the potentiation of *c-fos* by lithium is not clear; administration of lithium to humans is effective in the treatment of bipolar disorder and other affective disorders and does not result in seizures at therapeutic doses. An overstimulation of some neurons, mediated by enhanced 5-HT_{2A} receptor activity in the brain, for example, may contribute to some of the unwanted side effects of lithium, some of which occur at therapeutic plasma levels. For example, Hambrecht (1995) reported that lithium administration may be associated with "pseudohallucinations" in some patients, an effect that may be caused by 5-HT_{2A} receptor activation, because this receptor is thought to mediate the effects of hallucinogenic drugs such as lysergic acid diethylamide (LSD) and, indeed, DOI.

REFERENCES

Appel NM, Mitchell WM, Garlick RK, et al: Autoradiographic characterisation of (+/-)-1-(2,5-dimethoxy-4-[^{125}I]iodophenyl)-2-aminopropane ([^{125}I]DOI) binding to $5HT_2$ and $5HT_{1C}$ receptors in rat brain. J Pharmacol Exp Ther 255: 843–857, 1990

Arenada RC, Andrade R: 5-Hydroxytryptamine-2 and 5-hydroxytryptamine-1A receptors mediate opposing responses on membrane excitability in rat association cortex. Neuroscience 40:399–412, 1991

Baxter G, Kennet G, Blaney F, et al: 5-HT_2 receptor subtypes: a family re-united? Trends Pharmacol Sci 16:105–110, 1995

Bedard P, Pycock CJ: 'Wet-dog' shake behaviour in the rat: a possible quantitative model of central 5-hydroxytryptamine activity. Neuropharmacology 16:633–670, 1977

Belmaker RH, Bersudsky Y, Benjamin J, et al: Manipulation of inositol-linked second messenger systems as a therapeutic strategy in psychiatry, in Depression and Mania: From Neurobiology to Treatment. Edited by Gessa G, Fratta W, Pani L, et al. New York, Raven, 1995, pp 67–84

Berridge MJ, Irvine RF: Inositol phosphates and cell signalling. Nature 341:197–204, 1989

Berridge MJ, Downes CP, Hanley MR: Lithium amplifies agonist-dependent phosphatidyl-inositol responses in brain and salivary glands. Biochem J 206:587–595, 1982

Burnet PWJ, Eastwood, SL, Lacey K, et al: The distribution of 5-HT_{1A} and 5-HT_{2A} receptor mRNA in human brain. Brain Res 676:157–168, 1995

Davies MF, Deisz RA, Prince DA, et al: Two distinct effects of 5-hydroxytryptamine on single cortical neurons. Brain Res 423:347–352, 1987

Dragunow M, Robertson GS, Faull RLM, et al: D_2 dopamine receptor antagonists induce Fos and related proteins in rat striatal regions. Neuroscience 37:287–294, 1990

Duxon MS, Reavley AC, Flanigan TP, et al: Expression of the 5-HT$_{2B}$ receptor protein in the rat brain (abstract). Br J Pharmacol 115:105P, 1995

Elliott JM, Newberry NR, Bartrup JT, et al: 5-HT$_{2A}$ receptor-activated cascade in rat C6 glioma cells. Neuroscience 69:1119–1131, 1995

Flanigan TP, Reavley AC, Carey JE, et al: Evidence for expression of the 5-HT$_{2B}$ receptor mRNA in rat brain (abstract). Br J Pharmacol 114: 369P, 1995

Friedman E, Dallob A, Levine G: The effect of long-term lithium treatment on reserpine-induced supersensitivity in dopaminergic and serotonergic transmission. Life Sci 25:1263–1266, 1979

Godfrey PP, McClue SJ, White AM, et al: Potentiation by lithium of CMP-phosphatide formation in carbachol-stimulated rat cerebral-cortical slices and its reversal by myo-inositol. Biochem J 258:621–624, 1989a

Godfrey PP, McClue SJ, White AM, et al: Subacute and chronic in vivo lithium treatment inhibits agonist and sodium fluoride-stimulated inositol phosphate production in rat cortex. J Neurochem 52:498–506, 1989b

Goodwin GM, DeSouza RJ, Wood AJ, et al: Lithium decreases 5-HT$_{1A}$ and 5-HT$_2$ receptor and α-adrenoceptor mediated-function in mice. Psychopharmacology 90:482–487, 1986

Hallcher L, Sherman WR: The effects of lithium ion and other agents on the activity of myo-inositol-1-phosphatase from bovine brain. J Biol Chem 261:8100–8130, 1980

Hambrecht M: Lithium and pseudohallucinations: a rare side effect. Biol Psychiatry 37:120–121, 1995

Handley SL, Singh L: Neurotransmitters and shaking behaviour—more than a 'gutbath' for the brain. Trends Pharmacol Sci 7:324–328, 1986

Harrison-Read PE: Evidence from behavioural reactions to fenfluramine, 5-hydroxytryptophan and 5-methoxy-N,N-dimethyltryptamine for differential effects of short-term and long-term lithium on indolaminergic mechanisms in rats. Br J Pharmacol 66:144–145, 1979

Heninger GR, Charney DS, Sternberg DE: Lithium carbonate augmentation of antidepressant treatment; an effective treatment for treatment-refractory depression. Arch Gen Psychiatry 40:1335–1342, 1983

Hotta I, Yamawaki S, Segawa T: Long-term lithium treatment causes serotonin receptor down-regulation via serotonin presynapses in rat brain. Neuropsychobiology 16:19–26, 1986

Kalasapudi VD, Sheftel G, Divish MM, et al: Lithium augments c-*fos* protooncogene expression in PC12 pheochromocytoma cells: implications for therapeutic action of lithium. Brain Res 521:47–54, 1990

Kendall DA, Nahorski SR: Acute and chronic lithium treatments influence agonist and depolarization-stimulated inositol phospholipid hydrolysis in rat cerebral cortex. J Pharmacol Exp Ther 241:1023–1027, 1987

Kennett GA, Curzon G: Potencies of antagonists indicate that 5-HT$_{1C}$ receptors mediate 1–3(chlorophenyl)piperazine-induced hypophagia. Br J Pharmacol 103: 2016– 2020, 1991

Kofman O, Levin U: Myo-inositol attenuates the enhancement of the serotonin syndrome by lithium. Psychopharmacology 118:213–218, 1995

Leslie RA, Moorman JM, Coulson A, et al: Serotonin$_{2/1C}$ receptor activation causes a localized expression of the immediate-early gene c-fos in rat brain: evidence for involvement of dorsal raphe nucleus projection fibres. Neuroscience 53:457–463, 1993a

Leslie RA, Moorman JM, Grahame-Smith DG: Lithium enhances 5-HT$_{2A}$ receptor-mediated c-fos expression in rat cerebral cortex. Neuroreport 5:241–244, 1993b

Maggi A, Enna SJ: Regional alterations in rat brain neurotransmitter systems following chronic lithium treatment. J Neurochem 34:888–892, 1980

Maggio R, Lanaud P, Grayson DR, et al: Expression of *c-fos* mRNA following seizures evoked from an epileptogenic site in the deep prepiriform cortex: regional distribution in brain as shown by *in situ* hybridisation. Exp Neurol 119:11–19, 1993

Moorman JM, Leslie RA: Paradoxical effects of lithium on serotonergic receptor function: an immunocytochemical, behavioral and autoradiographic study. Neuropharmacology 37:357–374, 1998

Morilak DA, Garlow SJ, Ciaranello RD: Immunocytochemical localization and description of neurons expressing serotonin$_2$ receptors in the rat brain. Neuroscience 54:701–717, 1993

North RA, Uchimura N: 5-hydroxytryptamine acts at 5-HT$_2$ receptors to decrease potassium conductance in rat nucleus accumbens neurons. J Physiol 417:1–12, 1991

Olney JW, Collins RC, Sloviter RS: Excitotoxic mechanisms of epileptic brain damage. Adv Neurol 44:857–877, 1986

Ormandy GO, Song L, Jope RS: Analysis of the convulsant-potentiating effects of lithium in rats. Exp Neurol 111:356–361, 1991

Pazos A, Cortes R, Palacios JM: Quantitative autoradiographic mapping of serotonin receptors in the rat brain, II: serotonin-2 receptors. Brain Res 346: 231–249, 1985

Piredda S, Gale K: Evidence that the deep prepiriform cortex contains a crucial epileptogenic site. Nature 317:623–625, 1985

Popovici T, Represa A, Crépel V, et al: Effects of kainic acid-induced seizures and ischaemia on *c-fos*-like proteins in rat brain. Brain Res 536:183–194, 1990

Pranzatelli MR: Evidence for involvement of 5-HT$_2$ and 5-HT$_{1C}$ receptors in the behavioral effects of the 5-HT agonist 2,5-dimethoxy-4-iodophenylisopropylamine (DOI). Neurosci Lett 115:74–80, 1990

Price LH, Heninger GR: Lithium in the treatment of mood disorders. Drug Ther 331:591–598, 1994

Prien RF, Kupfer DJ, Mansky PA, et al: Drug therapy in the prevention of recurrences in unipolar and bipolar affective disorders. Arch Gen Psychiatry 41:1096–1104, 1984

Sheldon PW, Aghajanian GK: Excitatory responses to serotonin (5-HT) in neurons of the rat piriform cortex; evidence for mediation by 5-HT$_{1C}$ receptors in pyramidal cells and 5-HT$_2$ receptors in interneurons. Synapse 9:208–218, 1991

Sheng M, Greenberg ME: The regulation and function of c-fos and other immediate early genes in the nervous system. Neuron 4:477–485, 1990

Simonato M, Hosford DA, Labiner DM, et al: Differential expression of immediate early genes in the hippocampus in the kindling model of epilepsy. Mol Brain Res 11:115–124, 1991

Treiser SL, Cascio CS, O'Donohue TL, et al: Lithium increases serotonin release and decreases serotonin receptors in the hippocampus. Science 213:1529–1531, 1981

Wajda IJ, Banay-Schwartz M, Manigault I, et al: Modulation of the serotonin S2 receptor in brain after chronic lithium. Neurochem Res 11:949–957, 1986

Weiner ED, Kalasapudi VD, Papolos DF, et al: Lithium augments pilocarpine-induced *fos* gene expression in rat brain. Brain Res 553:117–122, 1991

Williams MB, Jope RS: Lithium potentiates phosphoinositol-linked 5-HT receptor stimulation in vivo. Neuroreport 5:1118–1120, 1994

Williams MB, Jope RS: Modulation by inositol of cholinergic- and serotonergic-induced seizures in lithium-treated rats. Brain Res 685:169–178, 1995

Wood AJ, Goodwin GM: A review of the biochemical and neuropharmacological actions of lithium. Psychol Med 17:579–600, 1987

CHAPTER 12

BEHAVIORAL CORRELATES OF THE EFFECTS OF LITHIUM ON SECOND MESSENGER SYSTEMS

Ora Kofman, Ph.D., Yuli Bersudsky, M.D., Ph.D., and Yardena Patishi, Ph.D.

Like most of the early psychoactive drugs, the clinical use of lithium antedated scientific investigation of its therapeutic mechanism. Lithium has a plethora of biochemical effects in vitro and ex vivo (Mørk 1990; Wood and Goodwin 1987); however, none of these has proven to be the basis of its therapeutic action. Because biochemical effects measured in vitro often can be the result of compensatory or secondary biochemical processes, our research strategy has focused on analysis of the behavioral effects of lithium. Antagonists are commonly used to reverse the biological effects of a drug to test its specificity and biological significance. In the case of lithium, a simple ion with multiple biochemical effects, we have attempted to reverse its behavioral effects by using agents that counteract one of its two major effects on signal transduction: either at the level of the phospholipase C (PLC)–linked second-messenger system or at the level of the adenylate cyclase second-messenger system.

LITHIUM- AND PHOSPHATIDYLINOSITOL-DERIVED SECOND MESSENGERS

Lithium reduces brain levels of inositol by inhibiting inositol monophosphatase, the enzyme that dephosphorylates inositol monophosphate to inositol in the brain (Allison and Stewart 1971; Hallcher and Sherman 1980). The K_i of lithium to inhibit the enzyme (Gee et al. 1988) is within its therapeutic range (K_i = 0.86 mM). Several neurotransmitters stimulate PLC, which leads to the breakdown of a membrane phospholipid, phosphatidylinositol 4,5-bisphosphate (PIP_2), into two second messengers—inositol 1,4,5-trisphosphate (IP_3), which enhances intracellular calcium flow, and diacylglycerol. Berridge et al. (1989) suggested that lithium inhibition of inositol monophosphatase could lead to a relative deficiency of inositol in overactive systems and to a dampening of the response of phosphatidylinositol (PI) to receptor activation.

Based on Berridge's theory, several groups have used inositol reversal to study the role of lithium on the PI system. Inositol can reverse many biological effects of lithium, including accumulation of cytidine monophosphate phosphatidic acid (Downes and Stone 1986; Godfrey 1989), lithium-induced reversal of desensitization of hippocampal neurons to carbachol (Pontzer and Crews 1990), and lithium-induced inhibition of photoreceptor firing in the *Limulus* (E. C. Johnson et al. 1998).

Applying the technique of inositol reversal to the behavioral effects of lithium seemed critical, because lithium clearly has multiple biochemical effects, and not all of them need be related to the therapeutic mechanism in mania and depression.

LITHIUM AND THE CYCLIC ADENOSINE MONOPHOSPHATE SECOND-MESSENGER SYSTEM

Cyclic adenosine monophosphate (cAMP) is another second messenger that is affected in vitro and ex vivo by lithium. Several neurotransmitter receptors are coupled to stimulatory (β- adrenergic, D_1 dopaminergic) or inhibitory (α_2-adrenergic, D_2 dopaminergic, 5-HT_{1A} serotonergic) guanine nucleotide binding proteins (G proteins), which are linked to adenylate cyclase. Reduced cAMP levels in both cerebrospinal fluid (CSF) and urine from patients with depression (reviewed in Belmaker et al. 1980) have been reported, and it has been hypothesized that dysbalance of second-messenger function may be involved in the pathophysiology of affective disorders (Wachtel 1989).

Many studies have reported that lithium inhibits cAMP generation (Andersen and Geisler 1984; Ebstein et al. 1976, 1980; Mrk and Geisler 1987a, 1987b; Newman and Belmaker 1987). Mørk and Geisler (1987b) found that lithium exerts an inhibitory effect directly on the catalytic subunit of adenylate cyclase purified from rat brain. Both calcium-calmodulin (Ca^{2+}-CaM)- and forskolin (colforsin)-stimulated, but not basal, activities were inhibited. The number of β-adrenoceptors was unaffected by chronic lithium treatment, indicating that the effect of lithium may be distal to the receptor (Gross et al. 1988). Lithium also may interfere with cAMP generation at the level of G proteins, because lithium is reported to inhibit agonist-mediated increases in guanosine triphosphate (GTP) binding in the cerebral cortex of rats (Avissar et al. 1988).

Behavioral studies of drugs that alter cAMP levels suggest that increases in noradrenaline (NA)-sensitive cAMP are correlated with decreases in spontaneous locomotion in mice (Hamburger-Bar et al. 1986; Stalvey et al. 1976). Moreover, forskolin, a diterpene compound that activates adenylate cyclase; rolipram, a cAMP phosphodiesterase inhibitor; and dibutyryl-cAMP all decrease spontaneous activity in rodents (Barraco et al. 1985; Kofman and Patishi, in press; Smith 1990; Wachtel 1982).

Although stimulation of the cAMP second-messenger system decreases spontaneous locomotion, drugs that lower cAMP, such as reserpine and lithium, also reduce motor activity (Belmaker et al. 1982). The explanation of this paradox may involve regional differences in brain cAMP activity. Skolnick and Daly (1974) found that accumulation of agonist-stimulated cAMP was positively correlated with spontaneous locomotion in the midbrain-striatum regions and inversely correlated with activity in the cortex. Although both drugs that enhance and those that diminish cAMP levels have similar effects on spontaneous locomotion, several studies have shown that hypoactivity induced by drugs that enhance cAMP levels (e.g., clenbuterol or rolipram) can be attenuated by lithium (Givant et al. 1990; Smith 1990) and, conversely, that rolipram can attenuate reserpine-induced hypokinesia (Wachtel and Schneider 1986). Thus, although hypoactivity per se is not a homologous model for clinical depression, drug-induced hypoactivity can be used as an assay model of pharmacological interactions between drugs that have opposing biochemical effects to cAMP.

Forskolin directly stimulates adenylate cyclase because it activates cAMP formation in the absence of functional receptors and G_s proteins (Bender and Neer 1983; Seamon et al. 1981). However, studies have also indicated that forskolin can potentiate the action of preactivated G_s proteins on cAMP formation (Krall and Jamgotchian 1987; Schimmer et al. 1987). Lithium has been shown to decrease forskolin-induced cAMP generation both in vitro and ex vivo (Andersen and Geisler 1984; Newman and Belmaker 1987) and in vivo in the dorsal hippocampus of freely moving rats (Mørk and Geisler 1995). We therefore used forskolin antagonism of lithium behavioral effects to test the adenylate cyclase theory of lithium action.

Suppression of locomotion and rearing is a well-described behavioral effect of lithium in rats (Belmaker et al. 1990; F. N Johnson 1972; Kofman and Belmaker 1990). The effects of inositol and forskolin were tested in a series of experiments to determine whether these agents alter the locomotor-suppressant effect of lithium.

REVERSAL OF LITHIUM-INDUCED SUPPRESSION OF REARING BY INOSITOL

Rats that were implanted with guide cannulae (Plastics One) in the dorsal part of the third ventricle via standard stereotaxic procedures received lithium chloride (LiCl) or sodium chloride (NaCl) (5 mEq/kg, intraperitoneally). Twenty-four hours later after inositol or vehicle ("artificial cerebrospinal fluid") was given intracerebroventricularly (10 mg/40 μL), activity was measured.

A significant interaction was found between lithium and inositol on the number of rears in the activity meter ($F_{1,34} = 4.18, P < 0.05$). Rats that received an acute injection of lithium showed less rearing than rats treated with NaCl. Intracerebroventricular administration of inositol dramatically reversed the lithium effect (Figure 12–1). This was the first finding suggesting that inositol could reverse a behavioral effect of lithium (Kofman and Belmaker 1990).

BLOCKING OF FORSKOLIN-INDUCED HYPOACTIVITY BY CHRONIC BUT NOT ACUTE LITHIUM

Acute Lithium and Forskolin

Male Sprague-Dawley rats were intraperitoneally injected with 6 mEq/kg of LiCl in isotonic solution or 6 mEq/kg of NaCl in isotonic solution 24 hours before the experiments. A 5-μL Hamilton microsyringe with an injection cannula protruding 0.5 mm below the guide cannula was used to inject half of the rats in each group with 5 μL containing forskolin (50 or 100 μg) in dimethylsulfoxide (DMSO) and half of the rats with DMSO only. Three minutes after the injection, rats were placed in the center of an automatic rat activity monitor (Opto-Varimex, Columbus Instruments, Columbus, OH) in a balanced order. Ambulatory, vertical, and total activity was measured. Acute lithium had no ef-

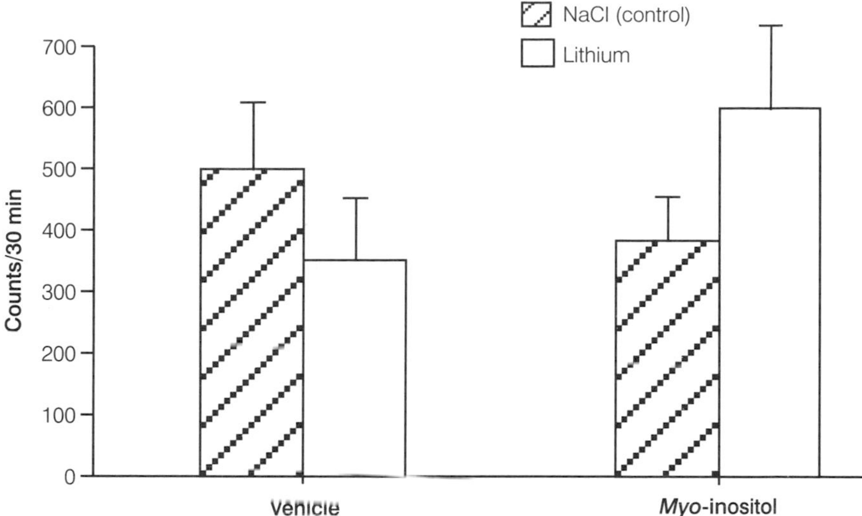

Figure 12–1. Rearing in rats during 30-minute period 24 hours after 5 mEq/kg intraperitoneal LiCl or NaCl and immediately after intracerebroventricular *myo*-inositol or cerebrospinal fluid (CSF).
Source. Adapted from Kofman O, Belmaker RH: "Intracerebroventricular *Myo*-Inositol Antagonizes Lithium-Induced Suppression of Rearing Behavior in Rats." *Brain Research* 534:345–347, 1990, with permission from Elsevier Science.

fect on hypoactivity induced by either a low or a moderate dose of forskolin (Bersudsky et al. 1997).

Chronic Lithium and Forskolin

Male Sprague-Dawley rats implanted with the cannulae as described in the previous paragraph were fed standard chow containing 47 mmol/kg of LiCl for 17–23 days. Control rats received a standard diet. After about 3 weeks of lithium diet or regular chow, rats were divided into four experimental groups (Reg-DMSO, Li-DMSO, Reg-forskolin, Li-forskolin), and activity was measured in balanced order as described in the previous paragraph. Table 12–1 shows that moderate blood levels of chronic lithium partially reversed the behavioral effects of forskolin (Bersudsky et al. 1997).

In summary, chronic but not acute lithium affected forskolin-induced behavior. This could suggest that lithium must accumulate slowly inside the cell before adenylate cyclase is inhibited in vivo (Frazer et al. 1975) or that adaptive changes caused by chronic lithium are important for the reversal of forskolin-induced behavior. The fact that we observed an interaction between forskolin

Table 12–1. Effects of chronic lithium on behavior in rats induced by intracerebroventricular forskolin (colforsin) (in dimethylsulfoxide [DMSO]) (mean ±SD)

			Activity (counts per 10 minutes) in automatic activity meter (100 μg/5 μL DMSO)		
Group	***n***	**Li^+**	**Total**	**Ambulatory**	**Vertical**
Control	9		1,227 ±420	821 ±339	255 ±162
Forskolin	8		672 ±326	391 ±231	125 ±129
Lithium	9	0.7 ±0.2	911 ±500	592 ±381	212 ±199
Lithium + forskolin	8	0.7 ±0.2	1,132 ±499	712 ±390	147 ±90

Note. Chronic LiCl, 0.2% in food for 16 days, caused 20%–25% lowering of all activity measures in an automated rat activity monitor. Forskolin, 100 μg icv, caused a 45% reduction (statistically significant [$P = 0.015$]) of total and ambulatory activity. Vertical activity was lowered (50%), but this was not significant ($P = 0.09$). However, Li pretreatment completely blocked the forskolin effect on total (interaction $F = 6.5$, $P = 0.016$) and ambulatory activity (interaction $F = 5.5$, $P = 0.026$). There was no interaction effect between lithium and forskolin on vertical activity of rats.

Source. Reprinted from Bersudsky Y, Patishi Y, Jensen J B, et al.: "The Effect of Acute and Chronic Lithium on Forskolin-Induced Reduction of Rat Activity." *Journal of Neural Transmission* 104:943–952, 1997. Used with permission.

and lithium after only chronic and not acute lithium treatment supports the concept that this interaction is related to lithium's therapeutic effect. Mørk and Geisler (1994,1995) reported that the reduction in forskolin-induced cAMP formation does not require chronic treatment because the reduction in stimulated cAMP formation observed after chronic lithium treatment is about the same magnitude as that found with lithium in situ (Mørk and Geisler 1994, 1995). The reason for this contrast between the time course of the biochemical (Mørk and Geisler 1995) and behavioral (present results) interaction between lithium and forskolin is not clear. However, in situ lithium via microdialysis may achieve more rapid intracellular lithium levels than does a 6-mM/kg intraperitoneal injection.

CHRONIC AND ACUTE LITHIUM DOES NOT BLOCK PHORBOL ESTER–INDUCED HYPOACTIVITY

Protein kinase C (PKC) is a major enzyme that interacts with both adenylate cyclase and PLC-linked second messengers (Cooper et al. 1995). Lenox (1988) and Manji and Lenox (1994) proposed that lithium may affect PKC (see Manji et al., Chapter 7 in this volume; Lenox et al., Chapter 9 in this volume). Bitran et al. (1990) reported that chronic lithium attenuated the effects of phorbol ester on stimulation of the Na^+/H^+ antiporter in leukemia cells in culture. Casebolt and Jope (1991) reported that chronic lithium had no effect on PKC activity in the hippocampus but altered in vitro phosphorylation mediated by PKC. Manji et al. (1993) reported that chronic but not acute lithium treatment in rats decreased the hippocampal membrane-associated PKCα isozyme. Microinjection of phorbol esters in the hypothalamic ventromedial nucleus facilitated lordosis (Kow et al. 1994), and a PKC agonist injected into the third ventricle reduced adrenocorticotropic hormone–induced grooming (Gispen et al. 1985). Because it seemed important to study whether stimulation of PKC might have specific behavioral effects that interact with lithium, we studied the effect of phorbol 12-myristate, 13-acetate (PMA) administered intracerebroventricularly to rats with indwelling intracerebroventricular cannulae after acute or chronic lithium treatment.

We fed 49 rats food containing 0.2% LiCl (n = 22) or regular rat food (n = 27) for 21 days. Separate bottles of water and 0.9% NaCl solution were provided ad libitum for both groups of animals. After 21 days, half of the rats in each group were intracerebroventricularly injected with either 5 nmol of PMA in a volume of 6 μL of DMSO or DMSO vehicle. Manual PMA injections were given over 2 minutes via an injection cannula that was attached with polyethylene tubing to a 50-μL Hamilton microsyringe that was left in place for 1 minute before being replaced by the stylet. Behavioral observation began 5 minutes after PMA injection in a photocell activity monitor (Opto-Varimax, Columbus Instruments). Total, vertical, and ambulatory activity was automatically monitored for 20 minutes, and then the animals were observed for 2 hours. After this automatic activity monitoring and observation, animals were sacrificed by decapitation, and lithium levels that were measured in trunk blood were 0.7 ± 0.3 mM. Total, ambulatory, and vertical activity was significantly decreased in PMA-injected rats compared with control rats. However, no difference was found between chronic lithium–treated animals and control animals in this effect (Table 12–2).

REVERSAL OF LITHIUM-PILOCARPINE SEIZURES BY INOSITOL

Both inositol and forskolin showed behavioral interaction with lithium when basic exploratory locomotor behavior in a novel environment was tested,

Table 12–2. Effects of 5 nmol phorbol 12-myristate, 13-acetate (PMA) and chronic lithium (3 weeks) on ambulatory, vertical, and total activity in rats during 20 minutes in an automatic activity meter (mean ± SD)

	Activity (counts per 20 minutes) in automatic activity meter (100 µg/5 µL DMSO)			
Group	**Total**	**Ambulatory**	**Vertical**	***n***
Control	1,624 ± 721	1,001 ± 498	291 ± 213	9
PMA	639 ± 636	413 ± 492	71 ± 130	18
Lithium	1,969 ± 817	1,343 ± 625	445 ± 271	8
Lithium and PMA	714 ± 536	401 ± 328	92 ± 139	14

Note. Analysis of variance (ANOVA) showed a significant effect of PMA on ambulatory, vertical, and total activity (ambulatory, $P < 0.001$, $F = 28$; vertical, $P < 0.001$, $F = 28$; total, $P < 0.001$, $F = 33$), but no effect of lithium (ambulatory, $F = 1.5$; vertical, $F = 1.5$; total, F = 1.2) and no interaction between PMA and lithium treatment (ambulatory, $F = 0.9$; vertical, $F = 0.5$; total, $F = 5$).

Source. Reprinted from Patishi Y, Bersudsky Y, Belmaker RH: "Phorbol Ester Intracerebroventricularly Induces a Behavioral Hypoactivity That Is Not Affected by Chronic or Acute Lithium." *European Neuropsychopharmacology* 6:39–41, 1996b. Used with permission from Elsevier Science.

whereas PKC activation, which interacts with both systems, did not show any behavioral interaction with lithium. Given the complex inputs involved in locomotion, it is not surprising to find behavioral effects of agents affecting both PI and adenylate cyclase systems. However, to investigate the behavioral effects of lithium, we sought other agonist-stimulated behaviors that are known to be robustly affected by lithium. The next series of experiments involved the interaction of lithium with cholinergic and serotonergic agonists. We hypothesized that if a particular system was stimulated excessively, as is proposed to be the case in bipolar disorder, lithium might act preferentially on either the PI or the adenylate cyclase second-messenger system.

Honchar et al. (1983) first described lithium-pilocarpine limbic seizures in rats, but not in mice. Tricklebank et al. (1991) found that acute intracerebroventricular inositol administration to mice could prevent lithium-pilocarpine seizures with a much higher dose of pilocarpine than was required to induce seizures in rats. Lithium does not have general proconvulsant effects in rats (Ormandy et al. 1991). However, rats pretreated with lithium have limbic seizures following subconvulsant doses of pilocarpine and other cholinergic agonists (Honchar et al. 1983; Persinger et al. 1988; Terry et al. 1990). The combined treatment with lithium and pilocarpine results in an accumulation of inositol monophosphate and a reduction in cortical inositol that are about 10 times greater than the effects obtained with either drug alone (Sherman et al. 1985, 1986). We tested the ability of intracerebroventricular inositol to postpone and prevent lithium-pilocarpine seizures.

The animals were rated for the progression of limbic seizures once every 5 minutes for 75 minutes according to a modified version of the scale used by Patel et al. (1988). The scoring was as follows: 0 = no response, 1 = gustatory movements and/or fictive scratching, 2 = tremor, 3 = head-bobbing, 4 = forelimb clonus, and 5 = rearing, clonus, and falling. In addition, the latency to attain forelimb clonus (a score of 4) was recorded for each rat.

Inositol significantly increased the latency to onset of clonus (Figure 12–2) and lowered the seizure score (Figure 12–3). Eight of 16 rats treated with inositol had no limbic seizures at all, whereas only 1 of the 14 vehicle-treated rats did not show clonus. All of the rats treated with L-*chiro*-inositol had limbic seizures. Inositol's ability to prevent seizures was highly significant ($\chi^2 = 6.53$, $P < 0.01$ for *myo*-inositol vs. vehicle). Inositol has no effect on seizures induced by high doses of pilocarpine alone and thus is specific to the lithium effect (Kofman et al. 1993).

We have since studied the time course and dose response of the inositol effect. Inositol was effective at 1, 4, and 8 hours before pilocarpine, preventing seizures in 8 of 10, 9 of 10, and 9 of 10 rats, respectively. When injected immediately before or 24 hours before pilocarpine, inositol did not prevent seizures in any rat, and when injected 12 hours before pilocarpine, 5 of 10 rats seized. This time course suggests that inositol must have time to distribute within brain and to enter cells and that it is extruded from brain or metabolized within 8–24 hours after injection (Bersudsky et al. 1993).

To obtain a dose-response curve for inositol effects, 35 lithium-treated rats were injected intracerebroventricularly with either 40 μL of vehicle ($n = 13$), 5 mg of inositol ($n = 16$), or 10 mg of inositol ($n = 6$) 1 hour before pilocarpine (20 mg/kg) administration. The prevention of seizures by 5 mg of intracerebroventricular inositol was almost significantly different from that in vehicle-treated rats ($\chi^2 = 3.77$, $P = 0.052$), but the moderate effect of this dose of inositol was significantly less than the dramatic effect of 10 mg of intracerebroventricular inositol ($\chi^2 = 6.14$, $P < 0.01$; 5 mg vs. 10 mg). When we compared the latency to onset of clonus between those rats that did attain stage 4 in the control and 5-mg groups, we found a significant protective effect of the lower dose of inositol. Mean latency to clonus was 28.3 ± 6.4 minutes (mean ± standard deviation [SD]) for the vehicle-treated group and 37.9 ± 11.8 minutes for the 5-mg inositol group (2-tailed t test = 2.57, $P < 0.02$). These data suggest that there is a dose response for the attenuation of behavioral effects of lithium (Bersudsky et al. 1993).

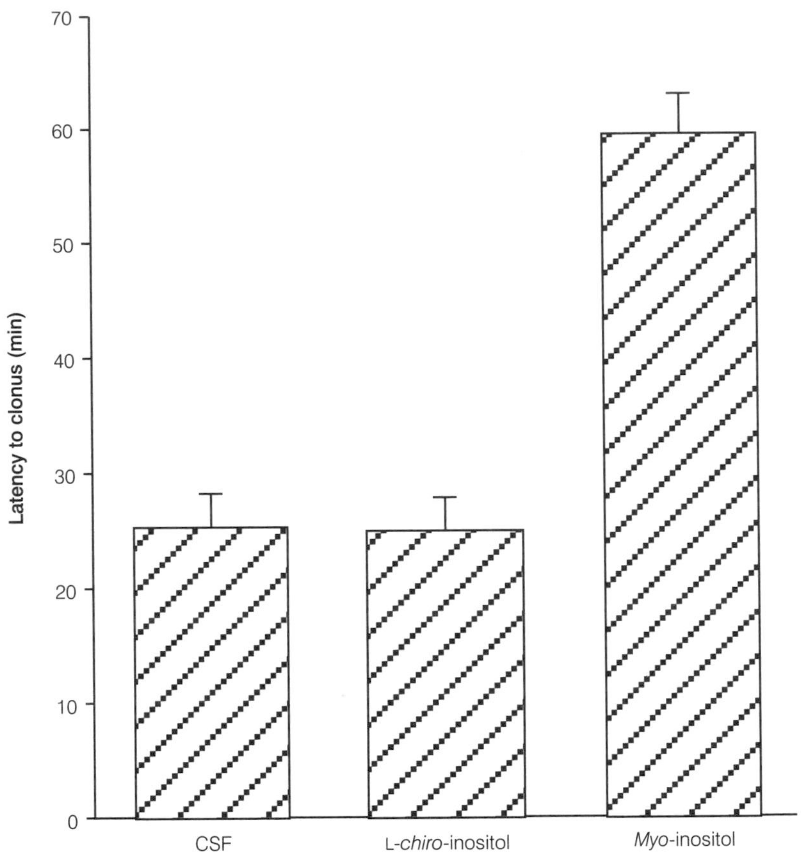

Figure 12–2. Latency to first exhibit forelimb clonus (behavioral score 4) following subcutaneous injection of pilocarpine, sc, in lithium-treated rats. Rats were injected 24 hours and 30 minutes before pilocarpine with artificial cerebrospinal fluid (CSF) (vehicle), L-*chiro*-inositol (10 mg/40 µL) or *myo*-inositol (10 mg/40 µL). The ordinate represents the latency to clonus in minutes following injection of pilocarpine (20 mg/kg, sc).
Source. Reprinted with permission from Kofman O, Sherman WR, Katz V, et al.: "Restoration of Brain *Myo*-Inositol Levels in Rats Increases Latency to Lithium-Pilocarpine Seizures." *Psychopharmacology (Berlin)* 110:229–234, 1993. Copyright 1993, Springer-Verlag.

Chronic Dietary Lithium and Intracerebroventricular *myo*-Inositol

To determine whether inositol reversal of lithium-pilocarpine seizures is possible after chronic lithium treatment, 14 rats, fed chronic dietary lithium for 21 days, were implanted with a guide cannula in the lateral ventricle. On the

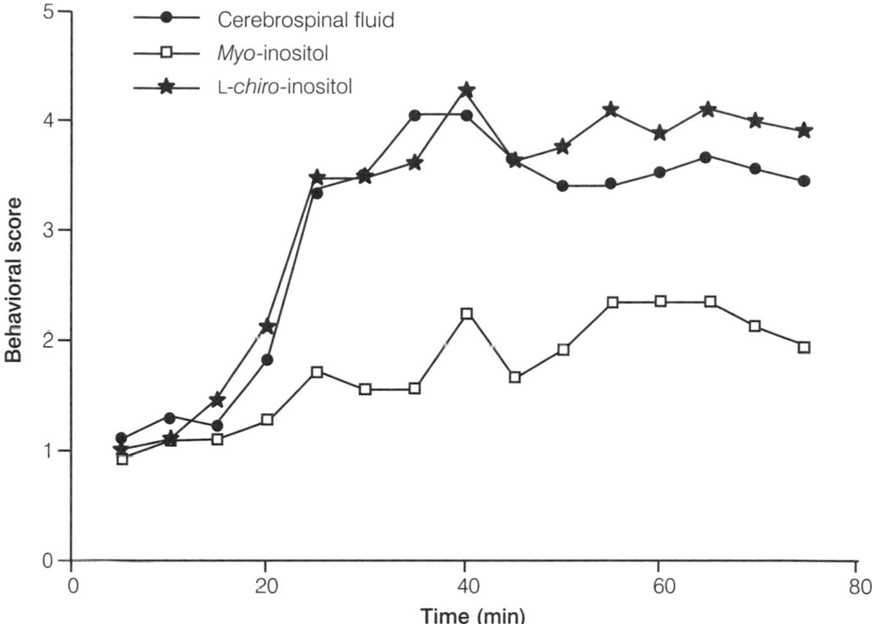

Figure 12–3. Score presenting the intensity of pilocarpine-induced behaviors (ordinate) in lithium-treated rats as described in the text. Abscissa represents the time in minutes following the injection of 20 mg/kg of pilocarpine. Kruskal-Wallis tests showed a significant effect of *myo*-inositol at 25–55 and 65–75 minutes.
Source. Reprinted with permission from Kofman O, Sherman WR, Katz V, et al.: "Restoration of Brain *Myo*-Inositol Levels in Rats Increases Latency to Lithium-Pilocarpine Seizures." *Psychopharmacology (Berlin)* 110:229–234, 1993. Copyright 1993, Springer-Verlag.

test day, 7 rats were injected with 10 mg/40 µL *myo*-inositol, and 7 were injected with 40 µL of artificial CSF (vehicle), 1 hour before 20 mg/kg of subcutaneous pilocarpine administration. All rats were rated for the progression of seizures with the scoring system described earlier in this chapter.

After chronic lithium treatment, only two of the seven rats pretreated with intracerebroventricular *myo*-inositol had lithum-pilocarpine seizures, whereas all seven of the vehicle-treated rats had seizures at a mean latency of 22.14 ± 8.49 (mean ± SD) minutes. The reduction in the incidence of forelimb clonus by *myo*-inositol was significant ($\chi^2 = 7.78$, $P < 0.01$). The serum lithium levels were 1.14 ± 0.78 mmol/L for the *myo*-inositol group and 1.59 ± 0.72 mmol/L for the vehicle-treated group (not significantly different). Thus, inositol reversal of lithium-pilocarpine seizures occurs after chronic as well as acute lithium treatment.

Species Specificity of Lithium-Pilocarpine Seizures

Sherman (1991) raised the question of whether lithium-pilocarpine seizures occurred in species other than rats, such as mice. Oppenheim et al. (1979) gave physostigmine to lithium-treated patients and did not observe lithium potentiation of the physostigmine effect. Hokin's group (Lee et al. 1992) studied the effects of cholinergic agonists on PI metabolism in cortical slices from several species, including monkeys, rats, and guinea pigs. They concluded that lithium-pilocarpine interactions occur only in species with low basal brain inositol levels, such as rats, and do not occur in monkeys or guinea pigs. The phenomenon can be elicited in vitro whenever cellular inositol levels are depleted in a low-inositol medium.

To test Hokin's (Lee et al. 1992) hypothesis in vivo, we attempted to elicit lithium-pilocarpine seizures in a wide variety of species. Rats (Sprague-Dawley, 300 g), mice (ICR, 25 g), guinea pigs (250 g), rabbits (500 g), chicks (70 g), frogs (10–40 g), and goldfish (30 g) were used. Animals were given intraperitoneal LiCl before the subcutaneous injection of the pilocarpine and were observed for 2 hours after pilocarpine administration. Control groups were given low-dose pilocarpine alone, after preliminary experiments determined the pilocparpine dose necessary to elicit seizures without lithium (Bersudsky et al. 1994).

Frogs did not have seizures with high doses of cholinergic agonists (pilocparpine 1 g/kg or carbachol 100 mg/kg). Consequently, there was also no seizure activity following lithium and low doses of cholinergic agonists.

Rats, mice, and goldfish showed a standard limbic seizure syndrome after lithium-pilocarpine administration but not with pilocarpine alone, with rhythmic contraction, loss of consciousness, fluctuating improvement, and eventual death. Of the nine guinea pigs, one given pilocarpine alone and one given lithium-pilocarpine had a tonic-clonic seizure and died immediately. One of two rabbits treated with lithium-pilocarpine died without seizures, but neither had a lithium-pilocarpine syndrome. Chicks had pilocarpine effects such as salivation, head-bobbing, and beak movements, but there was no difference between pilocarpine alone and lithium-pilocarpine; no loss of consciousness or rhythmic muscle contraction occurred.

The present results suggest that lithium-pilocarpine seizures are unique to rats, mice, and goldfish and do not occur in other mammals or birds, or even in other rodents such as guinea pigs. This supports Hokin's concept (Lee et al. 1992) that lithium-pilocarpine interactions are dependent on the low baseline inositol present in rat brain. The fact that goldfish show lithium-pilocarpine interactions and guinea pigs do not suggests that the property is not restricted to a specific evolutionary branch of brain development but is potentially present since at least teleost development (goldfish). It is interesting to speculate on the importance of interspecies variability for the use of lithium-pilocarpine seizures as a model for the testing of Berridge's inositol depletion hypothesis of lithium action.

Stereospecificity of the *myo*-Inositol Blockade of Lithium-Pilocarpine Seizures

The biologically inactive stereoisomers L-chiro-inositol (Kofman et al. 1993) and *scyllo*-inositol (Tricklebank et al. 1991) did not prevent lithium-pilocarpine seizures. However, Williams and Jope (1995) found that the stereoisomer *epi*-inositol, which was not incorporated into PI, did prevent lithium-pilocarpine seizures. This unexpected effect of a stereoisomer, which, in contrast to *myo*-inositol, did not reverse either the teratogenic effect of lithium in *Xenopus* oocytes (Busa and Gimlich 1989) or the suppression of neuronal firing of suprachiasmatic nucleus cells by lithium in vitro (Mason and Biello 1992), suggested that the mechanism of the reversal of behavioral effects of lithium by *myo*-inositol may be unrelated to the metabolism of PI-derived second messengers. However, Richards and Belmaker (1996) measured the effects of different inositol isomers on tritiated cytidine monophosphorylphosphatidate ([^{3}H]CMP-PA) in Chinese hamster ovary cells and in cross-chopped slices of rat cerebral cortex in the presence of carbachol and lithium. The effect of lithium to increase the accumulation of [^{3}H]CMP-PA was inhibited by *epi*-inositol and *myo*-inositol in a concentration-dependent fashion. *chiro*-Inositol had no effect, and *scyllo*-inositol elicited a slight inhibition. Recently, *epi*-inositol has been found to be behaviorally active in the plus-maze model of anxiety (Einat et al. 1998). Following the report by Williams and Jope (1995), we conducted a series of studies in an attempt to define the conditions under which the *epi*- and *myo*-inositol isomers reversed lithium-pilocarpine seizures.

Acute or Chronic Dietary Lithium and Intracerebroventricular *epi*-Inositol

We intraperitoneally injected 20 rats that had cannulae implanted in the lateral ventricle with 3 mEq/kg of LiCl 24 hours before intracerebroventricular administration of vehicle or inositol and subcutaneous pilocarpine. Rats were injected intracerebroventricularly with 40 μL of artificial CSF vehicle (n = 6),

10 mg/40 μL of *epi*-inositol (n = 7), or 10 mg/40 μL of *myo*-inositol (n = 7), followed 90 minutes later by subcutaneous pilocarpine (20 mg/kg). The rats were observed and rated for the progression of limbic seizures once every 5 minutes according to a modified version of the scale of Patel et al. (1988), as described earlier in this chapter. The latency to the onset of forelimb clonus also was noted. After acute lithium treatment, four of six control rats but only one of seven rats treated with *myo*-inositol and none of seven rats treated with *epi*-inositol had seizures.

Sixteen rats were fed chow containing 0.22% LiCl for 21 days and implanted with cannulae in the lateral ventricle, as described earlier in this chapter. On the test day, we injected rats intracerebroventricularly with either 10 mg/40 μL of *epi*-inositol or 40 μL of artificial CSF and rated them for seizures as described previously. After chronic lithium treatment, *epi*-inositol also reduced the number of rats showing clonus, preventing seizures in three of eight rats (χ^2 = 3.69, P = 0.055). All the control rats had seizures. The latency to onset of clonus was significantly longer in *epi*-inositol-treated rats (mean ± SD = 59.2 ± 8.04 minutes) than in control rats (27 ± 11.67 minutes) (t test = 5.38, P < 0.0005). The serum lithium levels were 1.24 ± 0.5 mmol/L for the *epi*-inositol group and 1.22 ± 0.4 mmol/L for the control group.

We implanted a single-guide cannula in the lateral ventricle of 22 rats, as described earlier in this chapter. After the rats recovered from surgery, we intraperitoneally injected them with 3 mEq/kg of LiCl. Twenty-four hours later, we intracerebroventricularly injected 12 rats with a solution of 9 mg of L-*chiro*-inositol and 1 mg of *myo*-inositol, dissolved in 40 μL of artificial CSF. Ten control rats were injected with artificial CSF. One hour later, we subcutaneously injected all of the rats with 20 mg/kg of pilocarpine and rated them for the progression of behavioral seizures, as described earlier. Two of the 12 rats treated with L-*chiro*-inositol and *myo*-inositol and 2 of the 10 rats treated with vehicle had no behavioral seizures. This difference was not statistically significant (χ^2 = 0.04). The latency to the onset of seizures was 33 ± 15.53 minutes (mean ± SD) in the control rats and 42.1 ± 12.71 minutes in the inositol-treated rats.

Forskolin Does Not Affect Lithium-Pilocarpine Seizures

Because lithium inhibits agonist-induced stimulation of cAMP as well (Belmaker 1981; Belmaker et al. 1980), we wanted to test the specificity of the inositol reversal of lithium-pilocarpine seizures by using intracerebroventricular forskolin as a pharmacological antagonist of lithium effects on adenylate cyclase. We injected 14 rats that had cannulae in the lateral ventricle with 3 mEq/kg of LiCl 20 hours before pilocarpine (20 mg/kg). One hour before administration of pilocarpine, we intracerebroventricularly injected the rats with forskolin (100 μg/5μL) or vehicle. There was no difference in the number of rats showing lithium-pilocarpine seizures (seven of seven forskolin-treated and five of seven control rats) and no difference in the latency to onset of clonus (mean ± SD = 36.71 ± 12.8 minutes for forskolin and 32.7 ± 8 minutes for control rats, t test = 0.69). Thus, antagonism of lithium inhibition of adenylate cyclase by forskolin does not reverse lithium-pilocarpine seizures.

INOSITOL EFFECTS ON LITHIUM MODULATION OF SEROTONERGIC BEHAVIORS

The antidepressant effect of lithium has been attributed to its ability to potentiate serotonin function, a hypothesis that is supported by reports that lithium enhances hormonal responses to serotonin agonists (Mühlbauer and Müller-Oerlinghausen 1985; Müller-Oerlinghausen 1985). However, others have reported that lithium does not potentiate hormonal responses to fenfluramine stimulation (Manji et al. 1991; Power et al. 1993; Shapira et al. 1992). In addition to its potentiation of therapeutic effects, the toxic *serotonin syndrome*, consisting of confusion, hypomania, restlessness, myoclonus, hyperreflexia, diaphoresis, shivering tremor, diarrhea, and incoordination, has been documented in patients receiving combined lithium and antidepressant treatment (Ohman and Spigset 1993; Sternbach 1991). The antidepressant and toxic interactions between lithium and serotoninergic agonists may be caused by a common biochemical mechanism of action.

Animal studies show that lithium enhances the serotonin syndrome elicited by 8-hydroxy-2-(di-*n*-propylamino) tetralin (8-OH-DPAT), a specific 5-HT_{1A} agonist, in rats. This effect distinguishes lithium from tricyclic antidepressants and monoamine oxidase inhibitors, which attenuate the syndrome (Goodwin et al. 1986a; Grahame-Smith 1988; Wood and Goodwin 1987), and from electroconvulsive shock, which attenuates the stereotypies but increases locomotion. The serotonin syndrome has been attributed to stimulation of brain stem and spinal cord 5-HT_{1A} receptors (Deakin and Green 1978; Tricklebank et al. 1985). Lithium potentiation is unaffected by pretreatment with the serotonin synthesis inhibitor para-chlorophenylalanine, suggesting that the site of potentiation is postsynaptic (Goodwin et al. 1986a). Because lithium attenuated the 5-HT_{1A}-mediated inhibition of forskolin-stimulated adenylate cyclase (Newman et al. 1991), the behavioral potentiation by lithium is perplexing. The 5-HT_{1A} receptor is negatively linked to adenylate cyclase through a G_i protein (Mørk et al. 1990; Peroutka 1993); however, evidence indicates that this may be a "promiscuous" receptor that stimulates PI hydrolysis (Peroutka 1993) as well. On the other hand, Claustre et al. (1988) reported that 8-OH-DPAT inhibited muscarinic-induced stimulation of PI hydrolysis in the hippocampus, suggesting that the 5-HT_{1A} receptor is negatively linked to PI hydrolysis. We therefore tested the effects of intracerebroventricular inositol and forskolin on lithium potentiation of the serotonin syndrome.

Standard stereotaxic procedures were used to implant 43 male Sprague-Dawley rats with a cannula in the lateral ventricle under pentobarbital anesthesia (50 mg/kg). On the test day, the rats were divided into two groups and injected intracerebroventricularly with either artificial CSF (40 μL) or *myo*-inositol (10 mg/40μL). Two and a half hours later, we injected the rats subcutaneously with 5-methoxy-*N*,*N*-dimethyltryptamine (5-MeODMT, 2.5 mg/kg), dissolved in 0.9% saline. Rats were placed in an open plastic cage and rated for components of the serotonin syndrome by an observer who was blind to the treatment condition.

Behavioral Rating

Five behaviors—forepaw treading, head-weaving, tremor, hindlimb abduction, and flat posture (Goodwin et al. 1986a)—were rated at 3, 5, 7, 9, 11, and 13 minutes after injection of 5-MeODMT as follows: 1 = not present, 2 = just noticeable, 3 = consistently present, and 4 = severe. Reactivity to a clap of the experimenter's hand was tested once after the 7-minute score was tabulated. Startle was scored as follows: 1 = no reaction, 2 = body jerk but no elevation of paws, 3 = elevation of forepaws, and 4 = jumps with all four paws off the ground. After the experiment, lithium-treated rats were decapitated under anesthesia, and trunk blood was collected in test tubes. Serum lithium levels were analyzed with an ion-selective electrode (Microlyte 3+2, Kone Ltd.). Data analysis was done only on those rats whose cannulae were found in the lateral ventricle.

Nonparametric Kruskal-Wallis analysis revealed a significant group difference for the total serotonin score ($H = 8.14$, $P = 0.043$) and for tremor ($H = 12.97$, $P < 0.005$). None of the other subscores had significant differences between groups. However, to examine the interaction between lithium and inositol, we conducted a two-way analysis of variance (ANOVA) for the effects of lithium and inositol for the total scores of each of the behavioral measures and for the sum of all the behavioral scores, excluding startle (total serotonin syndrome score). Analysis of simple main effects between the two CSF groups (regular vs. lithium) and the two inositol groups (regular vs. lithium) was conducted to determine whether lithium had a significant effect in both treatment conditions.

Lithium significantly enhanced total score ($F_{1,39} = 8.13$, $P = 0.007$), tremor ($F_{1,39} = 17.58$, $P < 0.0002$), hindlimb abduction ($F_{1,39} = 6.77$, $P < 0.02$), and flat posture ($F_{1,39} = 4.19$, $P < 0.05$). Lithium enhancement of forepaw treading was nearly significant ($F_{1,39} = 3.87$, $P = 0.056$). Headweaving and startle were not significantly enhanced by lithium (Figure 12–4).

Inositol had no main effect on any of the measures. There was a nonsignificant trend toward an interaction between inositol and lithium on the total serotonin score ($F_{1,39} = 3.23$, $P < 0.08$), suggesting that inositol mitigated the lithium effect. Examination of the individual behaviors confirmed that, with the exception of startle behavior, the lithium inositol group had consistently lower scores than the lithium-CSF group. In contrast, the scores of the lithium-inositol group were not significantly higher than those of the regular-inositol group, except in the case of tremor ($F_{1,21} = 4.57$, $P < 0.05$). However, the effect of lithium on tremor was still smaller in the inositol-treated rats than in the CSF-treated rats. Startle behavior was the only behavior measured that was unaffected by either lithium or inositol. Serum lithium levels were 0.45 ± 0.11 mmol/L (mean ± SD) for the CSF-lithium group and 0.6 ± 0.22 mmol/L for the inositol-lithium group and were not significantly different when compared by *t* test.

LITHIUM-FORSKOLIN INTERACTION ON THE SEROTONIN SYNDROME

We gave either chronic lithium food or regular laboratory chow to 35 male Sprague-Dawley rats implanted with a guide cannula in the lateral ventricle. On the test day, we divided the rats into two groups and injected them intracerebroventricularly with either DMSO (5 μL) or forskolin (100 μg/5 μL). Twenty minutes later, we injected the rats subcutaneously with 5-MeODMT (2.5 mg/kg), dissolved in 0.9% saline. Rats were placed in an open plastic cage and rated for components of the serotonin syndrome, as described earlier in this chapter. Eleven of the 17 lithium-treated rats had transient clonic or tonic-clonic seizures (5 forskolin- and 6 DMSO-treated rats). The behavior was not scored during the seizures, and average total scores were adjusted proportionally to account for the number of data points.

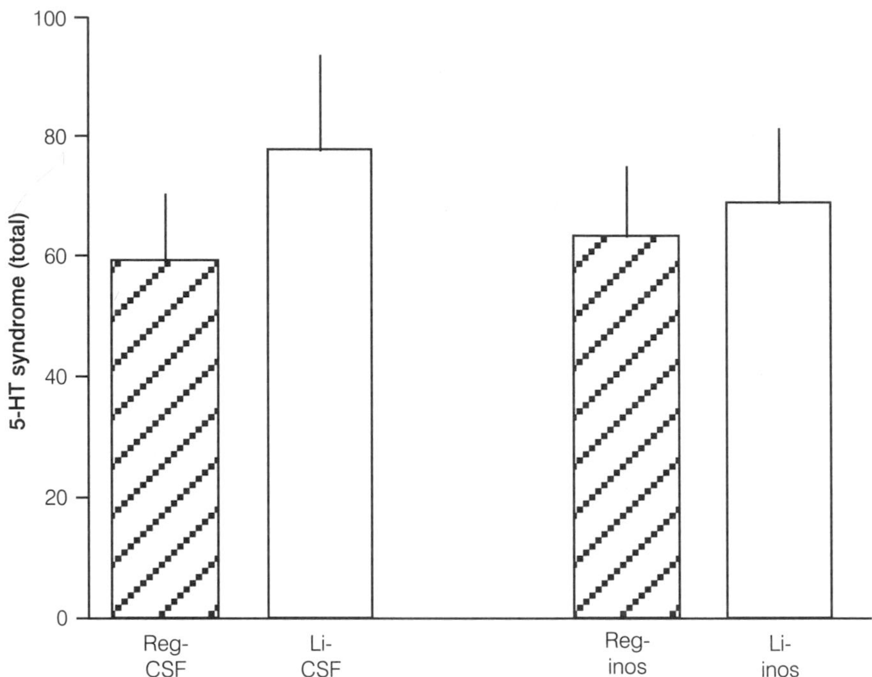

Figure 12–4. Behavioral severity score (mean ± SD) for the total serotonin (5-HT) syndrome following administration of 2.5 mg/kg 5-methoxy-*N*,*N*-dimethyltryptamine (5-MeODMT) in rats treated with regular food and intracerebroventricular (icv) artificial cerebrospinal fluid (CSF) (Reg-CSF, *n* = 11), regular food and icv inositol (Reg-inos, *n* = 14), lithium (Li) food and icv CSF (Li-CSF, *n* = 9), and lithium food and ICV inositol (Li-inos, *n* = 9).
Source. Adapted with permission from Kofman O, Levin U: "Lithium's Behavioural Interactions With Serotonin Agonists in Rats Are Differentially Affected by Intracerebroventricular *Myo*-Inositol." *Psychopharmacology (Berlin)* 118:213–218, 1995. Copyright 1995, Springer-Verlag.

The nonparametric Kruskal-Wallis analysis showed a significant between-group difference for tremor (H = 10.48, $P < 0.02$), but no significant differences were found for the other components of the serotonin syndrome or for the total score. Two-way ANOVA showed a significant lithium-induced enhancement of tremor ($F_{1,31}1 = 13.17$, $P = 0.01$) and a near-significant enhancement of the total serotonin syndrome score ($F_{1,31} = 3.62$, $P = 0.07$), flat posture ($F_{1,31} = 3.86$, $P < 0.06$), and startle behavior ($F_{1,31} = 3.38$, $P < 0.08$) (Figure 12–5). There was no main effect of forskolin and no interaction between lithium and forskolin. No difference in serum lithium levels was found between the DMSO- (mean ± SD = 0.52 ± 0.05 mmol/L) and forskolin (0.51 ± 0.14 mmol/L)-treated groups.

LITHIUM-INOSITOL INTERACTION WITH 5-HYDROXYTRYPTOPHAN–INDUCED WET DOG SHAKES

In contrast to its facilitative effects on 5-HT_{1A} behaviors, lithium attenuated 5-hydroxytryptophan (5-HTP)-induced head twitches in mice (Goodwin et al. 1986b) but did not affect wet dog shakes in rats (Goodwin et al. 1986a). These behaviors have been attributed to stimulation of brain stem 5-HT_2 receptors (Bedard and Pycock 1977; Blackshear and Sanders-Bush 1982; Tricklebank et al. 1985; Yap and Taylor 1983).

We gave either chronic lithium food or regular laboratory chow to 35 individually housed male Sprague-Dawley rats that were implanted with a guide cannula in the lateral ventricle, as described earlier in this chapter. On the test day (day 21 of the lithium diet), we injected half of each of the lithium and control groups with either *myo*-inositol (10 mg/40 µL) or artificial CSF vehicle (40 µL). Two and a half hours later, we intraperitoneally injected the rats with carbidopa (25 mg/kg) and 30 minutes later intraperitoneally injected them with 5-HTP (50 mg/kg). Observers who were blind to the treatment condition counted the number of wet dog shakes for a period of 5 minutes every 15 minutes over 2 hours.

Total wet dog shakes were analyzed by two-way ANOVA. Lithium significantly decreased the number of wet dog shakes ($F_{1,31} = 8.89$, $P = 0.006$), but inositol had no effect, and no significant interaction was found between lithium and inositol. There was no significant difference in the lithium levels between the rats pretreated with artificial CSF (mean ± SD = 0.56 ± 0.26 mmol/L) and those pretreated with inositol (0.52 ± 0.13 mmol/L).

CONCLUSION

Of the four centrally mediated behaviors that were found to be affected by lithium, three were reversed or attenuated by inositol. One behavior was also clearly affected by forskolin.

Inositol attenuated the ability of lithium to reduce rearing, to potentiate cholinergic seizures, and to potentiate the serotonin syndrome but did not affect the lithium-induced reduction of wet dog shakes following 5-HT_2 stimulation. It remains unclear why the *epi*-inositol stereoisomer was as effective as *myo*-inositol in the lithium-pilocarpine model and whether it would be effective in attenuating other lithum-induced effects. Although *epi*-inositol did not

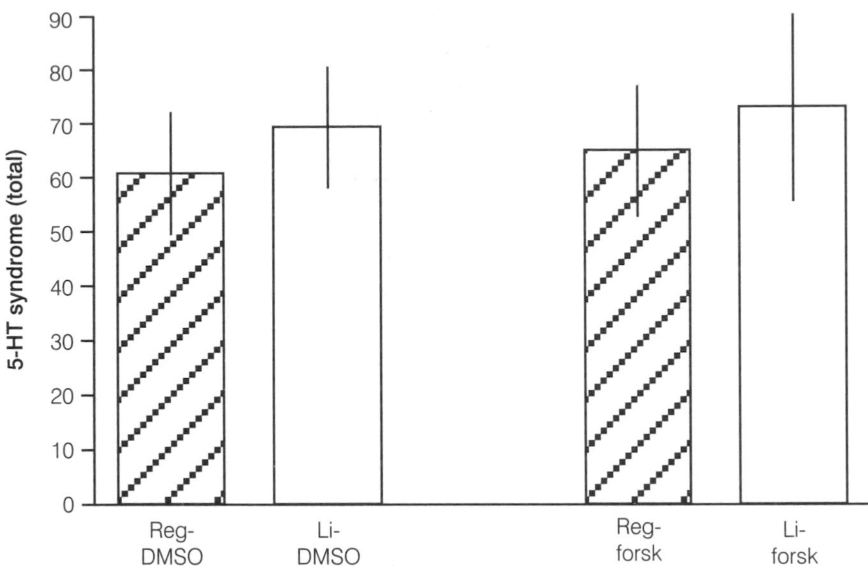

Figure 12–5. Behavioral severity score (mean ±SD) for the total serotonin (5-HT) syndrome following 2.5 mg/kg 5-methoxy-*N*,*N*-dimethyltryptamine (5-MeODMT) in rats treated with regular food and intracerebroventricular (icv) dimethylsulfoxide (DMSO) (Reg-DMSO, *n* = 9), regular food and icv forskolin (colforsin) (Reg-forsk, *n* = 9), lithium food and icv DMSO (Li-DMSO, *n* = 9), and lithium food and icv forskolin (Li-forsk, *n* = 8).
Source. Adapted with permission from Kofman O, Levin U: "Lithium's Behavioural Interactions With Serotonin Agonists in Rats Are Differentially Affected by Intracerebroventricular *Myo*-Inositol." *Psychopharmacology (Berlin)* 118:213–218, 1995. Copyright 1995, Springer-Verlag.

reverse the teratogenic effects of lithium (Busa and Gimlich 1989) or the lithium-induced suppression of suprachiasmatic nucleus cell firing in vitro (Mason and Biello 1992), both behavioral (Einat et al. 1998; Patishi et al. 1996a; Williams and Jope 1995) and biochemical studies (Richards and Belmaker 1996) suggested that this inositol isomer affects the PI cycle. Batty and Downes (1994) reported a secondary regulatory effect of inositol depletion on PLC activity. It is possible that *epi*-inositol is as effective as *myo*-inositol at another regulatory site. The search for a mechanism in which *epi*-inositol, but not *scyllo*- or *chiro*-inositol, is as active as *myo*-inositol could provide an important clue as to the exact site of action of lithium in the PI cycle. Forskolin interacted with lithium when locomotor activity was examined but not when specific lithium-cholinergic or lithium–5-HT_{1A} behaviors were tested. A similar interaction has been found between lithium and the cAMP analogue dibutyryl-cAMP (Kofman and Patishi, in press).

Our findings confirm that inositol replenishment can reverse some, but not all, of the behavioral effects of lithium. Behaviors that are regulated by multiple systems, such as locomotion, can be influenced by drugs that affect the PI or the cAMP system, whereas interactions between lithium and specific neurotransmitters may be affected by the second messenger linked to that particular receptor. Inositol reversed lithium-induced potentiation of cholinergic and serotonergic stimulation, whereas forskolin was ineffective in these paradigms.

It is interesting that recently accumulated evidence shows that inositol has behavioral and clinical effects when given alone. Inositol has been found in several clinical studies to have a therapeutic profile similar to that of serotonin reuptake inhibitors. Levine et al. (1993) found that 6 g/day of inositol alleviated symptoms of depression. The results of this open study were confirmed in a double-blind controlled study in which 12 g/day of inositol significantly reduced Hamilton Rating Scale for Depression scores after 4 weeks of treatment in 28 patients (Levine et al. 1995). Inositol was particularly effective on the subscales of psychic anxiety and depression. Controlled studies also have found significant clinical effects of inositol on obsessive- compulsive disorder (Fux et al. 1996) and panic disorder (Benjamin et al. 1995). Einat et al. (H. Einat, F. Clenet, A. Shaldevin, R. H. Belmaker, M. Bourin: "The Antidepressant Activity of Inositol in the Forced Swim Test Involves $5HT_2$ Receptors," manuscript submitted for publication) have shown that antidepressant effects of inositol in rat models of depression can be blocked by $5\text{-}HT_2$ receptor antagonists, supporting the hypothesis that inositol is acting via serotonergic receptors.

Many issues must be resolved before the role of lithium in second-messenger systems can be understood in behavioral terms. Because of the considerable evidence for cross-talk between second-messenger systems (Cooper et al. 1995), it is not surprising to find that a drug with multiple effects such as lithium can be antagonized at several different biochemical sites. Bipolar affective disorder is characterized by fluctuations in mood and level of activity, which may result from an imbalance in signal transduction beyond the receptor. Once the pathological process is initiated at any point within the signal transduction cascade, the intricate systems of regulatory feedback will become perturbed. At this point, a versatile drug such as lithium, which has the ability to act at more than one site in the signal transduction system, may be more efficacious than a very specific drug. Thus, an agent that is known to attenuate both facets of bipolar depression may be required to act on multiple mechanisms.

As our knowledge of signal transduction has expanded, the simplistic "specific pathophysiology" models have become obsolete. Both PKC and calcium, dual products of PLC stimulation via diacylglycerol and IP_3, respectively, stimulate different subtypes of adenylate cyclase (Cooper et al. 1995; Yoshimasa et al. 1987; Yoshimura and Cooper 1993). These subtypes of adenylate cyclase are differentially distributed in the rat brain and therefore are functionally diverse (Cooper et al. 1995). Moreover, phorbol esters can also enhance cAMP in cells lacking $G\alpha_s$ and may do so by inhibiting $G\alpha_i$ activity (Bell and Brunton 1986). Preliminary data (Patishi et al. 1996b) suggest that lithium neither enhances nor attenuates the behavioral effect of PKC; however, the specificity of the PKC effect in these paradigms has not yet been tested. Further research should take cross-talk mechanisms into account and focus on regional distribution of different signal transduction systems.

With the development of drugs that inhibit adenylate cyclase stimulation, such as SQ22,356 (Iannonee et al. 1989), and agents that act as inositol antagonists (Kozikowski et al. 1990), the effects of drugs that mimic particular aspects of lithium's biochemical effects can be tested on more sophisticated and valid animal models of mania and depression.

REFERENCES

Allison JH, Stewart MA: Reduced brain inositol in lithium-treated rats. Nature: New Biology 233:267–268, 1971

Andersen PH, Geisler A: Lithium inhibition of forskolin-stimulated adenylate cyclase. Neuropsychobiology 12:1–3, 1984

Avissar S, Schreiber G, Danon A, et al: Lithium inhibits adrenergic and cholinergic increases in GTP binding in rat cortex. Nature 331:440–442, 1988

Barraco RA, Phillis JW, Altman HJ: Depressant effect of forskolin on spontaneous locomotor activity in mice. Gen Pharmacol 16:521–524, 1985

Batty IH, Downes CP: The inhibition of phosphoinositide synthesis and muscarinic-receptor-mediated phospholipase C activity by Li^+ as secondary, selective, consequences of inositol depletion in 1321N1 cells. Biochem J 297:529– 537, 1994

Bedard P, Pycock CJ: 'Wet-dog' shake behaviour in the rat: a possible quantitative model of central 5-hydroxytryptamine activity. Neuropharmacology 16:663–670, 1977

Bell JD, Brunton LL: Enhancement of adenylate cyclase activity in S49 lymphoma cells by phorbol esters. J Biol Chem 261:12036–12041, 1986

Belmaker RH: Receptors, adenylate cyclase, depression and lithium. Biol Psychiatry 16:333–350, 1981

Belmaker RH, Zohar J, Ebstein RP: Cyclic nucleotides in mental disorder. Advances in Cyclic Nucleotide and Protein Phosphorylation Research 12:187–198, 1980

Belmaker RH, Lerer B, Klein E, et al: The use of behavioral methods in the search for compounds with lithium-like activity, in Behavioral Models and the Analysis of Drug Action. Edited by Levy A, Spiegelstein MY. Amsterdam, Elsevier, 1982, pp 343–356

Belmaker RH, Livne A, Agam G, et al: Role of inositol-1-phosphatase inhibition in the mechanism of action of lithium. Pharmacol Toxicol 66 (suppl III):76–83, 1990

Bender JL, Neer EJ: Properties of the adenylate cyclase catalytic unit from caudate nucleus. J Biol Chem 258:2432–2439, 1983

Benjamin J, Levine J, Fux M, et al: Inositol treatment for panic disorder: a double-blind placebo-controlled crossover trial. Am J Psychiatry 152:1084–1086, 1995

Berridge MJ, Downes CP, Hanley MR: Neural and developmental action of lithium: a unifying hypothesis. Cell 59:411–419, 1989

Bersudsky Y, Vinnitsky I, Grisaru N, et al: Dose-response and time curve of inositol prevention of Li-pilocarpine seizures. Eur Neuropsychopharmacol 3:428–429, 1993

Bersudsky Y, Mahler O, Kofman O, et al: Species differences in susceptibility to Li-pilocarpine seizures. Eur Neuropsychopharmacol 4:429–430, 1994

Bersudsky Y, Patishi Y, Jensen JB, et al: The effect of acute and chronic lithium on forskolin-induced reduction of rat activity. J Neural Transm 104:943–952, 1997

Bitran JA, Potter WZ, Manji HK, et al: Chronic Li^+ attenuates agonist- and phorbol ester-mediated Na^+/H^+ antiporter activity in HL-60 cells. Eur J Pharmacol 188: 193–202, 1990

Blackshear MA, Sanders-Bush E: Serotonin receptor sensitivity after acute and chronic treatment with mianserin. J Pharmacol Exp Ther 221:303–308, 1982

Busa WB, Gimlich RL: Lithium-induced teratogenesis in frog embryos prevented by a polyphosphoinositide cycle intermediate or a diacylglycerol analog. Dev Biol 132: 315–324, 1989

Casebolt TL, Jope RS: Effects of chronic lithium treatment on protein kinase C and cyclic AMP dependent protein phosphorylation. Biol Psychiatry 25:329–340, 1991

Claustre Y, Benavides J, Scatton B: 5-HT1A receptor agonists inhibit carbachol-induced stimulation of phosphoinositide turnover in rat hippocampus. Eur J Pharmacol 149:149–153, 1988

Cooper DMF, Mons N, Karpen JW: Adenylyl cyclases and the interaction between calcium and cAMP signaling. Nature 374:421–424, 1995

Deakin JFW, Green AR: The effects of putative 5-hydroxytryptamine antagonists on the behaviour produced by administration of tranylcypromine and L-tryptophan or tranylcypromine and L-DOPA to rats. Br J Pharmacol 64:201–209, 1978

Downes CP, Stone MA: Lithium induced reduction in intracellular inositol supply in cholinergically stimulated parotid gland. Biochem J 234:199–204, 1986

Ebstein RP, Belmaker RH, Grunhaus L, et al: Lithium inhibition of adrenaline-sensitive adenylate cyclase in humans. Nature 259:411–413, 1976

Ebstein RP, Hermoni M, Belmaker RH: The effect of lithium on noradrenaline-induced cyclic AMP accumulation in rat brain: inhibition after chronic treatment and absence of super-sensitivity. J Pharmacol Exp Ther 213:161–167, 1980

Einat H, Elkabaz-Shwortz Z, Cohen H, et al: Chronic epi inositol has an anxiolytic-like effect in the plus maze model in rats. International Journal of NeuroPsychopharmacology 1:31–34, 1998

Frazer A, Haugaard ES, Mandels J, et al: Effects of intracellular lithium on epinephrine-induced accumulation of cyclic AMP in skeleton muscle. Biochem Pharmacol 24:2273–2277, 1975

Fux M, Levine J, Aviv A, et al: Inositol treatment of obsessive-compulsive disorder. Am J Psychiatry 153:1219–1221, 1996

Gee NS, Ragan CI, Watling KJ, et al: The purification and properties of *myo*-inositol monophosphatase from bovine brain. Biochem J 249:883–889, 1988

Gispen WH, Schrama LH, Eichberg J: Stimulation of protein kinase C reduces ACTH-induced excessive grooming. Eur J Pharmacol 114:399–400, 1985

Givant Y, Zohar J, Lichtenberg P, et al: Chronic lithium attenuates clenbuterol-induced hypoactivity. Lithium 1:183–185, 1990

Godfrey PP: Potentiation by lithium of CMP-phosphatidate formation in carbachol-stimulated rat cerebral-cortical slices and its reversal by *myo*-inositol. Biochem J 258:621–624, 1989

Goodwin GM, de Souza RJ, Wood AJ, et al: The enhancement by lithium of the 5-HT1A mediated serotonin syndrome produced by 8-OH-DPAT in the rat: evidence for a post-synaptic mechanism. Psychopharmacology 90:488–493, 1986a

Goodwin GM, de Souza RJ, Wood AJ, et al: Lithium decreases 5-HT1A and 5-HT2 receptor and α2-adrenoreceptor mediated function in mice. Psychopharmacology 90:482–487, 1986b

Grahame-Smith DG: Neuropharmacological adaptive effects in the actions of antidepressant drugs, ECT and lithium, in New Concepts in Depression (Pierre Fabre Monograph Series, Vol 2). Edited by Briley M, Fillion G. Basingstoke, MacMillan, 1988, pp 1–14

Gross G, Dodt C, Hanft G: Effect of chronic lithium administration on adrenoceptor binding and adrenoceptor regulation in rat cerebral cortex. Naunyn Schmiedebergs Arch Pharmacol 337:267–272, 1988

Hallcher LM, Sherman WR: The effect of lithium ion and other agents on the activity of *myo*-inositol-1-phosphatase from bovine brain. J Biol Chem 255:10896–10901, 1980

Hamburger-Bar R, Robert M, Newman M, et al: Interstrain correlation between behavioral effects of lithium and effects on cortical cyclic AMP. Pharmacol Biochem Behav 24:9–13, 1986

Honchar MP, Olney JW, Sherman WR: Systemic cholinergic agents induce seizures and brain damage in lithium-treated rats. Science 220:323–325, 1983

Iannone, MA, Wolberg G, Zimmerman TP: Chemotactic peptide induces cAMP elevation in human neutrophils by amplification of the adenylate cyclase response to endogenously produced adenosine. J Biol Chem 264:20177–20180, 1989

Johnson EC, Gray-Keller MP, O'Day PM: Rescue of excitation by inositol following Li^+-induced block in *Limulus* ventral photoreceptors. Vis Neurosci 15:105–112, 1998

Johnson FN: Dissociation of vertical and horizontal components of activity in rats treated with lithium chloride. Experimenta 28:533–535, 1972

Kofman O, Belmaker RH: Intracerebroventricular *myo*-inositol antagonizes lithium-induced suppression of rearing behavior in rats. Brain Res 534:345–347, 1990

Kofman O, Patishi Y: Interactions of lithium and drugs that affect signal transduction on behaviour in rats. Eur Neuropsychopharmacol (in press)

Kofman O, Sherman WR, Katz V, et al: Restoration of brain *myo*-inositol levels in rats increases latency to lithium-pilocarpine seizures. Psychopharmacology (Berl) 110:229–234, 1993

Kow LM, Brown HE, Pfaff DW: Activation of protein kinase C in the hypothalamic ventromedial nucleus of the midbrain central gray facilitates lordosis. Brain Res 660:241–248, 1994

Kozikowski AP, Fauq AH, Powis G, et al: Efficient synthetic routes to fluorinated isoteres of inositol and their effects on cellular growth. Journal of the American Chemical Society 112:4528–4531, 1990

Krall JF, Jamgotchian N: Forskolin refractoriness: exposure to the diterpene alters guanine nucleotide-dependent adenylate cyclase and calcium-uptake activity of cells cultured from the rat aorta. Biochem J 241:463–467, 1987

Lee CH, Dixon JF, Reichman M, et al: Li+ increases accumulation of inositol 1,4,5-trisphosphate and inositol 1,3,4,5-tetrakisphosphate in cholinergically stimulated brain cortex slices in guinea pig, mouse and rat. Biochem J 282:377– 385, 1992

Lenox RH: Lithium interactions with the phosphoinositide system and protein kinase C in the nervous system, in Progress in Catecholamine Research. Edited by Belmaker RH, Sandler M, Dahlstrom A. New York, Alan R Liss, 1988, pp 327–335

Levine J, Gonzalves M, Barbur I, et al: Inositol 6 gm daily may be effective in depression but not in schizophrenia. Human Psychopharmacology 8:49–53, 1993

Levine J, Barak Y, Gonsalves M, et al: A double-blind controlled trial of inositol treatment in depression. Am J Psychiatry 152:792–794, 1995

Manji HK, Lenox RH: Long-term action of lithium: a role for transcriptional and posttranscriptional factors regulated by protein kinase C. Synapse 16:11–28, 1994

Manji HK, Hsiao JK, Risby ED, et al: The mechanism of action of lithium, I: effects of serotonergic and noradrenergic systems in normal subjects. Arch Gen Psychiatry 48:505–512, 1991

Manji HK, Etcheberrigaray R, Chen G, et al: Lithium decreases membrane-associated protein kinase C in hippocampus: selectivity for the α isozyme. J Neurochem 61:2303–2310, 1993

Mason R, Biello SM: A neurophysiological study of a lithium-sensitive phosphoinositide system in the hamster suprachiasmatic (SCN) biological clock in vitro. Neurosci Lett 144:135–138, 1992

Mørk A: Actions of lithium on second messenger activity in the brain: the adenylate cyclase and phosphoinositide systems. Lithium 1:131–147, 1990

Mørk A, Geisler A: Effects of lithium on calmodulin-stimulated adenylate cyclase activity in cortical membranes from rat brain. Pharmacol Toxicol 60:17–23, 1987a

Mørk A, Geisler A: Mode of action of lithium on the catalytic unit of adenylate cyclase from rat brain. Pharmacol Toxicol 60:241–248, 1987b

Mørk A, Geisler A: Lithium in situ decreases extracellular levels of cyclic AMP in the dorsal hippocampus of living rats. Pharmacol Toxicol 74:300–302, 1994

Mørk A, Geisler A: Effect of chronic lithium treatment on agonist-enhanced extracellular concentrations of cyclic AMP in the dorsal hippocampus of freely moving rats. J Neurochem 65:134–139, 1995

Mørk A, Klysner R, Geisler A: Effects of treatment with a lithium-imipramine combination on components of adenylate cyclase in the cerebral cortex of the rat. Neuropharmacology 29:261–267, 1990

Mühlbauer HD, Müller-Oerlinghausen B: Fenfluramine stimulation of serum cortisol in patients with major affective disorders and healthy controls: further evidence for a central serotonergic action of lithium in man. J Neural Transm 61:81–94, 1985

Müller-Oerlinghausen B: Lithium long term treatment—does it act via serotonin? Pharmacopsychiatry 18:214–217, 1985

Newman M, Belmaker RH: Effects of lithium *in vitro* and *ex vivo* on components of the adenylate cyclase system in membrane from the cerebral cortex of the rat. Neuropharmacology 26:211–217, 1987

Newman ME, Ben-Zeev, Lerer B: Chloroamphetamine did not prevent the effects of chronic antidepressants on 5-hydroxtryptamine inhibition of forskolin-stimulated adenylate cyclase in rat hippocampus. Eur J Pharmacol 207:209–213, 1991

Ohman R, Spigset O: Serotonin syndrome induced by fluvoxamine-lithium interaction. Pharmacopsychiatry 26:263–264, 1993

Oppenheim G, Ebstein RP, Belmaker RH: Effect of lithium on the physostigmine-induced behavioral syndrome and plasma cyclic GMP. J Psychiatry Res 15:133–138, 1979

Ormandy GC, Song L, Jope RS: Analysis of the convulsant-potentiating effects of lithium in rats. Exp Neurol 111:356–361, 1991

Patel S, Meldrum BS, Fine A: Susceptibility to pilocarpine-induced seizures in rats increases with age. Behav Brain Res 31:165–167, 1988

Patishi Y, Belmaker RH, Bersudsky Y, et al: A comparison of the ability of myo-inositol and epi-inositol to attenuate lithium-pilocarpine seizures in rats. Biol Psychiatry 40:656–659, 1996a

Patishi Y, Bersudsky Y, Belmaker RH: Phorbol ester intracerebroventricularly induces a behavioral hypoactivity that is not affected by chronic or acute lithium. Eur Neuropsychopharmacol 6:39–41, 1996b

Peroutka SJ: 5-Hydroxytryptamine receptors. J Neurochem 60:408–416, 1993

Persinger MA, Makarec K, Bradley JC: Characteristics of limbic seizures evoked by peripheral injections of lithium and pilocarpine. Physiol Behav 44:27–37, 1988

Pontzer NJ, Crews FT: Desensitization of muscarinic stimulated hippocampal cell firing is related to phosphoinositide hydrolysis and inhibited by lithium. J Pharmacol Exp Ther 253:921–929, 1990

Power AC, Dorkins CE, Cowen PJ: Effect of lithium on prolactin response to D-fenfluramine in healthy subjects. Biol Psychiatry 33:801–805, 1993

Richards MH, Belmaker RH: Epi inositol is biochemically active in reversing lithium effects on cytidine monophosphorylphosphatidate (CMP-PA). J Neural Transm103:1281–1285, 1996

Schimmer BP, Tsao J, Borenstein R, et al: Forskolin-resistant Y1 mutants harbor defects associated with the guanyl nucleotide-binding regulatory protein G_S. J Biol Chem 262:15521–15526, 1987

Seamon KB, Padget W, Daly JW: Forskolin: unique diterpene activator of adenylate cyclase in the membranes and in intact cells. Proc Natl Acad Sci U S A 78: 3363–3367, 1981

Shapira B, Yagmur MJ, Gropp C, et al: Effects of clomipramine and lithium on fenfluramine-induced hormone release in major depression. Biol Psychiatry 31: 975–983, 1992

Sherman WR: Lithium and the phosphoinositide signalling system, in Lithium and the Cell. Edited by Birch NJ. London, Academic Press, 1991, pp 121–157

Sherman WR, Honchar MP, Munsell LY: Detection of receptor-linked phosphoinositide metabolism in brain of lithium treated rats, in Inositol and Phosphoinositides: Metabolism and Regulation. Edited by Bleasdale JE, Eichborg J, Hauser C. Clifton, NJ, Humana Press, 1985, pp 49–65

Sherman WR, Gish BG, Honchar MP, et al: Effects of lithium on phosphoinositide metabolism in vivo. Federation Proceedings 45:2639–2646, 1986

Skolnick P, Daly JW: Norepinephrine-sensitive adenylate cyclases in rat brain: relation to behavior and tyrosine hydroxylase. Science 184:174–176, 1974

Smith DF: Effects of lithium and rolipram enantiomers on locomotor activity in inbred mice. Pharmacol Toxicol 66:142–145, 1990

Stalvey L, Daly JW, Dismukes RK: Behavioral activity and accumulation of cyclic AMP in brain slices of strains of mice. Life Sci 19:1845–1850, 1976

Sternbach H: The serotonin syndrome. Am J Psychiatry 148:705–713, 1991

Terry JB, Padzernik TL, Nelson SR: Effect of LiCl pretreatment on cholinomimetic-induced seizures and seizure-induced brain edema in rats. Neurosci Lett 114: 123–127, 1990

Tricklebank MD, Forler C, Middlemiss DN, et al: Subtypes of the 5-HT receptor mediating the behavioural responses to 5-methoxy-N,N-dimethyltryptamine in the rat. Eur J Pharmacol 117:15–24, 1985

Tricklebank MD, Singh L, Jackson A, et al: Evidence that a proconvulsant action of lithium is mediated by inhibition of *myo*-inositol phosphatase in mouse brain. Brain Res 558:145–148, 1991

Wachtel H: Characteristic behavioral alterations in rats induced by rolipram and other selective adenosine cyclic 3',5'-monophosphate phosphodiesterase inhibitors. Psychopharmacology 77:309–316, 1982

Wachtel H: Dysbalance of neural second messenger function in the aetiology of affective disorders: a pathophysiological concept hypothesizing defects beyond first messenger receptors. J Neural Transm 75:21–29, 1989

Wachtel H, Schneider HH: Rolipram, a novel antidepressant drug, reverses the hypothermia and hypokinesia of monoamine-depleted mice by an action beyond postsynaptic monoamine receptors. Neuropharmacology 25:1119–1126, 1986

Williams MB, Jope RS: Modulation by inositol of cholinergic- and serotonergic-induced seizures in lithium treated rats. Brain Res 685:169–178, 1995

Wood AJ, Goodwin GM: A review of the biochemical and neuropharmacological actions of lithium. Psychol Med 17:579–600, 1987

Yap CY, Taylor DA: Involvement of 5-HT2 receptors in the wet-dog shake behaviour induced by 5-hydroxytryptophan in the rat. Neuropharmacology 22:801–804, 1983

Yoshimasa T, Sibley DR, Bouvier M, et al: Cross-talk between cellular signalling pathways suggested by phorbol-ester-induced adenylate cyclase phosphorylation. Nature 327:67–70, 1987

Yoshimura M, Cooper DMF: Type-specific stimulation of adenylyl cyclase by protein kinase C. J Biol Chem 268:4604–4607, 1993

CHAPTER 13

GUANINE NUCLEOTIDE BINDING PROTEIN DISTURBANCES IN BIPOLAR DISORDER

Jerry J. Warsh, M.D., Ph.D., L. Trevor Young, M.D., Ph.D., and Peter P. Li, Ph.D.

During the past decade, a growing body of data has accrued from clinical and animal studies implicating disturbances in transmembrane and intraneuronal signaling in the pathophysiology of bipolar disorder (BD). Among the possible abnormalities considered to be particularly relevant to the pathophysiology of BD, considerable attention has focused on the potential role of elevated brain levels and functionality (hyperfunction) of the stimulatory guanine nucleotide binding protein (G protein) α-subunit (α_s) (Avissar and Schreiber 1992; Schreiber et al. 1991; Young et al. 1993). Not unexpectedly, observations indicating that the prototypical mood-stabilizing agent lithium, at therapeutically relevant concentrations, modulates G-protein–dependent transmembrane signal transduction at several sites in receptor-effector–second-messenger signaling chains have been seminal in directing investigators to scrutinize G proteins and their function in BD.

The framework of observations implicating signal transduction and G-protein disturbances in the pathophysiology of BD and as target sites for the action of mood-stabilizing agents has been the subject of several excellent

---

Aspects of this work were supported by grants from the Medical Research Council of Canada, the Stanley Research Foundation, the Ontario Mental Health Foundation, and the Ministry of Health of Ontario.

reviews (Dubovsky et al. 1992; Hudson et al. 1993; Manji 1992; Manji and Lenox 1994; Manji et al. 1995b; Warsh and Li 1996). In this chapter, we focus primarily on the application of the postmortem research strategy, which we have exploited to provide more direct evidence of G-protein–dependent signaling disturbances in BD. This is preceded by a very brief overview of the molecular biology and functions of G proteins, because this knowledge is critical to the interpretation of G-protein findings in these studies. We also describe observations from complementary clinical investigations of G proteins in mononuclear leukocytes (MNLs) from BD patients, which extend postmortem brain findings to the living patient. Finally, we consider the potential therapeutic implications of the G-protein signal transduction abnormalities identified in BD.

G PROTEINS AND SIGNAL TRANSDUCTION

The heterotrimeric G proteins are critical intermediates coupling membrane receptor activation to effector and intracellular responses. They are a family of homologous yet structurally diverse proteins composed of α-, β-, and γ-subunits. The functional diversity of G proteins may be ascribed to differences in both the primary structure of the $G\alpha_s$ subunit and the βγ-subunit composition with which the former pairs. Mammalian $G\alpha_s$ subunits have been grouped into four classes based on amino acid identity (and presumed evolutionary distance): 1) $G\alpha_s$ and $G\alpha_{olf}$; 2) $G\alpha_{t1\&2}$, $G\alpha_{i1,2\&3}$, $G\alpha_o$, $G\alpha_z$, and $G\alpha_g$; 3) $G\alpha_q$, $G\alpha_{11}$, $G\alpha_{14}$, and $G\alpha_{15/16}$; and 4) $G\alpha_{12}$ and $G\alpha_{13}$. Further structural and, in some cases, functional diversity results from formation of alternative splice variants in the case of $G\alpha_s$ (four splice variants; two major expressed proteins of 52 and 45 kDa) and $G\alpha_o$ (two splice variants and expressed proteins of ~39 kDa) (Birnbaumer et al. 1990; Helper and Gilman 1992; Simon et al. 1991). Other $G\alpha_s$ alternative splice transcripts have been identified by polymerase chain reaction (PCR)–based cloning, although mature α_s proteins have not been found for these transcripts (Crawford et al. 1993; Habecker et al. 1993; Ishikawa et al. 1990; Swaroop et al. 1991). All Gαsubunits show structural homology in terms of guanine nucleotide binding and guanosine triphosphate (GTP) hydrolysis sites and, within classes, receptor and effector recognition sites (Simon et al. 1991). Certain $G\alpha_s$ subunits are myristoylated (e.g., $G\alpha_o$ and $G\alpha_i$) or palmitoylated (e.g., $G\alpha_s$ and $G\alpha_q$), modifications that are critical for membrane attachment, high-affinity interaction with the βγ complex, and effector interaction (Wedegaertner et al. 1995).

The $G\alpha_s$ subunit binds guanine nucleotides with high affinity and specificity and hydrolyzes GTP to guanosine diphosphate (GDP). GTP hydrolysis, receptor interaction, and subunit dissociation are the key events thought to allow G proteins to alternate between inactive and active states. The α_s and $\beta\gamma$-subunits couple a large family of heptahelical receptors to an array of effectors, including adenylyl cyclase (AC), phospholipase C (PLC)-β, phospholipase A_2, mitogen-activated protein kinase, and ion channels (Clapham and Neer 1993; Helper and Gilman 1992; Inglese et al. 1995; Wickman and Clapham 1995). In addition, the $\beta\gamma$-complex maintains $G\alpha_s$ subunits in an inactive state by suppressing GDP dissociation, provides anchorage for $G\alpha_s$ subunits, promotes high-affinity coupling between holo–G protein and receptor, and stimulates phosphorylation of agonist-bound receptors during homologous desensitization (Clapham and Neer 1993).

G-protein regulation of AC activity is now recognized to be quite complex, involving $G\alpha_s$, $G\alpha_i$, and $\beta\gamma$-subunits, as well as cross-talk regulation by calcium and protein kinase C (PKC), and differs for specific AC subtypes (types I–IX) (Iyengar 1993; Sunahara et al. 1996). Reconstitution experiments with purified recombinant proteins have shown that activated $G\alpha_s$ interacts directly with AC isoforms to stimulate cyclic adenosine monophosphate (cAMP) formation. $G\alpha_s$-stimulated AC (types II and IV, calcium-calmodulin [Ca^{2+}-CaM] insensitive) activity can be conditionally augmented by $\beta\gamma$-subunits released from holo-G_i (or possibly other holo–G proteins). AC (types II and VII) activity also can be stimulated through phosphorylation by PKC (Iyengar 1993). The interaction of $G\alpha_i$- and $\beta\gamma$-subunits with specific isoforms of AC inhibits AC activity: the inhibitory effects of $G\alpha_i$ are AC-isoform and activator dependent (Sunahara et al. 1996). The inhibitory effect of $\beta\gamma$-subunits appears specific to type I (Ca^{2+}-CaM activated) AC (Iyengar 1993). $G\alpha_{olf}$ is expressed abundantly in olfactory epithelium, where it couples to AC type III (Menco et al. 1992), and in striatum and nucleus accumbens (Drinnan et al. 1991, Herve et al. 1993), where it appears to couple to other specific AC subtypes (e.g., AC type V).

Another major second-messenger system regulated by G proteins involves receptor-linked activation of PLC. Of the three major families of PLC (β, γ, and δ), the β-isozymes are regulated by either pertussis-toxin–sensitive or –insensitive mechanisms. The former is mediated through $\beta\gamma$-subunits (Sternweis and Smrcka 1992), whereas the $G\alpha$ members of the $G_{q/11}$ subfamily mediate the pertussis-toxin–insensitive stimulation of PLC-β (Rhee and Choi 1992).

Compelling evidence indicates that protein and messenger RNA (mRNA) transcript levels of $G\alpha$ subunits can be regulated by agonists (e.g., hormones and neurotransmitters), drugs, and pathophysiological states (pseudohypoparathyroidism, diabetes, heart failure) (for review, see Milligan and Wakelam 1992). Long-term sensitization and desensitization of heptahelical receptors are accompanied by changes in components of receptor-effector response pathways, including the Gα subunits with which the receptors normally interact (Milligan 1993). Also, cross-regulation between opposing receptor-effector systems, such as the stimulatory and inhibitory pathways regulating AC activity, is extensive (Hadcock and Malbon 1993). This provides a mechanism at the G-protein level to compensate for sustained changes in neurotransmitter release and receptor activation, in addition to the rapid sensitivity changes induced by receptor-effector protein phosphorylation. Agonist regulation of G-protein levels is mediated by alterations in gene transcription or mRNA stability, both of which affect steady-state mRNA levels (Hadcock and Malbon 1993). In addition, posttranslational mechanisms (e.g., adenosine 5′ -diphosphate [ADP] ribosylation) may regulate cellular G-protein levels (Milligan 1993). Thus, Gα subunit levels are regulated in a highly coordinated manner in response to agonist stimulation, and these orchestrated changes play a critical role in physiological regulation of receptor sensitivity.

POSTRECEPTOR SIGNAL TRANSDUCTION DISTURBANCES IN BIPOLAR DISORDER

The principal lines of evidence implicating postreceptor signal transduction disturbances in affective disorders are summarized in Table 13–1. Studies of norepinephrine- and isoproterenol-stimulated AC activity in MNLs from patients with affective disorders (reviewed in Warsh et al. 1988; Werstiuk et al. 1990) constitute one of the earliest lines of evidence implicating transmembrane signaling disturbances in mood disorders. MNLs contain β_2-adrenoceptors (Williams et al. 1976) coupled to AC through G_s, providing a readily accessible analogous cellular model for clinical studies. The observations of blunted noradrenergic agonist-stimulated AC responses in MNLs from depressed subjects first suggested that disturbances in the β_2-adrenoceptor–effector-coupled response in mood disorders may occur, but the abnormalities were initially ascribed to the noradrenergic receptor protein itself because this was central to the conceptualization of the psychobiological basis of mood disorders at that time. However, when taken together with the observations of blunted GTP analogue and forskolin (colforsin) stimulation of

Table 13–1. Evidence for signal transduction disturbances in affective disorders

Clinical studies
Decreased mononuclear leukocyte basal, adrenergic agonist- and forskolin-stimulated adenylyl cyclase activity occurs in depressed subjects.
Postreceptor (forskolin and NaF) and receptor-stimulated (prostaglandin E_1) adenylyl cyclase activity is decreased in platelets and mononuclear leukocytes from depressed patients.
Resting intracellular calcium concentrations are increased in platelets and lymphocytes in bipolar disorder.
Animal and cell models
Antidepressants and electroconvulsive shock (ECS) increase coupling between G-protein α-subunit $G\alpha_s$ and adenylyl cyclase in rat brain.
Lithium, carbamazepine, and ECS reduce noradrenergic- and muscarinic-agonist-stimulated guanosine triphosphate (GTP) binding in rat cerebral cortical membranes.
Lithium decreases the levels of messenger RNA encoding $G\alpha_s$, $G\alpha_{i1}$, and $G\alpha_{i2}$ subunits.
Lithium alters the cellular disposition and abundance of protein kinase C isoforms in rat brain and cultured cell lines.
Antidepressants modify $G\alpha_s$ immunoreactivities in selective rat brain regions.

AC activity in platelets and lymphocytes from patients with affective disorders, these findings suggested that, at least to some extent, altered receptor responses in mood disorders involved postreceptor mechanisms.

The findings of Schreiber and co-workers (1991) provided more important evidence that altered MNL receptor-effector responses, at least in BD, may involve disturbances at the level of the G protein. They reported increased agonist-stimulated [^{3}H]-5′-guanylylimidodiphosphate [Gpp(NH)p] binding in MNL membranes from untreated manic patients compared with control subjects, whereas this measure in lithium-treated euthymic BD patients was not different from control subjects. Along with the earlier report by these authors that administration of lithium and other mood stabilizers to rats reduced agonist-stimulated [^{3}H]-GTP binding in cerebral cortical membranes (Avissar et al. 1988, 1990), these observations point to the G proteins to which GTP binds as important postreceptor candidates contributing to the signaling abnormalities in BD.

POSTRECEPTOR PHARMACOLOGICAL EFFECTS OF MOOD STABILIZERS AND ANTIDEPRESSANTS

Results of studies on the molecular mechanisms of action of mood-stabilizing and antidepressant agents have provided a particularly important, although indirect, body of evidence to support the notion that postreceptor signaling disturbances occur in BD (Hudson et al. 1993; Jope and Williams 1994; Manji 1992). Substantial evidence now indicates that therapeutically relevant concentrations of lithium act at multiple sites in signal transduction and second-messenger systems (Manji et al. 1995b; see also Manji et al., Jope et al., and Lenox et al., Chapters 7, 8, and 9 in this volume, respectively). With respect to transmembrane G-protein–mediated signaling, lithium generally attenuates G_s-, G_i-, and $G_{q/11}$-mediated effector responses (Jope and Williams 1994; Manji et al. 1995b; Mork et al. 1992). The specific mechanisms by which lithium induces these effects, however, are less clear. On the one hand, evidence indicates that lithium has direct effects on G proteins (G_s and G_i) by displacing Mg^{2+} from its binding site on the α_s (Avissar et al. 1991). On the other hand, studies have reported indirect modifications of G proteins mediated through processes such as ADP ribosylation (Nestler et al. 1995) and possibly even transcriptional regulation and expression of genes encoding $G\alpha_s$ and $G\alpha_i$ (Colin et al. 1991; Lesch et al. 1991; Li et al. 1991, 1993b).

Lithium also may affect G-protein function through cross-talk regulation resulting from actions at more distal loci in signal transduction chains (Manji 1992; Manji et al. 1995b). Among several postreceptor actions, lithium alters PKC levels (Li et al. 1993a; Manji et al. 1995b) and affects the degree of rat brain protein phosphorylation (Casebolt and Jope 1991; Lenox et al. 1992; Vatal and Aiyar 1984) and Ca^{2+} flux in rat forebrain synaptosomes (Koenig and Jope 1988). Abundant evidence supports a complex array of receptor cross-talk regulation mediated through PKC, Ca^{2+}, and cAMP-dependent protein kinase A (PKA) (Asaoka et al. 1991; Hill and Kendall 1989; Port and Malbon 1993). In this regard, phosphorylation of both α_i and α_s by PKC (Pyne et al. 1992; Strassheim and Malbon 1994) may represent an important cross-talk mechanism (Asaoka et al. 1991) regulating the function of these G proteins and consequently signal integration and modulation through multiple diverse receptor-effector units.

POSTMORTEM BRAIN STRATEGY

Findings from clinical studies of peripheral blood cells and investigations of chronic mood-stabilizer treatment discussed earlier in this chapter provided the heuristic framework for the general hypothesis that disturbances in transmembrane signal transduction at the level of G_s and/or G_i are central to the pathophysiology of BD, but, until recently, little direct evidence supported this notion. In vivo neuroimaging techniques are not yet able to measure postreceptor mechanisms in brain. Accordingly, we decided to use an alternative strategy of examining the state of G-protein–mediated signal transduction systems in postmortem brain from BD subjects to test the signal transduction disturbance hypothesis. First, we posited that the disturbances might involve changes in G-protein abundance, structure, or factors regulating receptor–G protein–effector interactions. Alterations in abundance may result from abnormalities in the coordinated expression and/or turnover of G-protein subunits, effectors, and polypeptide regulators (e.g., phosducin, regulators of G-protein signaling [RGS] proteins) of these transducing proteins.

Autopsied brains were obtained from various brain banks (Canadian Brain Tissue Bank, Montreal Brain Bank, Boston Brain Bank, National Neurological Tissue Bank), and medical records were reviewed to retrospectively establish DSM-III-R (American Psychiatric Association 1987) criteria for the diagnosis of BD. The presence of concurrent medical illnesses, alcohol and drug abuse, and history of antemortem psychotropic and nonpsychotropic drug administration was determined by available medical records. The absence of neurological disorder was confirmed by neuropathological examination and chart review. BD subjects were compared with a control group matched as closely as possible on age and postmortem delay (the time from death until freezing of brain tissue). Control subjects had no neurological or psychiatric disorder, which was confirmed by chart review and neuropathology.

Details of these subjects have been reported previously (Young et al. 1993). Seven of 10 patients had symptoms that met full criteria for BD, and in 3 patients, all criteria, including major depressive episodes, were met, but the length of manic episodes could not be established with certainty because of incomplete records. In 1 patient, the differential diagnosis of schizoaffective disorder could not be ruled out, and in another patient the diagnosis of BD type II could not be excluded with certainty. Subject groups did not differ in mean age. Postmortem delay was less than 24 hours in all patients except 2 (33 and 39 hours) and was not different between BD and comparison subjects. Brain pH, which was measured as a parameter of agonal status (Butterworth and Tennant 1989), was not different between patient and control groups.

G-Protein Immunolabeling Studies in Bipolar Disorder

Established immunoblotting procedures were used to assay G-protein subunits from brain regions in crude membrane preparations, as previously described (Young et al. 1993). Figure 13–1 depicts a composite of the immuno-

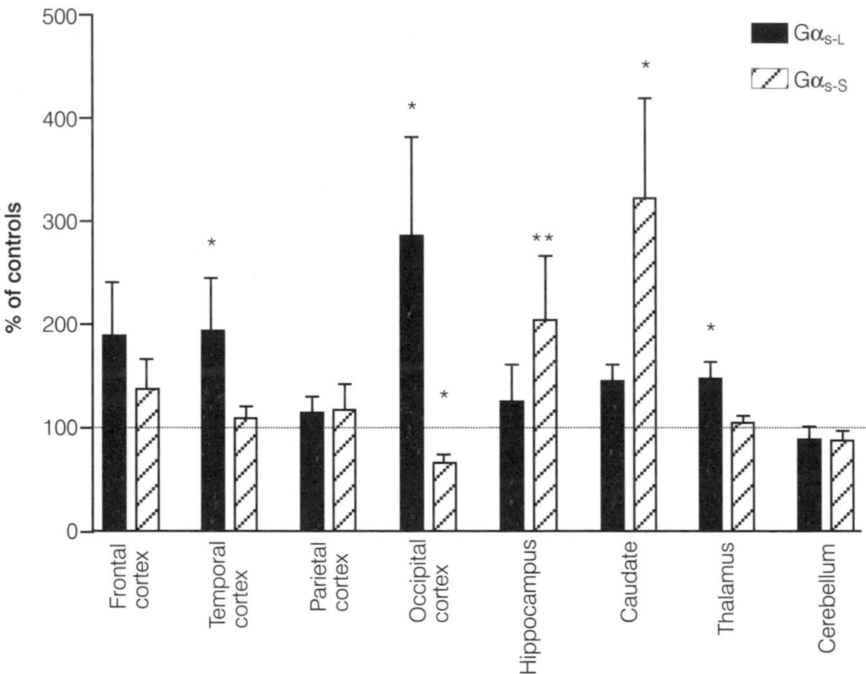

Figure 13–1. Immunolabeling of the long (52 kDa, $G\alpha_{s\text{-}L}$) and short (45 kDa, $G\alpha_{s\text{-}s}$) isoforms of $G\alpha_s$ in postmortem brain regions of individuals with bipolar disorder. $G\alpha_s$ isoforms were quantified as described in Young et al. (1993) after resolution on 12.5% polyacrylamide gels to separate $G\alpha_{s\text{-}s}$ from $G\alpha_{olf}$ (46 kDa). The data are expressed as a percentage of the respective paired control for 5 to 10 subjects. *$P < 0.05$ and **$0.05 < P < 0.1$ (paired t test), compared with matched control subjects.

assay results obtained to date on $G\alpha_s$ in BD and control brain regions. Compared with results in matched control subjects, $G\alpha_s$ (52-kDa species) immunoreactivity was higher in frontal, temporal, and occipital cortex and moderately elevated in thalamus in subjects with BD. Levels of the short form of $G\alpha_s$ (45 kDa) were also higher in BD than in control subjects in the hippocampus and caudate but were significantly reduced in occipital cortex. Although these observations suggest that the changes in immunoreactive $G\alpha_s$ levels may occur more diffusely throughout the brain in this illness than previously thought (Young et al. 1993), the lack of changes in $G\alpha_s$ levels in the parietal cortex and cerebellum is not consistent with this notion. In those brain regions showing altered $G\alpha_s$ immunolabeling, the $G\alpha_{s\text{-}L}$ and $G\alpha_{s\text{-}S}$ isoforms were differentially affected; that is, immunolabeling of either $G\alpha_{s\text{-}L}$ or $G\alpha_{s\text{-}S}$, but not both, was higher in BD compared with control subjects. This finding may reflect differential regulation of alternatively spliced $G\alpha_s$ subunit mRNA transcripts in affected BD brain regions, leading to an abundance of one isoform relative to the other. Also, factors affecting the turnover of these $G\alpha_s$ isoforms may account for the differential changes. Because the two $G\alpha_s$ species may have different coupling efficiencies to AC (Walseth et al. 1990) and receptors (Seifert et al. 1998), regulation of the differential expression of the two $G\alpha_s$ isoforms may be functionally significant with respect to the efficiency of the receptor-effector coupling.

An important issue that has surfaced recently is whether the expression of $G\alpha_{olf}$ is altered in BD. Berrettini et al. (1994) reported positive logarithm of odds (LOD) scores in three BD pedigrees by using microsatellite markers to the 18p11 region, a region to which $G\alpha_{olf}$ is mapped. $G\alpha_{olf}$ is expressed abundantly in the striatum, nucleus accumbens, olfactory epithelium, and olfactory bulb (Drinnan et al. 1991; Herve et al. 1993). Of additional interest, Herve and colleagues (1993) found low-level expression of $G\alpha_{olf}$ transcripts throughout the rat brain, raising the possibility that $G\alpha_{olf}$ may be expressed in other brain regions. $G\alpha_{olf}$ (46 kDa) is not separated from the short form of $G\alpha_s$ (45 kDa) on 10% polyacrylamide gels, as used previously (Young et al. 1993), and the antiserum to $G\alpha_s$ (RM/1) cross-reacts with $G\alpha_{olf}$. Consequently, $G\alpha_{olf}$ would not have been identified with the conditions used in our previous immunoblot assay.

We recently addressed this issue by demonstrating the complete separation of the immunoreactive species corresponding to $G\alpha_{olf}$ from $G\alpha_s$ (45 kDa) on 12.5% polyacrylamide gels, confirmed with $G\alpha_{olf}$ specific antisera (J. J. Warsh, P. P. Li, D. Sibony, S. J. Kish, unpublished data, 1999). We used this separation system with the RM/1 antiserum, which detects both $G\alpha_{olf}$ and $G\alpha_s$ with high sensitivity, to reassay these G-protein subtypes in the BD cerebral cortical regions in which $G\alpha_s$ isoforms were previously quantified. Relative to $G\alpha_s$, $G\alpha_{olf}$ immunolabeling was low in all these cerebral cortical regions, and no differences ($P > 0.1$) were found in $G\alpha_{olf}$ immunolabeling between BD and comparison subjects (frontal cortex: 31 ± 26% [mean ± standard error of the mean, SEM] above control; temporal cortex: 34 ± 28%), with the exception of a modest elevation in occipital cortex (54 ± 28%, paired t test = 2.8, $df = 6$, $P < 0.05$), whereas the differences in $G\alpha_s$ immunolabeling were essentially as reported previously (Young et al. 1993). These findings argue against a contribution from aberrant expression of $G\alpha_{olf}$ to the observed differences in $G\alpha_s$ immunolabeling in BD.

In contrast to the changes observed for $G\alpha_s$, no statistically significant differences were identified in $G\alpha_o$, $G\beta_{35}$, or $G\beta_{36}$ immunoreactivities between BD and comparison subjects. In a previous report in which we measured $G\alpha_i$ immunoreactivity with an antibody that did not distinguish individual $G\alpha_i$ subtypes, we noted a trend toward higher immunolabeling across cerebral cortical regions in BD compared with control subjects (Young et al. 1993). Recently, we reassayed these same brain regions by using polyacrylamide gel electrophoresis conditions optimized to separate $G\alpha_{i1}$ from $G\alpha_{i2}$. In this instance, no differences were observed in the levels of $G\alpha_{i1}$ or $G\alpha_{i2}$ between BD and comparison subjects (Table 13–2), thus ruling out any associated changes in $G\alpha_i$ levels as speculated previously (Young et al. 1993).

In comparison, $G\alpha_{q/11}$ levels were significantly elevated in the occipital cortex of BD compared with control subjects, but no statistically significant differences were observed in the frontal or temporal cortex (Figure 13–2). Interestingly, PLC-β_1 immunolabeling also showed a similar increase confined

Table 13–2. $G\alpha_{i1}$ and $G\alpha_{i2}$ immunoreactivity levels in cerebral cortical regions of bipolar disorder and control subjects

Region	Bipolar disorder	Control
$G\alpha_{i1}$		
Frontal cortex	3.18 ± 0.39	3.06 ± 0.69
Occipital cortex	3.38 ± 0.42	2.89 ± 0.48
Hippocampus	3.29 ± 0.43	2.07 ± 0.70
$G\alpha_{i2}$		
Frontal cortex	11.6 ± 0.71	11.8 ± 1.46
Occipital cortex	7.98 ± 0.78	7.69 ± 0.93
Hippocampus	13.4 ± 1.18	12.2 ± 1.56

Note. Data are expressed as the means ± SEM fmol/mg protein; $N = 8–10$ subjects per group.

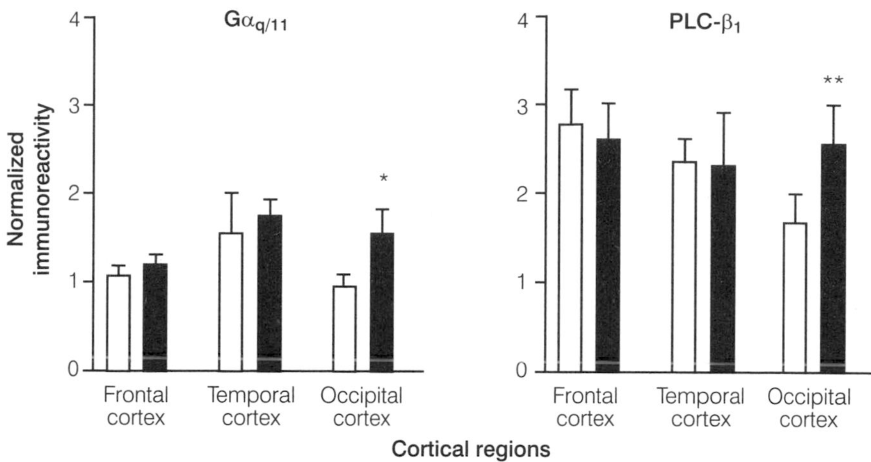

Figure 13–2. $G\alpha_{q/11}$ and phospholipase C (PLC)-β_1 immunolabeling in cerebral cortical regions of subjects with bipolar disorder compared with matched control subjects. The bars represent the means ± SEM for 5–10 subjects. Black bars = bipolar subjects; white bars = control subjects.
*$P < 0.05$ and **$0.05 < P < 0.1$ (paired *t* test), compared with matched control subjects.
Source. Modified by permission of Elsevier Science, Inc., from Mathews R, Li PP, Young LT, et al.: "Increased $G\alpha_{q/11}$ Immunoreactivity in Postmortem Occipital Cortex From Patients With Bipolar Affective Disorder." *Biological Psychiatry* 41: 649–656, 1997. Copyright 1997 by The Society of Biological Psychiatry.

to the occipital cortex in BD subjects, although this was only marginally statistically significant ($P = 0.07$). Furthermore, $G\alpha_{q/11}$ immunolabeling expressed as a percentage of matched control was significantly correlated ($r = 0.78$, $df = 8$, $P = 0.02$) with PLC-β_1 values in occipital but not temporal ($r = -0.47$, $df = 7$, $P > 0.1$) or frontal ($r = -0.62$, $df = 10$, $P > 0.05$) cortex (Mathews et al. 1997).

Because no differences in postmortem delay or age were found between BD patients and control subjects, and no patient had a coexistent neurodegenerative disease, the observed increased $G\alpha_s$ and $G\alpha_{q/11}$ levels in BD were not likely caused by age-related changes or neuronal cell death. Moreover, G-protein immunoreactivities were stable with respect to these variables (Cowburn et al. 1991; Mathews et al. 1997; Young et al. 1991), and brain pH, an index of agonal state (Butterworth and Tennant 1989), was similar between the two groups. The extent to which psychotropic medications, particularly lithium, contributed to the observed elevations in $G\alpha_s$ and $G\alpha_{q/11}$ immunoreactivities is uncertain. Six of the 10 BD subjects studied had no recent history of lithium intake based on available medical records, but temporal cortex lithium concentrations measured recently with a high-sensitivity assay based on inductively coupled argon plasma emission spectrometry revealed that 9 of the 10 subjects had detectable levels of lithium, although all were subtherapeutic, and in at least two cases were only trace levels at best (Rahman et al. 1997). By itself, the detection of lithium in brain samples from BD subjects is not sufficient evidence, however, to attribute the altered G-protein levels in BD cerebral cortex to the presence or history of administration of lithium. Indeed, no changes were found in the cerebral cortical levels of $G\alpha_s$ and $G\alpha_{q/11}$ in rats treated chronically with lithium or antidepressant drugs (Chen and Rasenick 1995; Emamghoreishi et al. 1996; Li et al. 1993a, 1993b). However, possible effects of other psychotropic (and nonpsychotropic) medications taken antemortem cannot be completely ruled out at present.

G-Protein Function in Bipolar Disorder

Initial attempts to determine the functional correlates of the elevated $G\alpha_s$ levels identified only associated statistically significant increases in forskolin- but not GTPγS-stimulated AC activity in occipital and temporal cortical regions in BD, although there was a trend toward elevated GTPγS-stimulated cAMP production in these areas (Young et al. 1993). No significant differences were apparent in basal AC activity. A significant correlation was observed between forskolin-stimulated cAMP formation and $G\alpha_{s\text{-}L}$ immunoreactivity when examined across these cortical regions. Tentative explanations for these observations have been discussed elsewhere (Young et al. 1993) and include the possibility that the enhanced forskolin-stimulated cAMP formation might reflect changes in activity of specific Ca^{2+}-CaM–insensitive AC (types II and IV) and/or increased concentrations of specific AC isotypes. The latter might be related to lithium treatment, which has been shown to increase the levels of rat brain AC, types I and II (Colin et al. 1991), and human platelet AC activity (Manji et al. 1995b), or to coregulated increases in AC with $G\alpha_s$ in this disorder.

The functional activity of $G\alpha_{q/11}$ in BD has been assessed recently by measuring the hydrolysis of [^{3}H]phosphatidylinositol in response to GTPγS (Jope et al. 1996; see also Jope et al., Chapter 8, in this volume). These authors found that the functional activity of $G\alpha_{q/11}$ is decreased selectively in the occipital cortex but not in the frontal and temporal cortex. This observation, and the regional specific increase in $G\alpha_{q/11}$ levels in BD (Mathews et al. 1997), raises an interesting possibility that compensatory changes (enhanced synthesis and/or stability) in $G\alpha_{q/11}$ occur consequent to a functional impairment in $G\alpha_{q/11}$ activity.

We have also shown that brain norepinephrine turnover is elevated in cerebral cortical, but not subcortical, regions of these same BD postmortem brains (Young et al. 1994c). These findings clearly suggest that the putative G-protein–mediated signal transduction disturbances in BD are linked to altered noradrenergic function in the brain implicated in a plethora of psychobiological studies of BD. Interestingly, β-adrenoceptor densities were not altered in BD cortex compared with control cortex (Young et al. 1994b), a finding reminiscent of the lack of downregulation in β-adrenoceptor density and blunted isoproterenol-stimulated AC responses in MNLs in depressed patients (Halper et al. 1988). This lack of change in receptor density in the face of altered G protein–effector responsivity suggests that coordinated regulation of receptor and G proteins (Hadcock and Malbon 1993; Milligan 1993) may be altered in BD.

Diagnostic Specificity

The specificity of the $G\alpha_s$ changes to BD is an important issue that has been directly assessed in only one study to date, although the results of an increasing number of G-protein studies of other neuropsychiatric disorders are clearly relevant to this issue. Young et al. (1993) found no significant differences in $G\alpha_s$ immunolabeling measured in the postmortem temporal cortex of schizophrenic and Alzheimer's disease subjects compared with control subjects, thus supporting the specificity of elevated $G\alpha_s$ levels to BD, at least for this brain region.

Measurement of G-protein immunolabeling and function in postmortem brain from subjects with histories or diagnoses of substance abuse and dependence (Escriba et al. 1994; Jope et al. 1998; Ozawa et al. 1993b), depression (Cowburn et al. 1994; Ozawa et al. 1993a), suicide (Cowburn et al. 1994; Pacheco et al. 1996), schizophrenia (Jope et al. 1998; Nishino et al. 1993; Okada et al. 1991, 1994; O'Neill et al. 1994; Yang et al. 1998), and Alzheimer's disease (Cowburn et al. 1992a, 1992b, 1993; McLaughlin et al. 1991; Ohm et al. 1991; Ross et al. 1993) (Table 13–3) lends further credence to the latter conclusion. With the exception of findings of a nonsignificant elevation in $G\alpha_s$ immunolabeling in the frontal cortex of depressed subjects who committed suicide (Cowburn et al. 1994), $G\alpha_s$ immunoreactivity levels were not elevated in any of the disorders studied.

The pattern of altered $G\alpha_s$ immunolabeling in the cerebral cortex in BD is not completely consistent with the bulk of evidence from both postmortem and in vivo brain imaging studies, which suggests abnormalities in receptor function and cerebral metabolism in the temporal and possibly frontal cortex

Table 13–3. Postmortem brain guanine nucleotide binding protein (G-protein) alterations in neuropsychiatric disorders

Disorder	G-protein immunolabeling	G-protein functionality	Reference
Alcohol dependence	↓ $G\alpha_{s\text{-}L}$ in temporal but not parietal cortex; unaltered $G\alpha_i$, $G\alpha_{q/11}$, $G\alpha_o$, or $G\beta$	↓ AAGTP binding to G_s and G_i in temporal and parietal cortex	Ozawa et al. 1993a
	↓ $G\alpha_{i1}$ in and $G\alpha_o$ but not $G\alpha_{s\text{-}L}$, $G\alpha_{s\text{-}S}$, $G\alpha_{i2}$, and $G\alpha_{q/11}$ in frontal cortex		Jope et al. 1998
Bipolar disorder	↑ $G\alpha_{s\text{-}L}$ in frontal, temporal, and occipital but not parietal cortex	↑ Forskolin-stimulated AC (trend for ↑ GTPγS-stimulated AC) in temporal and occipital cortex	Young et al. 1993
	↑ $G\alpha_{s\text{-}S}$ in caudate, ±↑ in hippocampus, ±↓in occipital cortex	↓ GTPγS-stimulated [^{3}H]PI hydrolysis in occipital cortex	Jope et al. 1996
	↑ $G\alpha_{q/11}$ in occipital cortex; no change in $G\alpha_{i1/2}$, $G\alpha_o$, or $G\beta$		Mattews et al. 1997
	↑ $G\alpha_{s\text{-}L}$ and $G\alpha_{s\text{-}S}$, but not $G\alpha_i$, $G\alpha_{q/11}$, $G\alpha_o$, $G\alpha_z$, or $G\beta$ in frontal cortex	↑ Receptor agonist-activated GTPγS binding to Gα proteins	Freidman and Wang 1996
Depression	No difference in $G\alpha_{s\text{-}L}$, $G\alpha_{s\text{-}S}$, $G\alpha_i$, $G\alpha_{q/11}$, $G\alpha_o$, or $G\beta$ in temporal and parietal cortex	↑ AAGTP binding to $G\alpha_s$ and $G\alpha_{i/o}$ in temporal and parietal cortex	Ozawa et al. 1993b
Opiate abuse/dependence	Small but significant ↑ in $G\alpha_{s\text{-}L}$, $G\alpha_{i1/2}$, $G\alpha_o$, and $G\beta$ in frontal cortex	—	Escriba et al. 1994
Suicide (violent death, depression)[a]	Nonsignificant ↑ in $G\alpha_{s\text{-}S}$ levels; no difference in $G\alpha_{s\text{-}L}$ or $G\alpha_i$ in frontal cortex	↓ Basal, GTPγS, and forskolin-stimulated AC	Cowburn et al. 1994
	↑ $G\alpha_{s\text{-}S}$ and ↓$G\alpha_{i2}$ but not $G\alpha_{s\text{-}L}$, $G\alpha_{q/11}$, $G\alpha_{i1}$, or $G\alpha_o$ in frontal cortex	↓ GTPγS-stimulated [^{3}H]PI hydrolysis in frontal cortex	Pacheco et al. 1996

Schizophrenia	↓ ADP ribosylated $G\alpha_{i/o}$ in left hippocampus	—	Okada et al. 1991
	↓ $G\alpha_i$, $G\alpha_{q/11}$, and $G\alpha_o$ but not $G\alpha_{s\text{-}L}$, $G\alpha_{s\text{-}S}$, and Gβ in left temporal cortex	—	Nishino et al. 1993
	↓ $G\alpha_o$ but not $G\alpha_i$ in right hippocampus and head of the caudate; no differences in other cortical regions	—	Okada et al. 1994
	↑ $G\alpha_o$ but not $G\alpha_{s\text{-}L}$, $G\alpha_{s\text{-}S}$, $G\alpha_{i1/2}$, and $G\alpha_{q/11}$ in frontal cortex	↓ GTPγS-stimulated [^{3}H]PI hydrolysis in frontal cortex	Jope et al. 1998
	↓ $G\alpha_i$ and $G\alpha_o$ but not $G\alpha_{s\text{-}L}$, $G\alpha_{s\text{-}S}$, $G\alpha_{q/11}$, and Gβ in left nucleus accumbens and amygdala		Yang et al. 1998
Alzheimer's disease	↓ Temporal cortex $G\alpha_{i1}$, no change in $G\alpha_{s\text{-}L}$, $G\alpha_{s\text{-}S}$, $G\alpha_o$, or Gβ in frontal cortex, hippocampus, or cerebellum; no differences in levels of the above α-subunits or $G\alpha_{q/11}$ in frontal cortex, hippocampus, and/or angular gyrus	± ↓ Basal and ↓ stimulated (isoprenaline, Gpp(NH)p, GTPγS, AlF_4) AC in hippocampus, frontal and temporal cortex, and/or cerebellum; ↓ high-affinity GTPase activity in frontal cortex and hippocampus; ↓ β_1 AR–G-protein coupling in temporal cortex; ↓ GTPγS and carbachol-stimulated [^{3}H]PI hydrolysis	Ohm et al. 1991; McLaughlin et al. 1991; Cowburn et al. 1992a, 1992b, 1993; Ross et al. 1993; Jope et al. 1994; O'Neill et al. 1994

Note. Empty cells indicate that the investigators cited did not do immunolabeling or functional measures (whichever column is blank).
AAGTP = azidoanilido guanosine triphosphate; AC = adenylyl cyclase; GTP = guanosine triphosphate; NaF = sodium fluoride;
PI = phosphatidylinositol; ADP = 5′-diphosphate; Gpp(NH)p = [^{3}H]-5′-guanylylimidodiphosphate; AR = adrenoceptor.
[a]Effects were most apparent in those who had committed suicide 1) who died by violent means or 2) who had had a history of depression.

of patients with affective disorders, including BD (Baxter et al. 1989; Gross-Isseroff et al. 1991; Jeste et al. 1988; Korpi et al. 1986; McKeith et al. 1987; Owen et al. 1986; Stanley and Mann 1983). Furthermore, the basis for the regionally selective differences in $G\alpha_{q/11}$ levels in BD brain is also somewhat enigmatic. Differences in $G\alpha_s$ levels between BD and control subjects were also evident in occipital cortex as was the forskolin-activated AC response (Young et al. 1993). However, a broader, and possibly lateralized-cortical (e.g., right frontotemporal or left parieto-occipital in maniclike symptoms, left frontotemporal and right parieto-occipital in depression) and caudate involvement has also been implicated in this disorder (Goodwin and Jamison 1990; Guze and Gitlin 1994). Thus, it is conceivable that disturbances in important functional connections in which the occipital region plays an integral role may form part of the neuoroanatomical basis for BD. Given the substantial evidence for cross-talk between cAMP- and phosphoinositide-signaling systems in the regulation of cellular functions (Hill and Kendall 1989; Port and Malbon 1993), the observed differences in occipital cortical $G\alpha_{q/11}$ levels may also reflect the consequences of relatively greater disturbances in signaling through the cAMP transduction pathway in this brain region in BD. Unfortunately, the limited availability of postmortem brain from BD subjects precluded our selecting cortical regions from the same hemispheres for analysis. This absence of control over laterality of sampling (i.e., left vs. right hemispheres) may have obscured important patterns of regional differences in biochemical measures that might otherwise have been elucidated. An interesting alternative theory is that the regionally selective changes in biochemical parameters within the phosphoinositide- and cAMP-signaling systems may reflect disease-related changes in the occipital cortex that persist despite lithium treatment, unlike other cerebral cortical regions in which $G\alpha_{q/11}$ levels normalized with treatment (Jope et al. 1996). These preliminary findings, however, clearly raise important questions about the extent and regional selectivity of the signal transduction disturbances occurring in the BD brain.

Downstream Signaling Targets Alteration in Bipolar Disorder

Another unanswered question that is directly pertinent to the hypothesis of G-protein hyperfunctionality in BD is, what is the nature of the changes in second-messenger signaling that actually occur in association with or consequent to the G-protein disturbances? More simply, is there evidence that the G-protein changes (abundance and/or function) in the BD brain are, indeed, associated with enhanced cAMP signaling in neurons, or are there protective cellular processes that compensate for or adapt to the former, thereby attenuating or "normalizing" the signaling disturbances? Unfortunately, this question cannot be addressed directly in postmortem tissue because brain cAMP levels change exceedingly rapidly postmortem, which confounds the use of such measurements to assess the state of cAMP signaling in brain (Jones and Stavinoha 1979). Alternatively, we reasoned that it may be possible to determine the state of cAMP signaling that existed antemortem by examining an important downstream target protein on which cAMP acts, that of PKA.

PKA is a tetrameric protein composed of a dimeric regulatory (R) and two monomeric catalytic (C) subunits, both of which exist in multiple isoforms (Francis and Corbin 1994). Each R subunit has two cAMP binding sites that show positive cooperativity in cAMP binding and activation. Upon binding of cAMP to each R subunit, the inactive holoenzyme dissociates into a dimeric R-subunit complex and two monomeric active C subunits (Spaulding 1993). Studies suggest that sustained elevations in intracellular cAMP levels not only modulate catalytic activity but also cause adaptive changes in the levels of PKA R subunits (for reviews, see Francis and Corbin 1994; Spaulding 1993). Measurement of R-subunit levels in membrane and/or cytosolic fractions from postmortem BD brain samples, estimated by [^{3}H]cAMP binding, might therefore reflect the effect of direct or indirect changes in response to altered cAMP signaling posited to occur in this disorder.

We measured [^{3}H]cAMP binding in cytosolic and membrane fractions from postmortem cerebral cortex, as described by Nishino et al. (1993). In the cytosolic fractions from representative postmortem frontal cerebral cortical samples of control subjects, [^{3}H]cAMP binding was saturable, specific, and best fit by a single-site binding model, with an affinity of 0.73 ± 0.04 nM and a density of 232 ± 7 fmol/mg protein (n = 3), which agrees with previous estimates for human cerebral cortex (Nishino et al. 1993). In a single-point assay, mean specific [^{3}H]cAMP binding was significantly reduced in the cytosolic but not membrane fractions across all regions of BD postmortem brain examined compared with control subjects matched on age and postmortem delay (Rahman et al. 1997). This suggests that PKA R-subunits are decreased in the BD brain, a change that may affect the functional activity of this protein kinase in this disorder because the molar ratio of R- to C-subunits influences this enzyme's activity (Schwechheimer and Hofman 1977). Recent findings of significantly higher basal and maximal stimulated PKA activity and lower apparent activation constant for cAMP in temporal cortex cytosolic fractions from BD brain (Fields et al., in press) support this notion. It remains to be established whether such changes lead to alterations in endogenous cAMP-dependent protein phosphorylation, similar to those recently reported in platelets from euthymic BD patients (Perez et al. 1995). Collectively, the postmortem brain findings clearly suggest that signal transduction disturbances in the BD brain may extend beyond the receptor–G-protein-effector complex in the neuronal membrane to important intracellular proteins regulating a variety of neuronal responses.

CLINICAL ASSESSMENT OF G PROTEINS IN BIPOLAR DISORDER

Although the observations of altered G-protein $G\alpha_s$ immunolabeling and functionality in postmortem BD brain provide compelling evidence for G-protein disturbances in the pathophysiology of BD, the inability to control for the many potential confounding variables that may influence the interpretation of postmortem brain findings highlights the need for additional evidence to support this hypothesis. As discussed earlier in this chapter, observations of altered agonist- and G-protein–stimulated AC activity in platelets and MNLs from depressed patients suggested that disturbances in transmembrane signal transduction processes in mood disorders also may be manifest in these peripheral blood cells. More specific to BD, the finding of increased isoproterenol- and carbachol-stimulated [^{3}H]Gpp(NH)p binding in MNL membranes from manic patients compared with control subjects and recovered BD subjects (Schreiber et al. 1991) supports the view that signal transduction disturbances similar to those implicated in the central nervous system may be coexpressed in such peripheral blood cells in BD. Such observations also underscore the potential utility of such peripheral cell models to assess the diagnostic specificity and mechanisms underlying G-protein changes with research designs that can control for the effects of potential confounding variables. Accordingly, we examined $G\alpha_s$ and $G\alpha_i$ immunolabeling and function in MNLs from medication-free (at least 10 days) depressed patients (Hamilton Depression Scale score of at least 16) meeting Research Diagnostic Criteria for the diagnosis of BD or major depressive disorder and age- and sex-matched healthy comparison subjects (Young et al. 1994a). Details of the subject demographics, clinical research methods, and quantification of immunolabeled $G\alpha_{s\text{-}S}$ have been described previously (Young et al. 1994a).

As shown in Figure 13–3, $G\alpha_s$ immunolabeling was significantly higher (160% above values in matched healthy comparison subjects; $P < 0.01$, one-tailed Wilcoxon signed rank test) in MNL membranes of BD subjects than in those of healthy subjects. Unlike the observations in the BD postmortem cortex, $G\alpha_i$ (mostly $G\alpha_{i2}$) immunolabeling was also significantly elevated in MNL membranes from BD subjects, although to a smaller magnitude (114% above

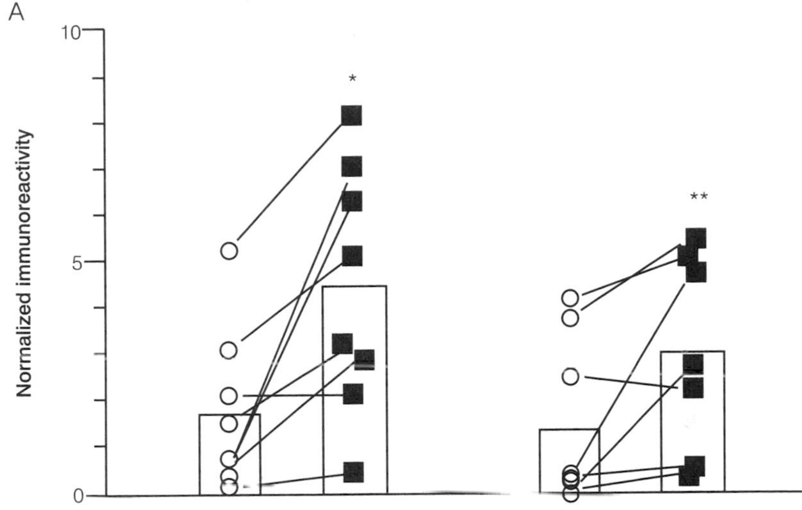

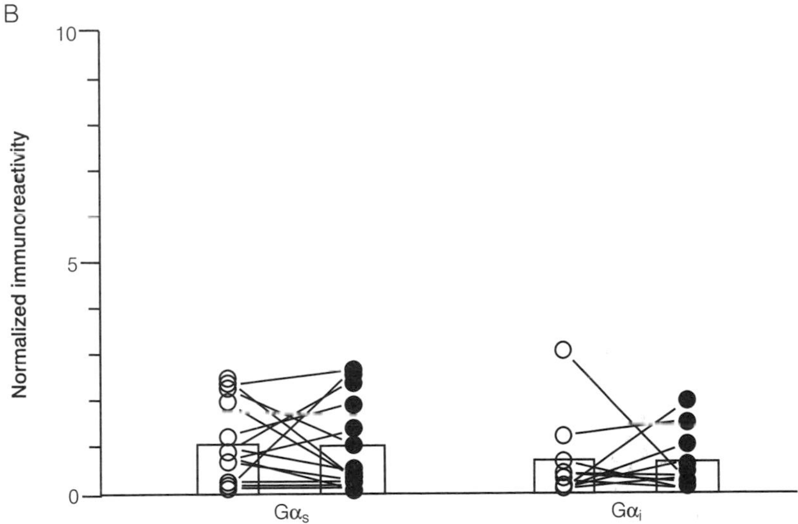

Figure 13–3. Mononuclear leukocyte $G\alpha_s$ and $G\alpha_i$ immunolabeling (normalized against a leukocyte membrane pool) in subjects with bipolar disorder (A, ■, $n = 8$) and major depressive disorder (B, ●, $n = 14$) versus age- and sex-matched psychiatrically healthy subjects (**O**). The open bars indicate the group mean values. $^*P = 0.009$, $^{**}P = 0.02$ (Wilcoxon signed rank test, one-tailed), comparing bipolar disorder patients with psychiatrically healthy subjects.

values in healthy control subjects; $P = 0.017$) than for $G\alpha_s$. In contrast to levels in BD subjects, $G\alpha_s$ and $G\alpha_i$ immunoreactivity levels in major depressive disorder patients were not statistically significantly different from those in healthy control subjects.

G-protein functionality was assessed in a subgroup of these same patients and age- and sex-matched control subjects by determining basal, GTPγS (10 mM)-, sodium fluoride (NaF; 10 mM)-, and forskolin (100 mM)-stimulated AC activity in MNL membranes. In BD subjects, MNL membrane GTPγS- and NaF-stimulated AC activity, expressed as a percentage of basal values, was significantly reduced, whereas forskolin-stimulated AC activity showed a nonsignificant trend toward reduction, and basal AC activity was not different (t test = 0.8, $df = 8$, $P = 0.4$) from that in healthy subjects (Figure 13–4). In comparison, basal MNL membrane AC activity was significantly reduced in major depressive disorder subjects (–26%, t test = 2.7, $df = 8$, $P = 0.027$) compared with matched control subjects, but GTPγS-, NaF-, and forskolin-stimulated activity did not differ (data not shown).

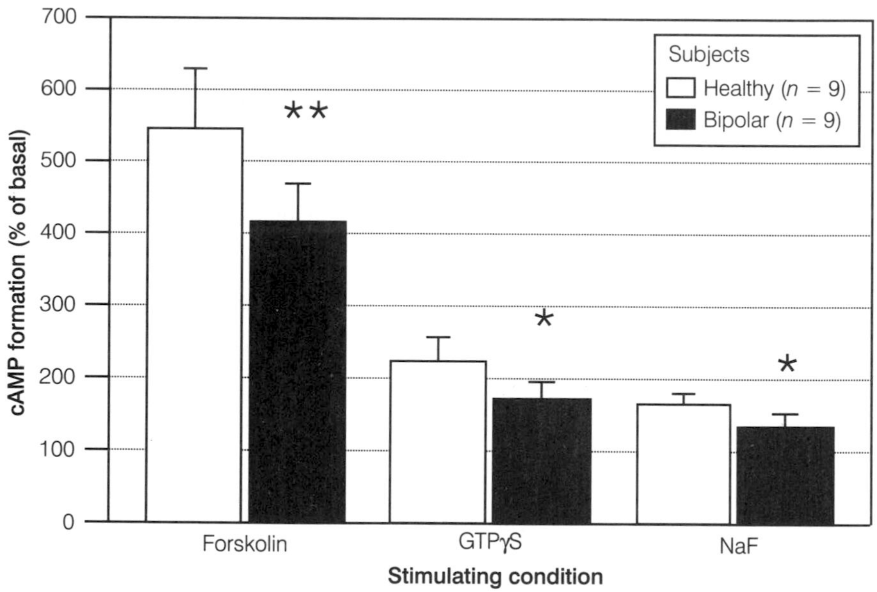

Figure 13–4. Cyclic adenosine monophosphate (cAMP) formation stimulated by forskolin (colforsin) (100 mM), GTPγS (10 mM), and sodium fluoride (NaF; 10 mM) in mononuclear leukocytes from subjects with bipolar disorder ($n = 9$) and age- and sex-matched psychiatrically healthy comparison subjects. *$P < 0.05$ and **$0.05 < P < 0.1$ (paired t test), compared with matched control subjects.

The interpretation of the MNL immunolabeling findings as reflecting G-protein abnormalities coexpressed in parallel with those in the brains of BD subjects was strengthened by the independent findings of Manji et al. (1995a) of higher (although of smaller magnitude) $G\alpha_{s\text{-}S}$ immunolabeling in MNL membranes from a group of both treated and untreated BD patients, compared with control subjects. A similar but nonsignificant trend toward elevated $G\alpha_{s\text{-}S}$ levels was also observed in platelets of BD subjects (Manji et al. 1995a). These authors did not, however, observe increased $G\alpha_i$ immunolabeling, as reported by our group, and $G\alpha_{q/11}$ levels were not altered in untreated BD subjects. The basis for the differences in the magnitude of the elevations in α_s immunolabeling between the two studies as well as for the discrepant findings regarding the presence or absence of changes in MNL membrane $G\alpha_i$ levels in BD may lie in confounding state-dependent effects. Patients in the Young et al. (1994a) study were all in the depressed phase of the illness, unlike those studied by Manji et al. (1995a), who were either manic or euthymic primarily. The observation of a modest correlation of Hamilton Rating Scale for Depression Scale score with MNL α_s ($r = 0.47$, $df = 20$, $P < 0.05$) but not α_i immunolabeling when examined across diagnostic groups (Young et al. 1994a) adds further support to this interpretation.

Of additional interest, the recent report of Avissar et al. (1997a, 1997b) (1995) of state-dependent changes in MNL membrane $G\alpha_s$ and $G\alpha_i$ levels (elevated in mania, decreased in depression) and G-protein function (increased and decreased agonist-stimulated [^{3}H]Gpp(NH)p binding, respectively) also appears to support the theory of confounding effects of state-dependent variables on MNL G-protein measures. However, the discordance between the observations of our group and those of Avissar et al. with regard to the direction of change in $G\alpha_s$ and $G\alpha_i$ levels in relation to affective state indicates a complex explanation for the differences in findings among these groups of investigators. The findings of reduced G-protein–coupled AC activation in MNLs from BD but not from major depressive disorder subjects compared with control subjects further complicate the interpretation of the functional changes and cellular specificity of the signal transduction disturbances attributable to the observed alterations in $G\alpha_s$ abundance. One possible explanation for the differences in immunolabeling and functional measures between brain and MNLs, however, is that compensatory adaptations occur in inhibitory control of AC activity and/or AC levels in MNLs, offsetting the effects of enhanced $G\alpha_s$ levels. The lack of or ineffective compensatory adaptations in cerebral cortical G-protein–mediated AC activation and/or AC levels, therefore, may be relevant to the pathophysiology of bipolar disorder.

MOLECULAR BASIS FOR G-PROTEIN α-SUBUNIT INCREASES IN BIPOLAR DISORDER

Because the mechanisms regulating G-protein subunit levels in the plasma membrane and the functional importance of such changes are still poorly understood, it is difficult to ascribe the alterations in postmortem brain G-protein immunolabeling and function in BD to specific molecular disturbances. Studies have excluded linkage between BD and the gene encoding $G\alpha_s$ (Ginns et al. 1992; Le et al. 1994; Ram et al. 1997). Thus, mechanisms other than mutations affecting the primary structure or upstream regulatory elements of the $G\alpha_s$ gene likely account for the G-protein changes observed in BD. G-protein levels may be regulated at multiple stages, including gene expression, mRNA stability, and protein turnover and degradation (Hadcock and Malbon 1993; Milligan 1993). The lack of concomitant changes in frontal, temporal, and occipital $G\alpha_s$ mRNA levels in postmortem BD brain (Young et al. 1996), however, suggests that processes other than alterations in $G\alpha_s$ gene expression may account for the changes in $G\alpha_s$ immunolabeling reported.

Recent findings regarding agonist-promoted regulation of $G\alpha_s$ levels during receptor desensitization and downregulation, as well as studies of the effects of constitutive $G\alpha_s$ activation on $G\alpha_s$ levels and turnover, highlight the critical significance of changes in G-protein levels and functionality in the latter processes (Milligan 1993; Mitchell et al. 1993; Mullaney et al. 1993) and suggest some possible sites of the molecular disturbances that might be operative in BD. In several cellular models, chronic agonist stimulation of G-protein–coupled receptors leads to decreased immunoreactive levels of the respective G proteins to which the receptors couple (reviewed in Milligan 1993). Interestingly, such changes appear to occur in connection with both homologous and heterologous receptor desensitization processes.

Constitutive activation of $G\alpha_s$ by cholera-toxin–catalyzed ADP ribosylation also leads to decreased immunolabeling of $G\alpha_s$ species without altering mRNA levels. Adrenergic denervation in rat pineal gland significantly increased levels of both $G\alpha_s$- and $G\beta$-subunits (Babila and Klein 1992), whereas cholera toxin treatment decreased the levels of both isoforms of $G\alpha_s$ (Babila and Klein 1994); these changes, interestingly, did not depend on cAMP-mediated mechanisms. Taken together, such observations clearly suggest that $G\alpha_s$ levels may be dynamically regulated at both transcriptional and post-translational stages as part of a series of coordinated changes effected to modulate transmembrane signaling through heptahelical membrane receptors. Furthermore, they emphasize that the molecular diathesis that accounts for the enhanced levels and functionality of $G\alpha_s$ in BD may lie in disturbances of the mechanisms coordinating production and/or turnover of the components of the membrane receptor–G protein–effector complexes. Potentially important candidate mechanisms in this regard include agonist-induced receptor activation (Milligan 1993) and ADP ribosylation (both of which appear to increase $G\alpha_s$ susceptibility to degradation), posttranslational acylation of $G\alpha_s$ (i.e., palmitoylation; Linder et al. 1993; Wedegaertner et al. 1995), Ca^{2+}-dependent (calpain) (Greenwood and Jope 1994; Sido et al. 1994) and adenosine triphosphate (ATP)–dependent (ubiquitin) (Madura and Varshavsky 1994; Obin et al. 1994) proteolysis, cytoskeletal interactions (Lieber et al. 1993; Yan and Rasenick 1990), and cross-talk regulatory mechanisms (reviewed in Hadcock and Malbon 1993).

SUMMARY: PATHOPHYSIOLOGICAL AND THERAPEUTIC IMPLICATIONS

The findings of changes in postmortem brain and peripheral signaling processes and proteins have provided a compelling argument that abnormalities in cellular signal transduction are central to the pathophysiology of BD, or at least a subgroup of this disorder. The initial excitement arising from findings suggesting that G-protein abnormalities might be the etiological lesion in BD has been tempered, however, by an increasing number of intracellular signaling alterations observed in this disorder. These changes may be either consequences of or antecedents to the G-protein abnormalities identified. The exclusion of linkage between polymorphic markers in the $G\alpha_s$ gene and BD and the lack of differences in $G\alpha_s$ mRNA levels in BD compared with control postmortem brain suggest one or more posttranslational processes modulating $G\alpha_s$ levels and function, either directly or indirectly, may more likely be causally related to the disorder.

Although substantial data suggest that lithium, at therapeutically relevant concentrations, alters signaling through G_s-coupled receptors (reviewed in Avissar and Schreiber 1992; Hudson et al. 1993; Manji 1992; Manji et al. 1995b), building evidence highlights the actions of lithium on several other important intracellular signaling proteins. These include modifications of the intracellular disposition of specific PKC isozymes, which may alter selective substrate proteins (Lenox et al. 1992; Manji et al. 1995b; Manji et al., Chapter 7, this volume); enhancement of endogenous ADP ribosylation, which may be linked to the nitric oxide signaling pathway (Nestler et al. 1995); and alteration of Ca^{2+}-calpain–mediated processes (Greenwood and Jope 1994). Such observations suggest that biochemical and molecular genetic explorations of these processes and agents that modulate their function may expand our knowledge of the mechanism of action of currently available mood stabilizers as well as identify novel and more efficacious antibipolar medications for future use. Regardless of the exact processes involved, the postmortem brain research strategy, as exemplified in our investigations, is and will likely continue to be an important complementary investigative tool to assist in unraveling the pathogenesis of BD.

REFERENCES

American Psychiatric Association: Diagnostic and Statistical Manual of Mental Disorders, 3rd Edition, Revised. Washington, DC, American Psychiatric Association, 1987

Asaoka Y, Shinomura T, Koide H, et al: The protein kinase-C family in cross-talk of cell signalling systems. Biotechnol Cell Reg 4:1–13, 1991

Avissar S, Schreiber G: The involvement of guanine nucleotide binding proteins in the pathogenesis and treatment of affective disorders. Biol Psychiatry 31:415–459, 1992

Avissar S, Schreiber G, Danon A, et al: Lithium inhibits adrenergic and cholinergic increases in GTP binding in rat cortex. Nature 331:440–442, 1988

Avissar S, Schreiber G, Aulakh CS: Carbamazepine and electroconvulsive shock attenuate β-adrenoceptor and muscarinic cholinoceptor coupling to G proteins in rat cortex. Eur J Pharmacol Mol Pharmacol 189:99–103, 1990

Avissar S, Murphy DL, Schreiber G: Magnesium reversal of lithium inhibition of β-adrenergic and muscarinic receptor coupling to G proteins. Biochem Pharmacol 41:171–175, 1991

Avissar S, Nechamkin Y, Barki-Harrington L, et al: Differential G protein measures in mononuclear leukocytes of patients with bipolar mood disorder are state dependent. J Affect Disord 43:85–93, 1997a

Avissar S, Nechamkin Y, Roitman G, et al: Reduced G protein functions and immunoreactive levels in mononuclear leukocytes of patients with depression. Am J Psychiatry 154:211–217, 1997b

Babila T, Klein D: Stimulus deprivation increases pineal $G\alpha_s$ and Gβ. J Neurochem 59:1356–1362, 1992

Babila T, Klein D: Cholera toxin-induced $G_s\alpha$ down-regulation in neural tissue. Brain Res 638:151–156, 1994

Baxter LRJ, Schwartz JM, Phelps ME: Reduction in prefrontal cortex glucose metabolism common to three types of depression. Arch Gen Psychiatry 46:243–250, 1989

Berrettini WH, Ferrado TN, Goldin LR, et al: Chromosome 18 DNA markers and manic-depressive illness: evidence for a susceptibility gene. Proc Natl Acad Sci U S A 91:5918–5921, 1994

Birnbaumer L, Abramowitz J, Brown A: Receptor-effector coupling by G proteins. Biochim Biophys Acta 1031:163–224, 1990

Butterworth J, Tennant MC: Postmortem human brain pH and lactate in sudden infant death syndrome. J Neurochem 53:1494–1499, 1989

Casebolt TL, Jope RS: Effects of chronic lithium treatment on protein kinase C and cyclic AMP-dependent protein phosphorylation. Biol Psychiatry 29:233–243, 1991

Chen J, Rasenick MM: Chronic antidepressant treatment facilitates G protein activation of adenylyl cyclase without altering G protein content. J Pharmacol Exp Ther 275:509–517, 1995

Clapham DE, Neer EJ: New roles for G-protein $\beta\gamma$-dimers in transmembrane signalling. Nature 365:403–406, 1993

Colin SF, Chang HC, Mollner S, et al: Chronic lithium regulates the expression of adenylate cyclase and Gi-protein alpha subunit in rat cerebral cortex. Proc Natl Acad Sci U S A 88:10634–10637, 1991

Cowburn RF, Garlind A, O'Neill C, et al: Characterization and regional distribution of adenylyl cyclase activity from human brain. Neurochem Int 18:389–398, 1991

Cowburn RF, O'Neill C, Ravid R, et al: Adenylyl cyclase activity in postmortem human brain: evidence of altered G protein mediation in Alzheimer's disease. J Neurochem 58:1409–1419, 1992a

Cowburn RF, O'Neill C, Ravid R, et al: Preservation of Gi-protein inhibited adenylyl cyclase activity in the brains of patients with Alzheimer's disease. Neurosci Lett 141:16–20, 1992b

Cowburn RF, Vestling M, Fowler CJ: Disrupted β_1-adrenoceptor G-protein coupling in the temporal cortex of patients with Alzheimer's disease. Neurosci Lett 155:163–166, 1993

Cowburn RF, Marcusson JO, Eriksson A, et al: Adenylyl cyclase activity and G-protein subunit levels in postmortem frontal cortex of suicide victims. Brain Res 633:297–304, 1994

Crawford JA, Mutchler KJ, Sullivan BE, et al: Neural expression of a novel alternatively spliced and polyadenylated Gsα transcript. J Biol Chem 268:9879–9885, 1993

Drinnan SL, Hope BT, Snutch TP, et al: G_{olf} in the basal ganglia. Mol Cell Neurosci 2:66–70, 1991

Dubovsky S, Murphy J, Christiano J, et al: The calcium second messenger system in bipolar disorders: data supporting new research directions. J Neuropsychiatry Clin Neurosci 4:3–14, 1992

Emamghoreishi M, Warsh JJ, Sibony D, et al: Lack of effect of chronic antidepressant treatment on Gs and Gi α-subunit protein and mRNA levels in the rat cerebral cortex. Neuropsychopharmacology 15:281–287, 1996

Escriba PV, Sastre M, Garcia-Sevilla JA: Increased density of guanine nucleotide-binding proteins in the postmortem brains of heroin addicts. Arch Gen Psychiatry 51:494–501, 1994

Fields A, Li PP, Kish SJ, et al: Increased cyclic AMP-dependent protein kinase activity in postmortem brain from patients with bipolar affective disorder. J Neurochem (in press)

Francis SH, Corbin JD: Structure and function of cyclic nucleotide-dependent protein kinases. Annu Rev Physiol 56:237–272, 1994

Friedman E, Wang HY: Receptor-mediated activation of G proteins is increased in postmortem brains of bipolar affective disorder subjects. J Neurochem 67:1145–1152, 1996

Ginns E, Egeland J, Allen C, et al: Update on the search for DNA markers linked to manic-depressive illness in the Old Order Amish. J Psychiatr Res 26:305–308, 1992

Goodwin FK, Jamison KR: Manic-Depressive Illness. New York, Oxford University Press, 1990, pp 503–524

Greenwood A, Jope R: Brain G-protein proteolysis by calpain: enhancement by lithium. Brain Res 636:320–326, 1994

Gross-Isseroff R, Dillon KA, Fieldust SJ, et al: Autoradiographic analysis of α_1-noradrenergic receptors in the human brain postmortem. Arch Gen Psychiatry 47:1049–1053, 1991

Guze BH, Gitlin MJ: The neuropathologic basis of major affective disorders: neuroanatomic insights. J Neuropsychiatry Clin Neurosci 6:114–121, 1994

Habecker BA, Martin JM, Nathanson NM: Isolation and characterization of a novel cDNA which identifies both neural-specific and ubiquitously expressed G_{sa} mRNAs. J Neurochem 61:712–717, 1993

Hadcock JR, Malbon CC: Agonist regulation of gene expression of adrenergic receptors and G-proteins. J Neurochem 60:1–9, 1993

Halper JP, Brown RP, Sweeney JA, et al: Blunted β-adrenergic responsivity of peripheral blood mononuclear cells in endogenous depression: isoproterenol dose response studies. Arch Gen Psychiatry 45:241–244, 1988

Helper J, Gilman A: G proteins. Trends Biochem Sci 17:383–387, 1992

Herve D, Levistrauss M, Mareysemper I, et al: G_{olf} and Gs in rat basal ganglia: possible involvement of G_{olf} in the coupling of dopamine-D_1 receptor with adenylyl cyclase. J Neurosci 13:2237–2248, 1993

Hill SJ, Kendall DA: Cross-talk between different receptor-effector systems in the mammalian CNS. Cell Signal 1:135–141, 1989

Hudson C, Young LT, Li PP, et al: CNS signal transduction in the pathophysiology and pharmacotherapy of affective disorders and schizophrenia. Synapse 13:278–293, 1993

Inglese J, Koch WJ, Touhara K, et al: Gβγ interactions with PH domains and Ras-MAPK signaling pathways. Trends Biochem Sci 20:151–156, 1995

Ishikawa Y, Bianchi C, Nadal-Ginard N, et al: Alternative promoter and 5′ exon generate a novel G_{sa} mRNA. J Biol Chem 265:8458–8462, 1990

Iyengar R: Molecular and functional diversity of mammalian G(s)-stimulated adenylyl cyclases. FASEB J 7:768–775, 1993

Jeste DV, Lohr JB, Goodwin FK: Neuroanatomical studies of major affective disorders: a review and suggestions for further research. Br J Psychiatry 153:444–459, 1988

Jones DJ, Stavinoha WB: Microwave inactivation as a tool for studying the neuropharmacology of cyclic nucleotides, in Neuropharmacology of Cyclic Nucleotides. Edited by Palmer GC. Munich, Germany, Urban & Schwarzenberg, 1979, pp 253–281

Jope RS, Williams MB: Lithium and brain signal transduction systems. Biochem Pharmacol 47:429–441, 1994

Jope RS, Song L, Li X: Impaired phosphoinositide hydrolysis in Alzheimer's brain. Neurobiol Aging 15:221–226, 1994

Jope RS, Song L, Li PP, et al: The phosphoinositide signal transduction system is impaired in bipolar affective disorder brain. J Neurochem 66:2402–2409, 1996

Jope RS, Song L, Grimes CA, et al: Selective increases in phosphoinositide signaling activity and G-protein levels in postmortem brain from subjects with schizophrenia or alcohol dependence. J Neurochem 70:763–771, 1998

Koenig ML, Jope RS: Effects of lithium on synaptosomal Ca^{2+} fluxes. Psychopharmacology 96:267–272, 1988

Korpi ER, Kleinman JE, Goodman SI, et al: Serotonin and 5-hydroxyindoleacetic acid in brains of suicide victims. Arch Gen Psychiatry 43:594–600, 1986

Le F, Mitchell P, Vivero C, et al: Exclusion of close linkage of bipolar disorder to the G_s-αsubunit gene in nine Australian pedigrees. J Affect Disord 32:187–195, 1994

Lenox RH, Watson DG, Patel J, et al: Chronic lithium administration alters a prominent PKC substrate in rat hippocampus. Brain Res 570:333–340, 1992

Lesch K P, Aulakh CS, Tolliver TJ, et al: Differential effects of long-term lithium and carbamazepine administration on $G_{s\alpha}$ and $G_{i\alpha}$ protein in rat brain. Eur J Pharmacol Mol Pharmacol 207:355–359, 1991

Li PP, Tam YK, Young LT, et al: Lithium decreases Gs, Gi-1 and Gi-2 α-subunit mRNA levels in rat cortex. Eur J Pharmacol Mol Pharmacol 206:165–166, 1991

Li PP, Sibony D, Green MA, et al: Lithium modulation of phosphoinositide signaling system in rat cortex: selective effect on phorbol ester binding. J Neurochem 61: 1722–1730, 1993a

Li PP, Young LT, Tam YK, et al: Effects of chronic lithium and carbamazepine treatment on G-protein subunit expression in rat cerebral cortex. Biol Psychiatry 34: 162–170, 1993b

Lieber D, Jasper J, Alousi A, et al: Alterations in G_s-mediated signal transduction in S49 lymphoma cells treated with inhibitors of microtubules. J Biol Chem 268:3833–3837, 1993

Linder M, Middleton P, Helper J, et al: Lipid modifications of G proteins: α subunits are palmitoylated. Proc Natl Acad Sci U S A 90:3675–3679, 1993

Madura K, Varshavsky A: Degradation of Gα by the N-end rule pathway. Science 265:1454–1458, 1994

Manji HK: G-proteins—implications for psychiatry. Am J Psychiatry 149:746–760, 1992

Manji HK, Lenox RH: Long-term action of lithium—a role for transcriptional and posttranscriptional factors regulated by protein kinase C. Synapse 16:11–28, 1994

Manji HK, Chen G, Shimon H, et al: Guanine nucleotide-binding proteins in bipolar affective disorder: effects of long-term lithium treatment. Arch Gen Psychiatry 52:135–144, 1995a

Manji HK, Potter WZ, Lenox RH: Signal transduction pathways: molecular targets for lithium's actions. Arch Gen Psychiatry 52:531–543, 1995b

Mathews R, Li PP, Young LT, et al: Increased $G\alpha_{q/11}$ immunoreactivity in postmortem occipital cortex from patients with bipolar affective disorder. Biol Psychiatry 41:649–656, 1997

McKeith IG, Marshall EF, Ferrier IN, et al: 5-HT receptor binding in postmortem brain from patients with affective disorder. J Affect Disord 13:74–76, 1987

McLaughlin M, Ross BM, Milligan G, et al: Robustness of G proteins in Alzheimer's disease: an immunoblot study. J Neurochem. 57:9–14, 1991

Menco BPM, Bruch RC, Dau B, et al: Ultrastructural localization of olfactory transduction components—the G-protein subunit G_{olf} and type-III adenylyl cyclase. Neuron 8:441–453, 1992

Milligan G: Agonist regulation of cellular G protein levels and distribution: mechanisms and functional implications. Trends Pharmacol Sci 14:413–418, 1993

Milligan G, Wakelam M: G Proteins: Signal Transduction and Disease. London, Academic Press, 1992

Mitchell F, Buckley N, Milligan G: Enhanced degradation of the phosphoinositidase C-linked guanine-nucleotide-binding protein $G\alpha_q/G\alpha_{11}$ following activation of the human M1 muscarinic acetylcholine receptor expressed in CHO cells. Biochem J 293:495–499, 1993

Mork A, Geisler A, Hollund P: Effects of lithium on 2nd messenger systems in the brain. Pharmacol Toxicol 71:4–17, 1992

Mullaney I, Dodd M, Buckley N, et al: Agonist activation of transfected human M1 muscarinic acetylcholine receptors in CHO cells results in down-regulation of both the receptor and the α subunit of the G-protein G_q. Biochem J 289:125–131, 1993

Nestler EJ, Terwilliger RZ, Duman RS: Regulation of endogenous ADP-ribosylation by acute and chronic lithium in rat brain. J Neurochem 64:2319–2324, 1995

Nishino N, Kitamura N, Hashimoto T, et al: Increase in [^{3}H]cAMP binding sites and decrease in $G_i\alpha$ and $G_o\alpha$ immunoreactivities in left temporal cortices from patients with schizophrenia. Brain Res 615:41–49, 1993

Obin M, Nowell T, Taylor A: The photoreceptor G-protein transducin (G_t) is a substrate for ubiquitin-dependent proteolysis. Biochem Biophys Res Commun 200:1169–1176, 1994

Ohm TG, Bohl J, Lemmer B: Reduced basal and stimulated (isoprenaline, GppNHp, forskolin) adenylate cyclase activity in Alzheimer's disease correlated with histopathological changes. Brain Res 540:229–236, 1991

Okada F, Crow TJ, Roberts GW: G proteins (Gi, Go) in the medial temporal lobe in schizophrenia: preliminary report of a neurochemical correlate of structural change. J Neural Transm 84:147–153, 1991

Okada F, Tokumitsu Y, Takahashi N, et al: Reduced concentrations of the α-subunit of GTP-binding protein Go in schizophrenic brain. J Neural Transm 95:95–104, 1994

O'Neill C, Wiehager B, Fowler CJ, et al: Regionally selective alterations in G protein subunit levels in the Alzheimer's disease brain. Brain Res 636:193–201, 1994

Owen F, Chambers DR, Cooper SJ, et al: Serotonergic mechanisms in brains of suicide victims. Brain Res 362:185–188, 1986

Ozawa H, Gsell W, Frolich L, et al: Imbalance of the G_s and $G_{i/o}$ function in post-mortem human brain of depressed patients. J Neural Transm 94:63–69, 1993a

Ozawa H, Katamura Y, Hatta S, et al: Alterations of guanine nucleotide-binding proteins in post-mortem human brain in alcoholics. Brain Res 62:174–179, 1993b

Pacheco MA, Stockmeier C, Meltzer HY, et al: Alterations in phosphoinositidie signaling and G-protein levels in depressed suicide brain. Brain Res 723:37–45, 1996

Perez J, Zanardi R, Mori S, et al: Abnormalities of cAMP-dependent endogenous phosphorylation in platelets from patients with bipolar disorder. Am J Psychiatry 152: 1204–1206, 1995

Port JD, Malbon CC: Integration of transmembrane signaling: cross-talk among G-protein-linked receptors and other signal transduction pathways. Trends in Cardiovascular Medicine 3:85–92, 1993

Pyne NJ, Freissmuth M, Palmer S: Phosphorylation of the spliced variant forms of the recombinant stimulatory guanine-nucleotide-binding regulatory protein (Gsa) by protein kinase-C. Biochem J 285:333–338, 1992

Ram A, Guedy F, Anibal C, et al: No abnormality in the gene for the G protein stimulatory α subunit in patients with bipolar disorder. Arch Gen Psychiatry 54:44–48, 1997

Rahman S, Li PP, Young LT, et al: Reduced [^{3}H]cyclic AMP binding in postmortem brain from subjects with bipolar affectiv disorder. J Neurochem 68:297–304, 1997

Rhee SG, Choi KD: Regulation of inositol phospholipid-specific phospholipase C isozymes. J Biol Chem 267:12393–12396, 1992

Ross BM, McLaughlin M, Roberts M, et al: Alterations in the activity of adenylate cyclase and high affinity GTPase in Alzheimer's disease. Brain Res 622:35–42, 1993

Schreiber G, Avissar S, Danon A, et al: Hyperfunctional G proteins in mononuclear leukocytes of patients with mania. Biol Psychiatry 29:273–280, 1991

Schwechheimer K, Hoffman F: Properties of regulatory subunit of cyclic AMP-dependent protein kinase (peak I) from rabbit skeletal muscle prepared by urea treatment of the holoenzyme. J Biol Chem 252:7690–7696, 1977

Seifert R, Wenzel-Seifert K, Lee TW, et al: Differential effects of Gsα splice variants on β_2-adrenoceptor-mediated signaling: the β_2-adrenoceptor coupled to the long splice variant of Gsα has properties of a constitutive active receptor. J Biol Chem 273:5109–5116, 1998

Sido T, Sorimachi H, Suzuki K: Calpain: new perspectives in molecular diversity and physiological pathological involvement. FASEB J 8:814–822, 1994

Simon M, Strathmann M, Gautam N: Diversity of G proteins in signal transduction. Science 252:802–808, 1991

Spaulding SW: The ways in which hormones change cyclic adenosine 3′, 5′-monophosphate-dependent protein kinase subunits, and how such changes affect cell behavior. Endocr Rev 14:632–650, 1993

Stanley M, Mann JJ: Increased serotonin-2 binding sites in frontal cortex of suicide victims. Lancet i:214–216, 1983

Sternweis PC, Smrcka AV: Regulation of phospholipase C by G proteins. Trends Biochem Sci 17:502–506, 1992

Strassheim D, Malbon CC: Phosphorylation of G_{ia2} attenuates inhibitory adenylyl cyclase in neuroblastoma/glioma hybrid (NG-108-15) cells. J Biol Chem 269: 14307–14313, 1994

Sunahara RK, Dessauer CW, Gilman AG: Complexity and diversity of ma,,alian adenylyl cyclases. Annu Rev Pharmacol Toxicol 36:461–480, 1996

Swaroop A, Agarwal N, Gruen JR, et al: Differential expression of novel Gs signal transduction protein cDNA species. Nucleic Acids Res 19:4725–4729, 1991

Vatal M, Aiyar AS: Phosphorylation of brain synaptosomal proteins in lithium-treated rats. Biochem Pharmacol 33:829–831, 1984

Walseth TF, Zhang H-J, Olson LK, et al: Increase in Gs and cyclic AMP generation in HIT cells: evidence that the 45-kDa α-subunit of G_s has greater functional activity than the 52-kDa α-subunit. J Biol Chem 264:21106–21111, 1990

Warsh JJ, Li PP: Second messenger systems and mood disorders. Curr Opin Psychiatry 9:23–29, 1996

Warsh JJ, Chiu AS, Li PP: Noradrenergic mechanisms in affective disorders: contributions of receptor research, in Receptors and Ligands in Psychiatry and Neurology. Edited by Sen AK, Lee T. Cambridge, England, Cambridge University Press, 1988, pp 271–302

Wedegaertner PB, Wilson PT, Bourne HR: Lipid modification of trimeric G proteins. J Biol Chem 270:503–506, 1995

Werstiuk ES, Steiner M, Burns T: Studies on leukocyte β-adrenergic receptors in depression: a critical appraisal. Life Sci 47:85–105, 1990

Wickman K, Clapham DE: Ion channel regulation by G proteins. Physiol Rev 75:865–885, 1995

Williams LT, Snyderman R, Lefkowitz RJ: Identification of beta-adrenergic receptors in human lymphocytes by (-)^{3}H dihydroalprenolol. J Clin Invest 57:149–155, 1976

Yan K, Rasenick M: Cytoskeletal participation in the signal transduction process: tubulin G protein interactions in the regulation of AC, in Biology of Cellular Transducing Signals. Edited by Vanderhoek J. New York, Plenum, 1990, pp 163–172

Yang CQ, Kitamura N, Nishino N, et al: Isotope-specific G protein abnormalities in the left superior temporal cortex and limbic structures of patients with chronic schizophrenia. Biol Psychiatry 43:12–19, 1998

Young LT, Li PP, Kish SJ, et al: Postmortem cerebral cortex Gs alpha-subunit levels are elevated in bipolar affective disorder. Brain Res 553:323–326, 1991

Young LT, Li PP, Kish SJ, et al: Cerebral cortex $G_s\alpha$ protein levels and forskolin-stimulated cyclic AMP formation are increased in bipolar affective disorder. J Neurochem 61:890–898, 1993

Young LT, Li PP, Kamble A, et al: Increased mononuclear leukocyte G-proteins in bipolar but not unipolar depression. Am J Psychiatry 151:594–596, 1994a

Young LT, Li PP, Kish SJ, et al: Cerebral cortex β-adrenoceptor binding in bipolar affective disorder. J Affect Disord 30:89–92, 1994b

Young LT, Warsh JJ, Kish SJ, et al: Reduced brain 5-HT and elevated NE turnover and metabolites in bipolar affective disorder. Biol Psychiatry 35:121–127, 1994c

Young LT, Asghari V, Li PP, et al: Stimulatory G-protein α-subunit mRNA levels are not increased in autopsied cerebral cortex from patients with bipolar disorder. Mol Brain Res 42:45–50, 1996

CHAPTER 14

CARBAMAZEPINE AND ADENOSINE RECEPTORS

Dietrich van Calker, M.D., Ph.D., Knut Biber, Ph.D., Jörg Walden, M.D., Peter Gebicke, Ph.D., and Mathias Berger, M.D.

The established antiepileptic drug carbamazepine (CBZ) is now also widely accepted as an alternative to lithium salts in the therapeutic and prophylactic treatment of bipolar affective disorders. It may even have advantages over lithium in the treatment and prophylaxis of schizoaffective disorder and rapid-cycling bipolar disorder (Goodwin and Jamison 1990; Solomon et al. 1995). CBZ's mode of action in these disorders, however, remains elusive.

Several neurobiological actions of CBZ could be involved in its therapeutic effects. The inhibitory effects of CBZ on voltage-dependent sodium (Na^+) channels are probably instrumental to its anticonvulsive properties (for review, see Catteral 1987). In addition, CBZ has been shown to potentiate the action of γ-aminobutyric acid B receptor ($GABA_B$) agonists (von Wegerer et al. 1998) to interfere with the function of peripheral benzodiazepine receptors (Weiss and Post 1991) and to act as a calcium (Ca^{2+}) antagonist (Walden et al. 1993). This latter function is of particular interest in the light of the accumulating evidence that disturbed intracellular Ca^{2+} regulation may be involved in the pathophysiology of affective disorders.

Ca^{2+} antagonists such as verapamil and nimodipine have been found to be efficacious in the treatment of both manic (for review, see Dubovsky 1993) and depressive (Walden et al. 1995) episodes, and several case reports have indicated nimodipine's value in the maintenance treatment of ultrarapid-cycling bipolar disorder and brief recurrent depression (Pazzaglia et al. 1993).

The most compelling evidence for a role of intracellular Ca^{2+} regulation in affective disorders relates, however, to the biological activities of lithium. The therapeutic and prophylactic effects of lithium are thought to result from a modulation of the inositol phosphate (IP)–Ca^{2+} second-messenger system, secondary to a lithium-induced depletion of intracellular inositol. The IP-Ca^{2+} system is an important intracellular signaling pathway that regulates cellular activity through a release of diacylglycerol (DAG) and inositol 1,4,5-trisphosphate (IP_3), two second-messenger molecules that activate various protein kinases either directly (DAG) or via the intracellular release of Ca^{2+} ions (IP_3) (for review, see Berridge and Irvine 1989; Berridge et al. 1989). The idea that lithium might act via a selective dampening of this system in neural circuits that are presumably overactive in affective disorders was originally based on in vitro studies (for review, see Berridge et al. 1989) and has been subsequently corroborated by experiments with slices from rat brain, which indeed showed a compromised agonist-stimulated accumulation of IPs after the animals were chronically treated with lithium salts (for review, see Nahorski et al. 1991).

However, recent reports have raised doubts about the validity of the rat brain slice system, which is prone to an artificially exaggerated inositol depletion. These effects of lithium could not be observed in other species, in which the supply of inositol is not compromised as readily (for review, see Atack et al. 1995; Jope and Williams 1994). Nevertheless, clinical studies have provided evidence that in patients chronically treated with lithium, the activity of the IP-Ca^{2+} system is compromised. Neutrophils from lithium-treated patients showed a significantly reduced intracellular accumulation of IP and Ca^{2+} ions after stimulation with an agonist as compared with control subjects (Förstner et al. 1994; Greil et al. 1991; van Calker et al. 1993). Moreover, evidence has accumulated that the sensitivity of the IP-Ca^{2+} second-messenger system is increased in patients with an acute manifestation of depression and mania, at least in peripheral cells such as platelets (Eckert et al. 1993; Kusumi et al. 1991; Mikuni et al. 1991) and neutrophils (Bohus et al. 1995; van Calker et al. 1993; for review, see Atack et al. 1995). Therefore, investigators hypothesized (Bohus et al. 1996; van Calker et al. 1993) that affective disorders are caused by an overactivity of certain neural circuits, which is secondary to an exaggerated sensitivity of the IP-Ca^{2+} system, and that prophylactic treatment with lithium and CBZ might act via a compensatory inhibition of this system. This idea would gain more credibility if CBZ could be shown to have dampening effects on the IP-Ca^{2+} system similar to those of lithium. However, effects of CBZ on the IP-Ca^{2+} system in the brain have been reported only for presumably already toxic concentrations (McDermott and Logan 1989) and have not been verified by other authors (Elphick et al. 1988).

Although CBZ, at therapeutically relevant concentrations, apparently does not directly influence the generation of second messengers from inositol phospholipids, it may do so via indirect mechanisms (e.g., by an influence on the modulatory actions of some neuroactive substances). Adenosine appears to be a likely candidate for such a substance because effective treatments of affective disorders, such as electroconvulsive therapy and sleep deprivation, are associated with an upregulation of adenosine A_1 receptors (Durcan and Morgan 1990). Furthermore, adenosine inhibits the release of several neurotransmitters in the brain (e.g., noradrenaline and acetylcholine) (Dunwiddie 1985) that are likely involved in the pathophysiology of affective psychosis and modulates the accumulation of IPs and Ca^{2+} ions triggered by these and other agents (see section, "Modulation of the Neurotransmitter-Stimulated Generation of Second Messengers From Inositol Phospholipids in the Brain by Adenosine Receptors," later in this chapter).

In this chapter, we review results of our group's studies, which indicate that CBZ via a blockade of adenosine A_1 receptors can modulate adenosine's potentiating effect on the activation by neurotransmitters of the IP-Ca^{2+} second-messenger system.

ATTENUATION OF NEURONAL OVERACTIVITY AND MODULATION OF THE LONG-TERM REGULATION OF NEURONAL EXCITABILITY BY ADENOSINE

Adenosine, as a metabolite of adenosine triphosphate (ATP), has already (very early in evolution) acquired a role as a "retaliatory metabolite" (Newby 1984), which signals to the surrounding cells an imbalance of energy supply and demand. Increased adenosine concentrations induce, by activation of adenosine receptors, compensating activities such as increased blood flow (and thereby oxygen supply) and/or diminished cellular activity, such as reduced heart rate or inhibition of neuronal firing. In accordance with this general biological function are the sedative, anxiolytic, and sleep-promoting behavioral properties of adenosine, which reduce energy consumption by the brain and elsewhere in the body. In the brain, activation of adenosine receptors probably has an important adaptive function in situations of exaggerated neuronal activity, such as epileptic seizures (Dragunow 1988), or excessive energy depletion, such as ischemia and hypoxia (for review, see Rudolphi et al. 1992). In these conditions, large amounts of adenosine are released into the extracellular space, where it acts both pre- and postsynaptically to inhibit neurotransmitter release and neuronal excitability (for review, see Greene and Haas 1991).

Adenosine is therefore considered the brain's "endogenous anticonvulsive" (Dragunow 1988) and neuroprotective agent (Rudolphi et al. 1992). The regulatory interplay between adenosine and excitatory amino acids appears to be important in these activities. Adenosine inhibits the release of glutamate from presynaptic terminals. However, its own release is evoked by activation of glutamate receptors either directly and in a Ca^{2+}-independent manner via non–*N*-methyl-D-aspartate (NMDA) receptors as adenosine per se or via NMDA receptors and in a Ca^{2+}-dependent manner as a nucleotide that is subsequently converted extracellularly to adenosine (Craig and White 1993). In addition to these acute activities, adenosine appears to contribute to phenomena associated with the long-term regulation of neuronal excitability, such as synaptic plasticity (Alzheimer et al. 1993; Mendonca and Ribeiro 1993).

MODULATION OF THE NEUROTRANSMITTER-STIMULATED GENERATION OF SECOND MESSENGERS FROM INOSITOL PHOSPHOLIPIDS IN THE BRAIN BY ADENOSINE RECEPTORS

The inhibitory effects of adenosine on neurotransmitter release and neuronal excitability reviewed briefly in the previous section appear to be mediated predominantly by adenosine receptors of the A_1 type (Greene and Haas 1991). A_1 receptors are widely distributed in the brain and are particularly prominent in the hippocampus, striatum, and neocortex (for review, see Williams 1995). A_2 receptors, in contrast, are largely restricted to dopamine-rich areas such as the caudate, putamen, nucleus accumbens, and olfactory tubercle and are likely to be involved in the regulation of dopamine signaling in the basal ganglia (for review, see Williams 1995). The adenosine A_1- and A_2-receptor subtypes were originally distinguished by their differential effects on adenylate cyclase (Londos et al. 1980; van Calker et al. 1979) but are now classified according to the structure-activity relation of various adenosine analogues, including selective agonists and antagonists of either receptor type (for review, see Fredholm et al. 1994). A_2 receptors were further subdivided into A_{2a} and A_{2b} receptors. These three receptors and a fourth, the A_3 receptor, which are all coupled to guanine nucleotide binding proteins (G proteins), have been cloned (for review, see Fredholm et al. 1994).

In addition to adenylate cyclase, various effector systems are now known to be regulated by A_1 receptors, including potassium (K^+) and Ca^{2+} channels (Greene and Haas 1991). Direct stimulatory effects of adenosine on the IP-Ca^{2+} second-messenger system are known from cell lines that express high amounts of A_1 receptors (for review, see Dickenson and Hill 1994). In brain cells, adenosine alone does not seem to influence the IP-Ca^{2+} system. However, in slices from guinea pig cerebral cortex, adenosine agonists potentiated the histamine H_1 receptor–mediated increase in IP accumulation, whereas in cerebral cortical slices from mice and humans, they inhibited histamine-stimulated inositol phospholipid hydrolysis (for review, see Dickenson and Hill 1994).

The responses of other neurotransmitters such as noradrenaline, serotonin, and carbachol were neither inhibited nor potentiated by adenosine agonists in slices of cerebral cortex of these species. However, in slices of the rat striatum, adenosine agonists inhibited the histamine-induced accumulation of IPs (Petcoff and Cooper 1987), whereas the response to carbachol and noradrenaline was potentiated (El-Etr et al. 1989a). Synergistic (for review, see Glowinski et al. 1994) and inhibitory effects also were observed in various cell cultures (for review, see Dickenson and Hill 1994). In astrocytes cultured from various areas of embryonic mouse brain, region- and neurotransmitter-specific differences in the synergistic effects of adenosine agonists were observed (Delumeau et al. 1991; El-Etr et al. 1989b). These modulatory actions of adenosine appear to be mediated by adenosine receptors that pharmacologically resemble the A_1 subtype.

An A_1 receptor–induced release of arachidonic acid that requires a prior activation of phospholipase C (PLC) has been suggested as a possible mechanism of the synergistic effects of adenosine on the activity of the IP-Ca^{2+} second-messenger system (Glowinski et al. 1994). However, we have provided evidence that at least in rat astrocytes release of arachidonic acid is not involved in the synergistic effects of A_1-receptor activation but that this synergism is mediated most probably by recruitment of G-protein $\beta\gamma$-subunits for activation of PLC (Biber et al 1997). Similarly, $\beta\gamma$-subunits may also mediate the synergistic effects observed in other systems (Dickenson and Hill 1994). It is not known whether the A_1 receptors that mediate respectively the inhibitory and the synergistic effects belong to different subclasses of A_1 receptors or represent a single class of receptors that can, for example, couple differentially to distinct G proteins.

INHIBITION OF THE SYNERGISTIC EFFECTS OF ADENOSINE ON THE IP-CA^{2+} SYSTEM BY CARBAMAZEPINE

Because therapeutically relevant concentrations of CBZ inhibit in vitro ligand binding to adenosine receptors, a possible involvement of adenosine receptors in CBZ's therapeutic efficacy has been discussed for more than a decade (for review, see Durcan and Morgan 1990). Because the clinical properties of CBZ are similar to the anticonvulsive, sedative, and anxiolytic effects of adenosine agonists and are in sharp contrast to the opposite actions of adenosine antagonists such as caffeine, an adenosine-agonistic activity of CBZ has been expected. However, as already suggested on the basis of indirect evidence (Durcan and Morgan 1990), we showed that CBZ acts as a specific antagonist of A_1 receptors (van Calker et al. 1991).

In the rat pituitary cell line GH_3, A_1 receptors mediate an inhibition of the vasoactive intestinal peptide (VIP)-stimulated accumulation of cyclic adenosine monophosphate (cAMP). This inhibitory effect of adenosine antagonists is competitively antagonized by CBZ at a therapeutically relevant concentration. In contrast, A_{2a} receptor–mediated responses such as the inhibition of IP formation and Ca^{2+} influx in human neutrophils stimulated with the chemotactic tripeptide formylmethionylleucylphenylalanin are not influenced by CBZ (van Calker et al. 1991; D. van Calker, unpublished data, 1991). The selective interaction of CBZ with A_1 but not A_{2a} receptors was further verified by binding studies that used highly selective radioligands (van Calker et al. 1991). Because the dampening of the IP-Ca^{2+} second-messenger system is believed to underlie the therapeutic efficacy of lithium (see earlier discussion in this chapter), we were particularly interested in whether CBZ could by its A_1-antagonistic activity attenuate the synergistic effects of adenosine on the neurotransmitter-evoked formation of IP in brain cells.

We used cultured astrocytes from newborn rat brain to establish a model system in which the potentiating effects of adenosine on the neurotransmitter-induced accumulation of IPs could be reliably studied. Astrocytes cultured from various brain regions showed an increase in the intracellular formation of IPs when stimulated with the α_1-adrenergic agonist phenylephrine (Figure 14–1) or with noradrenaline (not shown). This effect is potentiated in astrocytes from all brain regions except the striatum and cerebellum (Figure 14–1) by adenosine agonists such as R-phenylisopropyladenosine (R-PIA) (Figure 14–2), cyclopentyladenosine (CPA) (Figure 14–1), and 5′-N-ethylcarboxamidoadenosine (NECA) (not shown), which do not show any effects on their own. The dose-response curves show an order of potency of

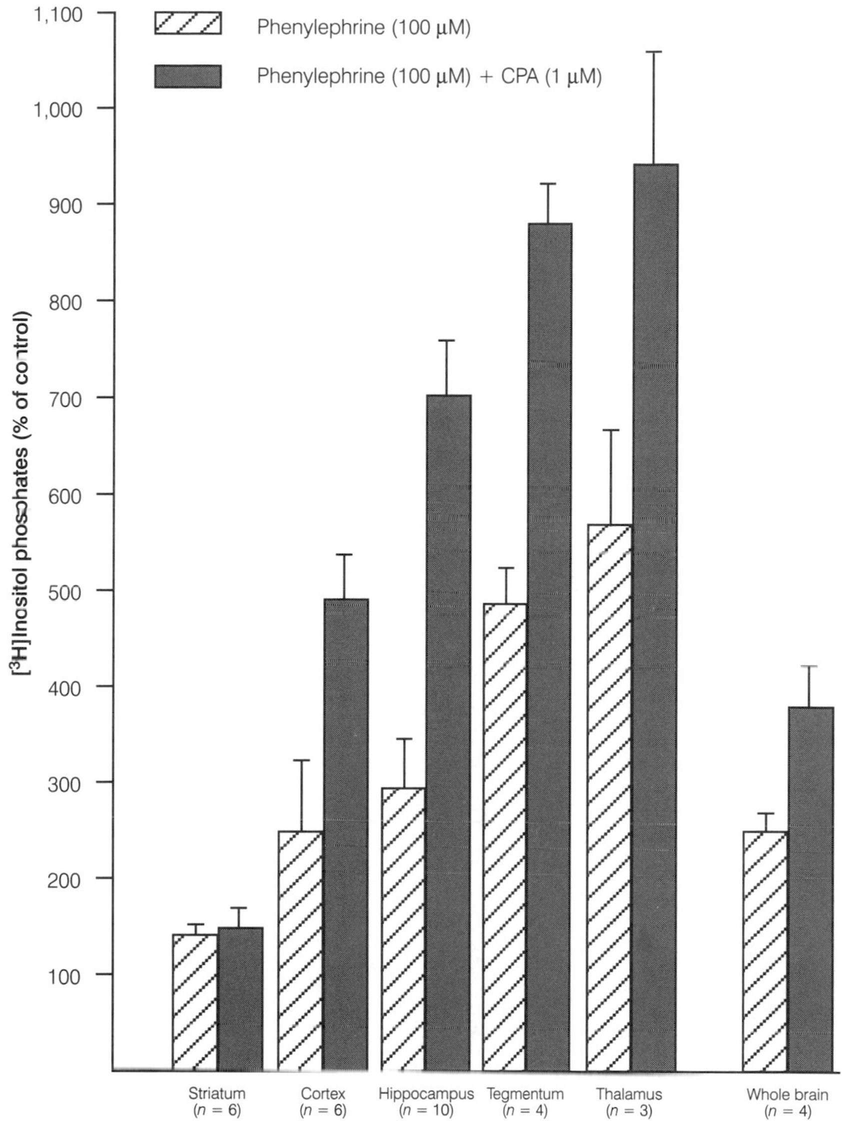

Figure 14–1. Influence of the adenosine agonist cyclopentyladenosine (CPA) on the phenylephrine-induced accumulation of inositol phosphates in astrocytes cultured from various areas of newborn rat brain. n = number of experiments.

CPA = R-PIA > NECA (Biber et al. 1996) in accordance with a mediation of this effect by an A_1 receptor. Indeed, the effects of R-PIA and CPA are antagonized by low (100 nM) concentrations of the A_1-specific antagonist 8-cyclopentyl-1,3-dipropylxanthin (DPCPX) (Biber et al. 1996). As expected

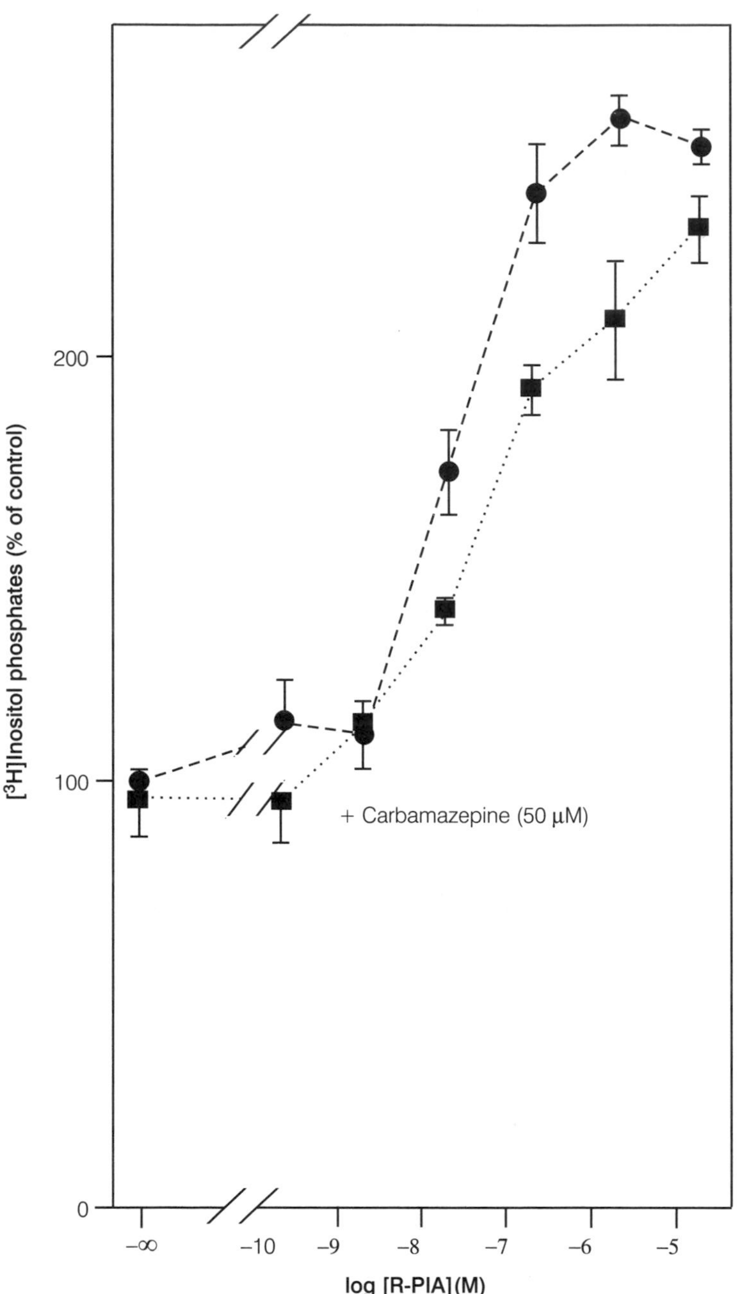

Figure 14–2. Inhibition by carbamazepine of the potentiation by R-phenylisopropyladenosine (R-PIA) of the phenylephrine-induced accumulation of inositol phosphates in rat hippocampal astrocyte cultures. Black squares and dotted lines = carbamazepine group; black circles and dashed lines = control group.

from its A_1-antagonistic activity, this potentiating effect is antagonized by a therapeutically relevant concentration of CBZ (50 μM) (Figure 14–2) (Biber et al. 1996; van Calker et al. 1991).

It is important to note that the synergistic action of adenosine is not found in striatal cultures of newborn rat brain (see Figure 14–1), whereas a pronounced potentiating effect in striatal cultures of embryonic mouse brain has been reported (El-Etr et al. 1989a, 1989b). This discrepancy is most likely due to the well-known (see section, "Modulation of the Neurotransmitter-Stimulated Generation of Second Messengers From Inositol Phospholipids in the Brain by Adenosine Receptors," earlier in this chapter) pronounced variability of the modulatory actions of adenosine among both different species and distinct brain areas. No inhibitory effect of adenosine on the agonist-stimulated IP response was found in astrocyte cultures from various brain areas. It is also surprising that in GH_3 cells, which have been reported to express A_1 receptors that mediate an inhibition of thyrotropin-releasing hormone–induced IP formation (Delahunty et al. 1988), no such effect could be reliably identified. Other investigators also have been unable to reproduce these inhibitory effects of adenosine in GH_3 cells (Cooper and Boyajian 1989). The reasons for these discrepancies are unclear.

DIFFERENTIAL MODIFICATION OF THE MODULATORY ACTIONS OF ADENOSINE IN DISTINCT BRAIN AREAS BY CARBAMAZEPINE VIA UPREGULATION OF A_1 RECEPTORS

The antagonism by CBZ of the A_1 receptors that mediate the potentiation of the neurotransmitter-induced formation of IPs should attenuate intracellular signaling via the IP-Ca^{2+} pathway in neural circuits, whose IP-Ca^{2+} system is synergistically regulated by adenosine. Thus, in these pathways, CBZ's acute effects would resemble the postulated mechanism of action of lithium. However, the time course of the clinical response to CBZ in affective disorders suggests that the biochemical effects of prolonged treatment with CBZ rather than those of acute treatment must be considered as related to its mechanism of action. Chronic treatment with CBZ in vivo has been reported to induce upregulation of adenosine A_1 receptors in the brain (Daval et al. 1989). These supersensitive A_1 receptors are probably functional, because at least the A_1 supersensitivity induced by chronic treatment with theophylline results in an increased sensitivity to adenosine in hippocampal slices (Lupica et al. 1991).

Upregulation of A_1 receptors by chronic CBZ treatment is also observed in cultured astrocytes. However, this effect is seen only in astrocyte cultures that express very low basal levels of A_1-receptor mRNA like those derived from cerebellum or striatum, whereas astrocyte cultures that express high levels of A_1-receptor mRNA (derived from cortex, hippocampus, tegmentum, and thalamus) show no substantial upregulation of A_1 receptors by chronic CBZ treatment (Biber et al. 1999). Astrocyte cultures with low basal A_1-receptor expression, which show no A_1-receptor–mediated potentiation of PLC activity (exemplified for striatum in Figure 14–1), are induced to exhibit this property by chronic CBZ treatment. On the other hand, the potentiation of PLC activity in cultures with high basal A_1-receptor expression (Figure 14–1) is not influenced by chronic CBZ treatment (Biber et al. 1999). In contrast, chronic CBZ treatment does not alter A_1-mediated inhibition of cAMP formation in cultures with low or high basal A_1 expression (Biber et al. 1999). These (Biber et al. 1999) and additional data (Biber et al. 1997) indicate that potentiation of PLC activity via A_1 receptors requires activation of many more A_1 receptors than does inhibition of adenylate cyclase. This is a result of the much lower affinity of $\beta\gamma$-subunits, which mediate the effect of A_1 activation on PLC, as compared with α-subunits (Biber et al. 1997). Consequently, upregulaton of A_1 receptors by CBZ might profoundly alter their signal transduction in areas of the brain in which A_1-receptor expression is low.

Upregulation of the A_1 receptors that cause the synergistic effect on the IP-Ca^{2+} system would tend to compensate the antagonistic effect of CBZ. Thus, under normal conditions and in the further presence of CBZ, its antagonistic effect should be approximately balanced by the upregulation of the A_1 receptors.

We have argued previously (van Calker and Berger 1993) that pathologically exaggerated neuronal activity, which is presumably involved in the pathophysiology of affective disorders, might lead to an increased extracellular accumulation of adenosine to concentrations high enough to totally override the antagonistic effect of CBZ. Thus, adenosine's activity at A_1 receptors would be selectively increased only in pathologically overactive neural pathways (van Calker and Berger 1993). Such a mechanism would, however, if applicable to the A_1 receptors that mediate the synergistic response, imply an increased rather than a decreased signaling via the IP-Ca^{2+} system after chronic treatment with CBZ, in direct contrast to the postulated mode of action of lithium.

To explain this apparent paradox, several points must be kept in mind. The results reviewed above were obtained with cultured astrocytes. It is not known how A_1 receptors regulate PLC activity in neurons and how this might be influenced by chronic CBZ treatment. Furthermore, activation of A_1 receptors not only potentiates but also inhibits the neurotransmitter-induced activation of the IP-Ca^{2+} system. The effect of these two opposite actions varies with the species, the brain region, and even the neurotransmitter involved (see section, "Modulation of the Neurotransmitter-Stimulated Generation of Second Messengers From Inositol Phospholipids in the Brain by Adenosine Receptors," earlier in this chapter). Whether CBZ also antagonizes the inhibitory action of adenosine is currently unknown. If it does, chronic CBZ treatment would, via upregulation of A_1 receptors, induce an attenuation of the IP-Ca^{2+} signaling in those brain areas and pathways in which the inhibitory effect of A_1 receptors predominates. This effect, by the same reasoning, would be restricted to pathologically overactive pathways. It is therefore tempting to speculate that chronic treatment with CBZ might induce an increase in signaling via the IP-Ca^{2+} system in some brain areas and neuronal pathways but a decrease in others. Indeed, indications suggest that the lithium-induced depletion of inositol (and, by inference, its dampening effect on the IP-Ca^{2+} system) after chronic treatment may be restricted to confined areas such as hypothalamus (Lubrich et al. 1997) or even neural pathways of the brain (for review, see Jope and Williams 1994; van Calker 1999).

CONCLUSION

The two properties of adenosine in the brain—its action as the brain's endogenous inhibitor of pathologically exaggerated neuronal activity and its presumed role as a modulator of neuronal plasticity—appear to be uniquely designed to fulfill an antibipolar function. Overactivity of certain neural pathways presumably causes some of the symptoms of affective disorders, and a progressive sensitization of certain neural pathways is thought to be instrumental to the increase in the frequency and severity of episodes, which occurs during the course of affective illness (Post 1992). Thus, adenosine and adenosine receptors might be envisaged as candidate targets for the action of antibipolar treatments. We have shown that at least one established antibipolar drug, CBZ, acts as a specific antagonist of adenosine A_1 receptors. We have postulated that chronic treatment with CBZ should, via consequent upregulation of A_1 receptors, increase the effect of adenosine in a manner selective for pathologically overactive neural circuits. The two opposite effects of A_1 receptors, which vary depending on the brain region and the neurotransmitter involved, imply that CBZ might differentially affect the function of the IP-Ca^{2+} system in distinct neural pathways. This highlights the need to conduct further studies on the mechanism of action of antibipolar drugs, with an enhanced consideration of possible region-specific actions, as already noted in the case of lithium's effects on IP-Ca^{2+} signaling (for review, see van Calker 1999; van Calker and Belmaker, in press).

REFERENCES

Alzheimer C, Sutor B, ten Bruggencate G: Disinhibition of hippocampal CA3 neurons induced by suppression of an adenosine A_1 receptor-mediated inhibitory tonus: pre- and postsynaptic components. Neuroscience 57:565–575, 1993

Atack JR, Broughton HB, Pollack SJ: Inositol monophosphatase—a putative target for Li^+ in the treatment of bipolar disorder. Trends Neurosci 18:343–349, 1995

Berridge MJ, Irvine RF: Inositol phosphates and cell signalling. Nature 341:197–205, 1989

Berridge MJ, Downes CP, Hanley MR: Neural and developmental actions of lithium: an unifying hypothesis. Cell 59:411–419, 1989

Biber K, Walden J, Gebicke-Härter P, et al: Carbamazepine inhibits the potentiation by adenosine analogues of agonist-induced inositol phosphate formation in astrocyte cultures. Biol Psychiatry 40:563–567, 1996

Biber K, Gebicke-Härter P, Berger M, et al: Adenosine A_1-receptor-mediated second-messenger responses in rat astrocyte cultures depend on the levels of receptor mRNA. J Neurosci 17:4956–4964, 1997

Biber K, Fiebich B, Gebicke-Härter PJ, et al: Carbamazepine-induced upregulation of adenosine A_1-receptors in astrocyte cultures affects coupling to the phosphoinositol signaling pathway. Neuropsychopharmacology 20:271–278, 1999

Bohus M, Förstner U, Kiefer C, et al: Increased sensitivity of the inositol-phospholipid-system in neutrophils from patients with acute major depressive episodes. Psychiatry Res 65:45–51, 1996

Catteral WA: Common modes of drug action on Na^+ channels: local anesthetics, antiarrhythmics and anticonvulsants. Trends Pharmacol Sci 8:57–65, 1987

Cooper DMF, Boyajian CL: Regulatory properties of adenosine A_1 receptors in the CNS and peripheral tissue, in Adenosine Receptors in the Nervous System. Edited by Ribeiro JA. London, Taylor & Francis, 1989, pp 103–112

Craig CG, White TD: N-methyl-D-aspartate– and non-N-methyl-D-aspartate–evoked adenosine release from rat cortical slices: distinct purinergic sources and mechanisms of release. J Neurochem 60:1073–1080, 1993

Daval JL, Deckert J, Weiss SRB, et al: Upregulation of adenosine A_1-receptors and forskolin binding sites following chronic treatment with caffeine or carbamazepine. Epilepsia 30:26–31, 1989

Delahunty TM, Cronin MJ, Linden J: Regulation of GH3-cell function via adenosine A_1-receptors: inhibition of prolactin release, cyclic AMP production and inositol phosphate generation. Biochem J 255:69–77, 1988

Delumeau JC, Tencé M, Marin P, et al: Synergistic regulation of cytosolic Ca^{2+} concentration by adenosine and α1-adrenergic agonists in mouse striatal astrocytes. Eur J Neurosci 3:593–650, 1991

Dickenson JM, Hill SJ: Interactions between adenosine A1-receptors and histamine H1-receptors. Int J Biochem 26:959–969, 1994

Dragunow M: Purinergic mechanisms in epilepsy. Prog Neurobiol 31:85–108, 1988

Dubovsky SL: Calcium antagonists in manic depressive illness. Neuropsychobiology 27:184–192, 1993

Dunwiddie TV: The physiological role of adenosine in the central nervous system. Int Rev Neurobiol 27:63–139, 1985

Durcan MJ, Morgan PF: Prospective role of adenosine and adenosinergic systems in psychiatric disorders. Psychol Med 20:475–486, 1990

Eckert A, Gann H, Riemann D, et al: Elevated intracellular calcium levels after 5-HT_2 receptor stimulation in platelets of depressed patients. Biol Psychiatry 34:565–568, 1993

El-Etr M, Cordier J, Glowinski J, et al: A neuroglial cooperativity is required for the potentiation by 2-chloroadenosine of the muscarinic-sensitive phospholipase C in the striatum. J Neurosci 9:1473–1480, 1989a

El-Etr M, Cordier J, Torrens Y, et al: Pharmacological and functional heterogeneity of astrocytes: regional differences in phospholipase C stimulation by neuromediators. J Neurochem 52:981–984, 1989b

Elphick M, Taghavi Z, Powell T, et al: Alteration of inositol phospholipid metabolism in rat cortex by lithium but not carbamazepine. Eur J Pharmacol 156:411–414, 1988

Förstner U, Bohus M, Gebicke-Härter PJ, et al: Chronic lithium treatment decreases the agonist-stimulated accumulation of cytosolic free calcium in neutrophils from manic depressive patients. Eur Arch Psychiatry Clin Neurosci 243:240–243, 1994

Fredholm B, Abbracchio M, Burnstock G, et al: Nomenclature and classification of purinoceptors. Pharmacol Rev 46:143–156, 1994

Glowinski J, Marin P, Tence M, et al: Glial receptors and their intervention in astrocyto-astrocytic and astrocyto-neuronal interactions. Glia 11:201–208, 1994

Goodwin FK, Jamison KR: Manic-Depressive Illness. New York, Oxford University Press, 1990

Greene R, Haas H: The electrophysiology of adenosine in the mammalian central nervous system. Prog Neurobiol 36:329–341, 1991

Greil W, Steber R, van Calker D: The agonist-stimulated accumulation of inositol phosphates is attenuated in neutrophils from male patients under chronic lithium therapy. Biol Psychiatry 30:443–451, 1991

Jope R, Williams M: Lithium and brain signal transduction systems. Biochem Pharmacol 47:429–441, 1994

Kusumi I, Koyoma T, Yamashita I: Serotonin-stimulated Ca^{++} response is increased in the blood platelets of depressed patients. Biol Psychiatry 30:310–312, 1991

Londos C, Cooper DM, Wolff J: Subclasses of external adenosine receptors. Proc Natl Acad Sci U S A 77:2551–2555, 1980

Lubrich B, Patishi Y, Kofman O, et al: Lithium-induced inositol depletion in rat brain after chronic treatment is restricted to the hypothalamus. Mol Psychiatry 2:407–412, 1997

Lupica CR, Jarvis MF, Berman RF: Chronic theophylline treatment in vivo increases high affinity adenosine A_1 receptor binding and sensitivity to exogenous adenosine in the in vitro hippocampal slice. Brain Res 542:55–62, 1991

McDermott EE, Logan SD: Inhibition of agonist-stimulated inositol lipid metabolism by the anticonvulsant carbamazepine in rat hippocampus. Br J Pharmacol 98:581–589, 1989

Mendonca de A, Ribeiro JA: Adenosine inhibits the NMDA receptor-mediated excitatory postsynaptic potential in the hippocampus. Brain Res 606:351–356, 1993

Mikuni M, Kusumi I, Kagaka A, et al: Increased 5-HT-2 receptor function as measured by serotonin-stimulated phosphoinositide hydrolysis in platelets of depressed patients. Biol Psychiatry 15:49–56, 1991

Nahorski SR, Ragan CI, Challiss RAJ: Lithium and the phosphoinositide cycle: an example of uncompetitive inhibition and its pharmacological consequences. Trends Pharmacol Sci 12:297–303, 1991

Newby AC: Adenosine and the concept of "retaliatory metabolites." Trends Biochem Sci 3:42–44, 1984

Pazzaglia PJ, Post RM, Ketter TA, et al: Preliminary controlled trial of nimodipine in ultra rapid cycling affective dysregulation. Psychiatry Res 49:257–272, 1993

Petcoff D, Cooper D: Adenosine receptor agonists inhibit inositol phosphate accumulation in rat striatal slices. Eur J Pharmacol 137:269–271, 1987

Post RM: The transduction of psychosocial stress into the neurobiology of recurrent affective disorder. Am J Psychiatry 149:999–1010, 1992

Rudolphi KA, Schubert P, Parkinson FE, et al: Neuroprotective role of adenosine in cerebral ischaemia. Trends Pharmacol Sci 13:439–445, 1992

Solomon DA, Keitner GI, Miller IW, et al: Course of illness and maintenance treatments for patients with bipolar disorders. J Clin Psychiatry 56:5–13, 1995

van Calker D: Lithium and cellular signal transduction, in Lithium: 50 Years of Psychopharmacology. Edited by Birch NJ, Becker RW, Gallicio VS. Cheshire, CT, Weidner Publishing, 1999, pp 136–153

van Calker D, Belmaker RH: The high affinity inositol transport system—implications for the pathophysiology and treatment of bipolar disorders. Bipolar Disorders (in press)

van Calker D, Berger M: Possible role of adenosine receptors in psychiatric diseases. Drug Development Research 28:354–358, 1993

van Calker D, Müller M, Hamprecht B: Adenosine regulates via two different types of receptors the accumulation of cyclic AMP in cultured brain cells. J Neurochem 33:999–1005, 1979

van Calker D, Steber R, Klotz K, et al: Carbamazepine distinguishes between adenosine receptors that mediate different second messenger responses. Eur J Pharmacol Mol Pharmacol Sect 206:285–290, 1991 van Calker D, Förstner U, Bohus M, et al: Increased sensitivity to agonist stimulation of the Ca^{++} response in neutrophils of manic depressive patients: effect of lithium therapy. Neuropsychobiology 27:180–183, 1993

von Wegerer J, van Calker D, Berger M, et al: Augmentation of GABA-B induced field potential changes by carbamazepine in the hippocampus. Comp Biochem Physiol 116C:227–232, 1998

Walden J, Grunze H, Mayer A, et al: Calcium antagonistic effects of carbamazepine in epilepsies and affective psychoses. Neuropsychobiology 27:171–175, 1993

Walden J, Fritze J, van Calker D, et al: A calcium antagonist for the treatment of depressive episodes: single case reports. J Psychiatr Res 29:71–76, 1995

Weiss SRB, Post RM: Contingent tolerance to carbamazepine: a peripheral benzodiazepine mechanism. Eur J Pharmacol 193:159–163, 1991

Williams M: Purinoceptors in central nervous system function, in Psychopharmacology: The Fourth Generation of Progress. Edited by Bloom FE, Kupfer DJ. New York, Raven, 1995, pp 643–655

CHAPTER 15

CLINICAL AND BIOLOGICAL INVESTIGATION OF MANIA FOLLOWING LITHIUM WITHDRAWAL

G. M. Goodwin, D.Phil., F.R.C.P.Edin., F.R.C.Psych.

It is conventional to start lithium treatment in bipolar patients after two illnesses within 2 years or three illnesses in 5 years. The factors inhibiting its use are the acknowledged danger in overdose, side effects and associated inconveniences to the patient, and uncertainty about the subsequent course of the illness (F. K. Goodwin and Jamison 1990). What is not commonly considered are the implications of stopping treatment prematurely and whether this may do harm (G. M. Goodwin 1994).

MANIC RELAPSE AFTER LITHIUM WITHDRAWAL IN BIPOLAR PATIENTS

Whether early manic relapse occurs after lithium discontinuation has been controversial, but early recurrence of affective illness after lithium discontinuation in stable patients was reviewed in detail by Suppes et al. (1991). This study offers a quantitative analysis of all of the existing reports, with additional unpublished data. Such analyses are preferable to selective, qualitative reviews of the research literature, which can be highly misleading and deflect argument away from the evidence and toward differences of opinion (Mann 1990). The

compared with that of clinically similar control subjects not given lithium showed no advantage of the intention to treat with lithium in the first 2 years, although some advantage did appear at 2–10 years after starting lithium (Markar and Mander 1989). By this time, however, most patients in the original sample from both groups had had recurrences. The simplest explanation is that many patients discontinue lithium within 2 years, have recurrences on withdrawal, and negate the advantages conferred on those who do persevere long term with adequate treatment.

The present argument appears not to apply as strongly to the use of lithium in recurrent unipolar depression, because no comparable evidence exists for a withdrawal syndrome (Souza et al. 1990; Suppes et al. 1991), or indeed in bipolar patients who do not have bipolar I type illness with clear-cut, clinically significant manic episodes (Sashidaran and McGuire 1983; Suppes et al. 1991). Withdrawal may nevertheless be associated with a return to an increased risk of depressive recurrence over time.

Three years is probably the minimum length of time that should be used to treat bipolar I disorder with lithium. Discontinuation after that time will depend on the usual balance of clinical judgments, but even when bipolar patients are treated successfully for long periods, are definitely compliant with treatment, and experience mood stability, withdrawal is still very likely to precipitate a manic recurrence (Mander and Loudon 1988). In addition, withdrawal in stable patients may carry the more deleterious additional risk of subsequent lithium refractoriness (Post et al. 1992). It is understandable that physicians are ambivalent about persuading patients to accept lithium treatment indefinitely. Unfortunately, to compromise with a treatment strategy that is too short term may be worse than useless.

BIOLOGICAL INVESTIGATION OF MANIA FOLLOWING LITHIUM WITHDRAWAL

The state of mania is probably the least studied and most poorly understood of the major psychiatric disorders. Withdrawal mania offers an important experimental opportunity because consent to and understanding of any proposed investigation can be obtained prospectively when subjects are euthymic.

Our first study in this area was guided by the association between endocrine disease and affective illness. Hyperthyroidism may precipitate affective illness (Lishman 1978), as indeed may exogenous or endogenous steroid excess (Boston Collaborative Drug Surveillance Program 1972). It follows that changes in hormone secretion after lithium withdrawal may, in fact, provoke mania. Lithium prophylaxis in bipolar patients appears to be associated with a direct inhibitory effect on the secretion of thyroxine (T_4) by the thyroid gland. Many studies have shown that this inhibition results in abnormal laboratory findings, with reduced plasma levels of T_4 and thyroid-stimulating hormone (TSH) in patients who are clinically euthyroid (Myers et al. 1985; Perrild et al. 1984; Schou 1976; Transbol et al. 1978; Villeneuve et al. 1974). The effects of long-term lithium treatment on cortisol secretion are much less established, with reports of either increases (Noyes et al. 1971; Platman and Fieve 1968), no change (Brooksbank and Coppen 1967; Sachar et al. 1970), or decreases in plasma cortisol levels during lithium treatment (Muehlbauer and Mueller-Oerlinghausen 1985; Smigan and Perris 1984). Most studies examined the effects of starting lithium and may have been confused by the hormonal effects of acute illness.

Our group (Souza et al. 1991) found that T_4 concentrations increased, TSH levels decreased, and cortisol levels also declined after lithium withdrawal (Table 15–1). The changes in T_4 and TSH were within the reference range (T_4 = 60–145 nmol/L; TSH = 0.1–5.6 mU/L). When T_4, TSH, and cortisol levels in those patients who relapsed (change in Modified Mania Rating Scale score greater than 20) were compared with levels in those who did not relapse, no differences were discernible (Table 15–1). The rebound increase in T_4 levels and reduced TSH levels in bipolar patients after lithium withdrawal is the corollary of many other studies describing decreased thyroid function during lithium treatment. This investigation allowed for the first time a direct comparison between the appearance of symptoms following lithium withdrawal and endocrine levels. No evidence supports the view that the absolute changes in endocrine levels predict relapse. However, changes in thy-

Table 15–1. Plasma thyroxine (T_4), thyroid-stimulating hormone (TSH), and cortisol concentrations [mean ± (SD)] in groups of bipolar patients who relapsed or remained well before and after lithium discontinuation

	Before discontinuation				**After discontinuation**			
	Relapsed		**Well**		**Relapsed**		**Well**	
T_4 (nmol/L)	84	(9)	100	(19)	102	(19)	123	(39)
TSH (mU/L)	1.9	(0.3)	2.1	(1.6)	1.4	(0.9)	0.9	(0.9)
Cortisol (nmol/L)	315	(176)	240	(40)	222	(70)	261	(80)

Note. There were statistically significant increases in T_4 and decreases in TSH after lithium withdrawal. The cortisol changes were not statistically significant.
Source. Data from Souza et al. 1991.

roid levels and indeed cortisol levels may contribute to the increased risk of relapse in those patients who are more sensitive to their psychotropic actions.

RELATIONSHIP BETWEEN BRAIN PERFUSION AND MANIC SYMPTOMS

We published one of the first descriptions of the uptake into brain of ^{99m}Tc-exametazime in patients younger than 65 years with major depression (Austin et al. 1992). ^{99m}Tc-exametazime is an intravenous ligand taken up in proportion to regional cerebral blood flow and trapped nonreversibly (Neirinckx et al. 1987). This allows single photon emission computed tomography examination of regional brain uptake of the tracer, which under normal conditions will be closely yoked to substrate demand or regional brain metabolism. The method is important because of its potential application in relatively large samples of patients with psychiatric disorders.

Imaging with a single-slice multidetector dedicated head scanner (Multi-X 810, Strichman Medical Equipment Inc., Boston, MA) was used in bipolar subjects. The maximal in-slice resolution of the scanner is 7.5 mm (full-width half-maximum) by 15-mm slice thickness. An indwelling intravenous catheter was inserted into an arm vein 15–30 minutes before the injection of 250–500 MBq of ^{99m}Tc-exametazime over 30 seconds. During and for 5 minutes after injection, patients were required to lie still and silent with eyes patched and ears unplugged; background noise was kept to a minimum. The subject's head was then placed in a molded headrest, positioned with the help of two crossed light beams, and fixed with two pressure pads over the zygomatic arches. Slices were acquired parallel to the orbitomeatal line. Two slices were chosen for analysis approximately 4 and 6 cm above the orbitomeatal line. All analyses were performed blind to the clinical details and indifferent to the biological findings but not to the order of the pairs of scans that were analyzed together. Regions of interest were drawn in advance from a standard brain atlas (Talairach et al. 1988); the method has been illustrated previously in Figure 1 of Austin et al. (1992). The regions outlined in the lower slice were anterior cingulate, frontal, anterior temporal, middle temporal, and posterior cingulate cortex; and caudate, putamen, and thalamus on the right and left sides of the brain. A symmetrical region including the occipital and calcarine cortex bilaterally was drawn as a reference area. A corresponding template for the higher slice identified anterior cingulate, frontal, parietal, and posterior cingulate areas with a bilateral reference area in the occipital region. Templates could be linearly deformed to fit the cortical rim, which was defined as 40% maximum counts in the slice. The mean uptake for each slice was chosen for normalization so that uptake into each individual region of interest was expressed as a ratio. Correlations between the tracer uptake and the severity of manic symptoms were calculated with Spearman's test. All significance levels are given two-tailed. Correlations are presented uncorrected for multiple comparisons because this is an essentially exploratory study.

The patients were required to be clinically euthymic and on lithium prophylaxis for at least 1 year. Patients with physical illness and physical complications of lithium treatment were not included in the study. The study consisted of three phases, each lasting 4 weeks. During the first phase, patients were stabilized on lithium carbonate (Camcolit, 400-mg tablets), and baseline clinical ratings were obtained. During the second and third phases, patients were randomized double-blind to receive either 4 weeks of lithium followed by 4 weeks of placebo or 8 weeks of placebo. Clinical assessment of patients was done every week, and symptoms of mania were rated with the Modified Mania Rating Scale; this was a separate study from that of Mander and Loudon (1988) but followed a similar design (see Mander and Loudon 1988 for more complete details). Patients were scanned in the first phase of the study while still taking lithium. Eight of 14 patients developed manic symptoms during the placebo phase of the study, confirming the findings of Mander and Loudon (1988).

Figure 15–2 illustrates the preliminary findings for brain regions of interest showing significant correlations between tracer uptake and mania. A pattern of positive correlations is seen in the upper brain slice involving parietal regions bilaterally and frontal and occipital areas on the left side only for scans conducted before lithium withdrawal; an additional negative correlation is seen on the right caudate nucleus. These findings carry the interesting implication that the risk for mania after lithium withdrawal correlates with increased brain activity, especially in parietal areas, in the scan before lithium withdrawal. The scan suggests that the activity of the brain before withdrawal is a guide to subsequent events of clinical significance. In any case, imaging studies are likely to cast further light on the relation between mood disorder and its associated behavioral disturbance. Extension of this methodology to the investigation of ligand displacement in different mood states will allow pharmacological and tographical mapping of mania.

CONCLUSION

The investigation of lithium withdrawal mania has both theoretical and practical implications. The investigation of the biology of mania is only really feasi-

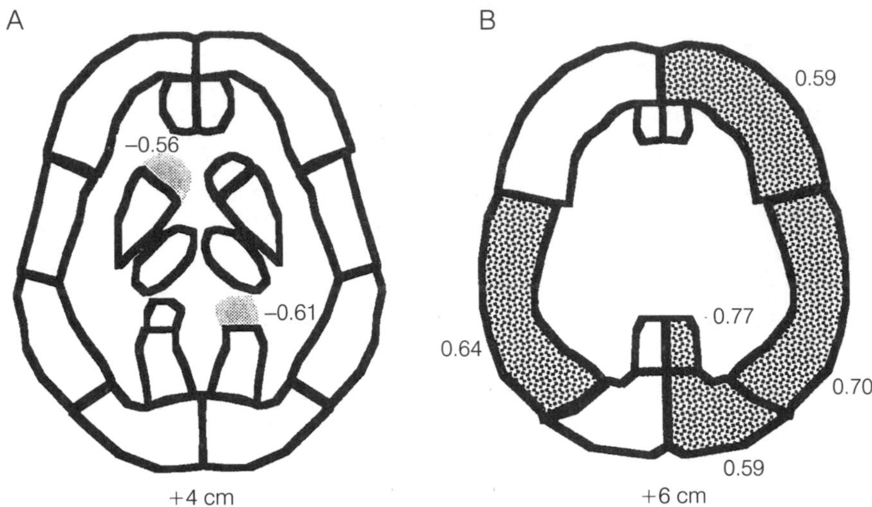

Figure 15–2. Significant correlations ($P < 0.05$) in the preliminary comparison of region of interest data from prewithdrawal ^{99m}Tc-exametazime uptake and subsequent manic severity. Heavy stippling shows positive associations, and light stippling shows negative associations, in two selected slices, (A) 4 cm and (B) 6 cm above the orbitomeatal line. Further experimental details of how the template was employed are given in the text and in Austin et al. 1992.

ble as the predictable aftermath of lithium withdrawal. It promises to be fruitful but is now underutilized. More practically, it may be argued that lithium should not be introduced for the prophylactic treatment of bipolar illness unless or until the physician and patient understand that it must be used for a minimum of 2 years (G. M. Goodwin 1994). Without such agreement, no worthwhile benefit is likely to result for the individual patient treated for a shorter time. Instead, premature recurrence of mania may be the unwanted result when lithium is abruptly discontinued.

REFERENCES

Austin M-P, Dougall N, Ross M, et al: Single photon emission tomography with ^{99m}Tc-Exametazime in major depression and the pattern of brain activity underlying the psychotic/neurotic continuum. J Affect Disord 26:31–44, 1992

Boston Collaborative Drug Surveillance Program: Acute adverse reactions to prednisone in relation to dosage. Clin Pharmacol Ther 13:694–698, 1972

Brooksbank BWL, Coppen A: Plasma 11-hydroxycorticosteroids in affective disorders. Br J Psychiatry 113:395–404, 1967

Dickson WE, Kendell RE: Does maintenance lithium therapy prevent recurrences of mania under ordinary clinical conditions? Psychol Med 16:521–530, 1986

Goodwin FK, Jamison KR: Manic-Depressive Illness. New York, Oxford University Press, 1990

Goodwin GM: The recurrence of mania after lithium withdrawal: implications for the use of lithium in the treatment of bipolar affective disorder. Br J Psychiatry 164:149–152, 1994

Lishman WA: Organic Psychiatry. Oxford, England, Blackwell Scientific, 1978

Mander AJ: Is there a lithium withdrawal syndrome? Br J Psychiatry 149:498–501, 1986

Mander AJ, Loudon JB: Rapid recurrence of mania following abrupt discontinuation of lithium. Lancet 2:15–17, 1988

Mann C: Meta-analysis in the breech. Science 249:476–480, 1990

Markar HR, Mander AJ: Efficacy of lithium prophylaxis in clinical practice. Br J Psychiatry 155:496–500, 1989

Muehlbauer HD, Mueller-Oerlinghausen B: Fenfluramine stimulation of serum cortisol in patients with major affective disorders and healthy controls: further evidence for a central serotonergic action of lithium in man. J Neural Transm 61:81–94, 1985

Myers DH, Carter RA, Burns BH, et al: A prospective study of the effects of lithium on thyroid function and on the prevalence of antithyroid antibodies. Psychol Med 15:55–61, 1985

Neirinckx RD, Canning LR, Piper IM, et al: Technetium-99m D,1-HMPAO: a new radiopharmaceutical for SPECT imaging of regional cerebral blood perfusion. J Nucl Med 28:191–202, 1987

Noyes R, Ringdahl IC, Andreasen NJC: Effect of lithium citrate on adrenocortical activity in manic depressive illness. Compr Psychiatry 12:337–347, 1971

Perrild H, Hegedius L, Arnung K: Sex related goitogenic effect of lithium carbonate in healthy young volunteers. Acta Endocrinologica 106:203–208, 1984

Platman SR, Fieve RR: Lithium carbonate and plasma cortisol response in affective disorders. Arch Gen Psychiatry 18:591–594, 1968

Post RM, Leverich GS, Altshuler L, et al: Lithium discontinuation induced refractoriness: preliminary observations. Am J Psychiatry 149:1727–1729, 1992

Sachar EJ, Hellman L, Kream J, et al: Effects of lithium carbonate therapy on adrenocortical activity. Arch Gen Psychiatry 22:304–307, 1970

Sashidaran SP, McGuire RJ: Recurrence of affective illness after withdrawal of long-term lithium treatment. Acta Psychiatr Scand 68:126–133, 1983

Schou M: Pharmacology and toxicology of lithium, in Annual Review of Pharmacology and Toxicology. Edited by Elliot HW, George G, Okun R. Palo Alto, CA, Annual Reviews, 1976, pp 231–243

Smigan L, Perris C: Cortisol changes in long-term lithium therapy. Neuropsychobiology 11:219–223, 1984

Souza FGM, Mander AJ, Goodwin GM: The efficacy of lithium in prophylaxis of unipolar depression: evidence from its discontinuation. Br J Psychiatry 157:718–722, 1990

Souza FGM, Mander AJ, Foggo M, et al: The effects of lithium discontinuation and the non-effect of oral inositol upon thyroid hormones and cortisol in patients with bipolar affective disorder. J Affect Disord 22:165–170, 1991

Suppes T, Baldessarini RJ, Faedda GL, et al: Risk of recurrence following discontinuation of lithium treatment in bipolar disorder. Arch Gen Psychiatry 48:1082–1088, 1991

Symonds RL, Williams P: Lithium and the changing incidence of mania. Psychol Med 11:193–196, 1981

Talairach J, Zilkha G, Tournoux P, et al: Atlas d'Anatomie Stereotactique du Telencephale. Paris, Masson, 1988

Transbol I, Christiansen C, Baastrup PC: Endocrine effects of lithium, 1: hypothyroidism, its prevalence in long-term treated patients. Acta Endocrinologica 87:759–767, 1978

Villeneuve A, Gautier J, Jus A, et al: The effect of lithium on thyroid in man. International Journal of Clinical Psychology 9:75–80, 1974

CHAPTER 16

VALPROATE IN MANIA

Charles L. Bowden, M.D.

Valproate has been established as an effective treatment of mania in well-designed and executed studies (Bowden et al. 1994; Pope et al. 1991). In this chapter, I review the evidence of efficacy and safety from clinical trials, the spectrum of disorders in which valproate may be effective, and the pharmacodynamic properties of valproate.

Valproate was developed as an organic solvent by Burton (1881) and so used until a serendipitous observation of its ability to prevent experimentally induced seizures in laboratory rats (Meunier et al. 1975). First released as an antiepileptic drug in the 1960s, valproate was quickly observed to have antimanic and mood-stabilizing properties in persons with manic depression. Valproate was first reported as effective in the treatment of manic-depressive illness, or bipolar disorder, in 1966 (Lambert et al. 1966). Subsequent consistently positive clinician-driven reports were published over the next 20 years. Most studies focused on acute episode response in mania, although maintenance phase results also were consistently positive. A parallel development was that several studies made clear that the poor tolerability of lithium substantially impairs social and role function in more than 25% of patients and contributes to the poor compliance with lithium observed in more than one-third of lithium-treated patients and that long-term outcomes with lithium were unsatisfactory in one-third to one-half of patients, even when compliance and dosage were adequate (Goldberg et al. 1995; Murray et al. 1983; Swearer et al. 1988).

ACUTE MANIA

These intersecting developments contributed to the planning and conduct of two randomized, parallel-group, placebo-controlled trials of the divalproex form of valproate in hospitalized acutely manic patients. These studies had similar strengths of design. Diagnosis was determined by structured interviews, and behavioral rating of manic symptoms was done by trained raters. No neuroleptic drugs were allowed, and ancillary lorazepam was limited to the first week of the randomized trials and not allowed within 12 hours before behavioral ratings. The studies enrolled adults between ages 18 and 65 years.

The two studies also differed in important ways. The smaller study of 36 patients took place in one hospital, used one rater, and was limited to patients previously nonresponsive to or intolerant of lithium. Because of Institutional Review Board constraints, women of childbearing potential were excluded; thus, the sex distribution was atypical. Only 8 patients completed the trial, in part because of a priori criteria that allowed early termination of patients whose manic symptoms resolved or whose manic symptoms deteriorated (Pope et al. 1991). The second study of 179 patients is the largest randomized, placebo-controlled study of any treatment for mania and is the only randomized, blinded trial of lithium in acute mania (Bowden et al. 1994). Patients were enrolled regardless of prior response to lithium or carbamazepine. The study was conducted at eight academic medical centers to ensure that no unusual characteristics of patients associated with a single center contributed to the outcome.

Both studies found that divalproex was highly statistically superior to placebo, with evidence of responsiveness by day 5 of treatment in the Bowden et al. (1994) study. The magnitude of divalproex's superiority over placebo widened over the 3-week trial in both studies. The drug-placebo differences were quite large, representing both clinical and statistically significant differences (Bowden et al. 1996).

In the Bowden et al. (1994) study, the overall response of mania to divalproex and lithium did not differ. Equivalent and adequate dosages of divalproex and lithium were used, and adequate serum levels were attained. However, response was somewhat earlier in divalproex-treated patients, and the effect sizes of early and last visit changes in mania were larger for divalproex than for lithium (Bowden et al. 1996). Secondary analyses indicated that previous response to lithium was not associated with response to divalproex, whereas a recent poor response to lithium was associated with a poor response to lithium in the study, and a previous good response was associated with a good response (Bowden et al. 1994).

A higher percentage of lithium-treated patients than divalproex-treated patients dropped out of the Bowden et al. (1994) study because of drug intolerance (lithium, 11%; divalproex, 6%; placebo, 3%). Divalproex was generally better tolerated than lithium. The better tolerability of valproate compared with lithium was also observed in a recent 18-month trial by Lambert and Venaud (1992).

The results of these two well-designed studies are quite consistent with those of open studies or non-placebo-controlled studies of valproate in acute mania and indicate, at least for valproate, that open study data provide a relatively reliable indicator of the effects of treatment (Bowden et al. 1995). One factor contributing to the consistency of results is that the symptoms of acute mania are so specific that false-positive diagnostic cases are unlikely to be enrolled for study, and nonspecific symptom change is unlikely to be confused with recovery. The results do suggest, at least for valproate, that the preponderance of evidence regarding the effectiveness in mania will be reliable, but both open and much more methodologically difficult to conduct blinded, placebo-controlled studies are needed to advance the field.

SUBTYPES OF MANIA

Although patients with mixed manic features did significantly less well with lithium treatment, mixed and pure manic patients who received divalproex did equally well (Bowden 1995a). These favorable results with divalproex in mixed manic patients are consistent with those of other studies (Calabrese and Delucchi 1990; Freeman et al. 1992). The poor response of mixed mania to lithium is also consistent with results of other studies in both treatment of acute mania (Himmelhoch and Garfinkel 1986; Prien et al. 1988) and continuation treatment (Keller et al. 1986). The differences between mixed and pure mania are of scientific and practical interest, given evidence that biological characteristics may differ in these two equally common forms of mania. Hypercortisolism, especially morning elevations of cortisol following dexamethasone suppression, is consistently characteristic of mixed, but not pure, mania (Evans and Nemeroff 1983; Swann et al. 1992). Also, relatively higher excretion of norepinephrine characterizes mixed compared with pure manic patients (Swann et al. 1991). Clinically, manic episodes in youth, secondary mania, mania in the elderly, and mania comorbid with substance abuse all tend to have mixed features. Mixed mania is recognizable behaviorally by dysphoric mood, irritability, sadness, and pessimism, while reduced need for sleep, grandiosity, increased rate of speech, increased motor activity, and impaired judgment continue. That is, the patient has all of the clinical features of a manic episode plus concurrent depression. Although operational criteria are proffered in DSM-IV (American Psychiatric Association 1994), different criteria are likely to yield more prognostically useful groupings (McElroy et al. 1992).

Divalproex has been reported effective in open trials of patients with bipolar disorder who have concurrent substance abuse disorders, who are elderly, or who are adolescent (Brady and Sonne 1995; Kahn et al. 1988; McFarland et al. 1990; Papatheodorou et al. 1995). Lithium is generally less effective in such forms of bipolar disorder (Goodwin and Jamison 1990; Himmelhoch and Garfinkel 1986; Papatheodorou et al. 1995).

MAINTENANCE THERAPY

Maintenance studies to assess for ability to prevent relapse to new episodes and long-term function are more difficult to conduct. One factor contributing to this difficulty is the risk of relapse on placebo, which may realistically discourage study participation by patients with more severe forms of bipolar disorder and requirements for strict protocol adherence, which is inherently difficult given bipolar symptomatology. The longer the duration of a trial, the greater the likelihood that factors unrelated to the randomly assigned treatment conditions will affect results. Add to this the difficulty in capturing the multiple negative outcomes (e.g., mania, hypomania, mixed states, rapid cycling), which make choice of any single outcome criterion only partially satisfactory. Open maintenance trials generally report effectiveness in approximately 50%–55% of patients taking valproate for periods of 6–24 months (Calabrese and Delucchi 1990; Puzynski and Klosiewicz 1984).

The study of Calabrese and Delucchi is particularly thorough, describing 1-year follow-up of patients initially selected for rapid-cycling bipolar disorder. More than 90% did well in the trial, with approximately 50% treated with divalproex alone and 50% treated with divalproex plus lithium. A randomized, open comparison of valproate and lithium reported generally good efficacy for both drugs over an 18-month period. However, the average number of episodes favored valproate (Lambert and Venaud 1992). Among the 4 patients changed to lithium for either clinical deterioration or adverse effects, 5 new illness episodes occurred subsequently, whereas among the 10 patients changed to valproate, only 1 new episode occurred.

BIPOLAR DEPRESSIVE EPISODES

Few studies have been reported of valproate's effectiveness in the depressed phase of bipolar disorder, but the percentage of responsive patients has been consistently less than 40%, suggesting that any benefits are infrequent and modest (Bowden 1995b). Some patients who have frequently recurring depressive episodes without clear-cut manic episodes are thought to have atypical forms of bipolar disorder (Goodwin and Jamison 1990). Case reports of response to valproate in such patients have been published (Mitchell 1991).

RELATIONSHIP OF SERUM LEVEL TO RESPONSE

Patients who achieved serum levels of valproate of 45 μg/mL or greater were 3–7 times as likely to respond on key behavioral dimensions as were patients who did not achieve such levels (Bowden et al. 1996). The multicenter study of divalproex, lithium, and placebo from which these results were obtained provided a strong test of serum level–response relationships. All patients were hospitalized to allow control of dosing and timing of venipuncture. During the first 5 days of the 21-day study, patients received fixed-dose regimens, thereby avoiding the confound of dosage increase in nonresponding patients, which vitiates results from flexible-dose trials. Results from analyses at day 5 and at the last evaluation were similar. The results also indicated that onset of three characteristic adverse effects associated with divalproex (nausea, vomiting, sedation) was strongly linked to serum valproate concentrations of 125 μg/mL or greater. For example, 2.9% of patients with levels in the range of 100–125 μg/mL reported nausea, compared with 27% of patients with levels greater than 125 μg/mL. These results are consistent with those of small studies of patients with bipolar disorder (Pope et al. 1991) and epilepsy (Hendriksen and Johannessen 1995).

The evidence of relatively early response of manic patients to divalproex prompted studies to assess the effectiveness and tolerability of an initial loading-dose strategy. An initial dose of 20 μg/kg body weight resulted in improvement within 1–4 days in a small open trial of hospitalized manic patients (Keck et al. 1993).

SPECTRUM OF EFFICACY OF VALPROATE

The remarkable effectiveness of valproate as an antimanic and mood-stabilizing drug has led to interest in assessing its effectiveness for other disorders that are comorbid with bipolar disorder or that share some of the phenomenological characteristics of bipolar disorder (e.g., episodicity, relatively rapid onset and offset of episodes, and relatively high frequency of recurrences). Migraine headache is present approximately 6 times as often in patients with bipolar disorder as would be expected by chance. Divalproex significantly reduces the frequency of migraine headaches and has received U.S. Food and Drug Administration (FDA) approval for this indication (Jensen et al. 1994). Divalproex has been reported as effective in patients with impulsive aggression (Lott et al. 1995; Sovner 1989). This episodic display of threats and violence is characteristic of patients with dementia, severe developmental disabilities, and mental retardation. Divalproex has been reported as effective in patients with panic attacks, although data are limited to case reports. Valproate also has aided in relieving bulimia. Substitution with lithium led to recrudescence, and reinstitution of valproate again controlled the bulimia (Herridge and Pope 1985). Cases of cyclothymia and mild but rapid-cycling forms of bipolar disorder also have been reported as effectively treated with divalproex (Jacobsen 1993; Lambert and Venaud 1992).

COMPARATIVE ISSUES

Valproate has several comparative advantages over lithium, which are likely to increase valproate's role in treatment of mania. Divalproex is better tolerated than lithium (Bowden et al. 1994; Lambert and Venaud 1992). Valproate is easier to prescribe than lithium, with earlier onset and a greater spread between the usually beneficial serum levels needed for response and the levels at which adverse effects become more problematic. Valproate may be prescribed in a loading-dose strategy, which is not feasible with either lithium or carbamazepine (Keck et al. 1993). Valproate appears to be effective in a broader spectrum of bipolar conditions compared with lithium. Valproate has particular advantages in the very young and the elderly, which are linked to both the more common occurrence of mixed mania in these age groups and the consequences of adverse effects of lithium in youth and the elderly. More studies of the role for valproate in maintenance treatment and studies of the relative efficacy of divalproex in combination with other mood stabilizers, which is strongly supported by case reports (Pope et al. 1991) and open trials (Calabrese and Delucchi 1990), are needed.

PHARMACODYNAMIC MECHANISMS

Pharmacodynamic mechanisms associated with the clinical effectiveness of valproate are not conclusively established. Valproate alters γ-aminobutyric acid (GABA)ergic function by its effects on aldehyde dehydrogenase, GABA release, and GABA uptake (Godin et al. 1969). The possible mechanism of GABA in alleviating mania or in stabilizing mood is not known. Disturbance in circadian biological rhythms has been suggested as a factor in precipitating manic episodes. GABA has inhibitory input into the suprachiasmatic nucleus, which is a primary chemical locus of melatonin activity, which in turn varies in relation to day-night cycles. In manic patients in the randomized comparison of divalproex with lithium and placebo reviewed earlier in this chapter, increased pretreatment serum GABA levels were significantly positively correlated with greater reduction in manic symptomatology among divalproex- but not lithium- or placebo-treated patients (Petty et al. 1995). Over the 3-week period of treatment, GABA levels decreased significantly among divalproex- but not lithium- or placebo-treated patients. The reduction in serum GABA levels was not significantly correlated with change in manic symptomatology from baseline to the end of treatment.

As discussed elsewhere in this volume (see Manji et al. and Lenox et al., Chapters 7 and 9, this volume), valproate alters several intraneuronal signaling systems, including protein kinase C activity, protein kinase C isozymes, and myristoylated alanine-rich C kinase substrate (MARCKS) protein. Several of these changes are also observed in similar systems in response to added lithium. It is of interest that the rapidity of the changes appears greater in divalproex- than in lithium-treated patients. The effects with valproate appear to be of somewhat greater magnitude than those with lithium. It is interesting to conjecture that these changes may contribute to the more rapid onset of clinical effectiveness of valproate.

REFERENCES

American Psychiatric Association: Diagnostic and Statistical Manual of Mental Disorders, 4th Edition. Washington, DC, American Psychiatric Association, 1994

Bowden CL: Predictors of response to divalproex and lithium. J Clin Psychiatry 56(S4):25–30, 1995a

Bowden CL: Treatment of bipolar disorder, in The American Psychiatric Press Textbook of Psychopharmacology. Edited by Schatzberg A, Nemeroff C. Washington, DC, American Psychiatric Press, 1995b, pp 603–614

Bowden CL, Brugger AM, Swann AC, et al: Efficacy of divalproex vs lithium and placebo in the treatment of mania. JAMA 271:918–924, 1994

Bowden CL, Calabrese JR, Wallin BA, et al: Who enters therapeutic trials? Illness characteristics of patients in clinical drug studies of mania. Psychopharmacol Bull 31:103–109, 1995

Bowden CL, Janicak PG, Orsulak P, et al: Relation of serum valproate concentration to response in mania. Am J Psychiatry 153:765–770, 1996

Brady KT, Sonne SC: The relationship between substance abuse and bipolar disorder. J Clin Psychiatry 56 (suppl 3):19–24, 1995

Burton BS: On the propyl derivatives and decomposition products of ethyl acetoacetate. American Chemical Journal 3:385–395, 1881

Calabrese JR, Delucchi GA: Spectrum of efficacy of valproate in 55 patients with rapid-cycling bipolar disorder. Am J Psychiatry 147:431–434, 1990

Evans DA, Nemeroff CB: The dexamethasone suppression test in mixed bipolar disorder. Am J Psychiatry 140:615–617, 1983

Freeman TW, Clothier JL, Pazzaglia P, et al: A double-blind comparison of valproate and lithium in the treatment of acute mania. Am J Psychiatry 149:108–111, 1992

Godin Y, Heiner L, Mark J, et al: Effect of di-N-propyl-acetate, an antiepileptic compound, on GABA metabolism. J Neurochem 16:869–873, 1969

Goldberg JF, Harrow M, Grossman LS: Recurrent affective syndromes in bipolar and unipolar mood disorders at follow-up. Br J Psychiatry 166:382–385, 1995

Goodwin FK, Jamison KR: Manic-Depressive Illness. New York, Oxford University Press, 1990

Hendriksen O, Johannessen SI: Clinical and pharmacokinetic observations on sodium valproate: a five year follow-up study on 100 children with epilepsy. Acta Neurol Scand 65:504–523, 1995

Herridge PL, Pope HG Jr: Treatment of bulimia and rapid-cycling bipolar disorder with sodium valproate: a case report. J Clin Psychopharmacol 5:229–230, 1985

Himmelhoch JM, Garfinkel ME: Sources of lithium resistance in mixed mania. Psychopharmacol Bull 22:613–620, 1986

Jacobsen FM: Low dose valproate: a new treatment for cyclothymia, mild rapid cycling disorders, and premenstrual syndrome. J Clin Psychiatry 54:229–234, 1993

Jensen R, Brinck T, Olesen J: Sodium valproate has a prophylactic effect in migraine without aura: a triple-blind, placebo-controlled crossover study. Neurology 44:647–651, 1994

Kahn D, Stevenson E, Douglas CJ: Effect of sodium valproate in three patients with organic brain syndromes. Am J Psychiatry 145:101–111, 1988

Keck PE Jr, McElroy SL, Tugrul KC, et al: Valproate oral loading in the treatment of acute mania. J Clin Psychiatry 54:305–308, 1993

Keller MB, Lavori PW, Coryell W, et al: Differential outcome of pure manic, mixed/cycling, and pure depressive episodes in patients with bipolar illness. JAMA 255:3138–3142, 1986

Lambert PA, Venaud G: Comparative study of valpromide versus lithium in the treatment of affective disorders. Nervure 5:57–65, 1992

Lambert PA, Cavaz G, Borselli S, et al: Action neuropsychotrope d'un nouvel anti-epileplique: Le Depamide. Annales Medico-Psychologiques 1:707–710, 1966

Lott AD, McElroy SL, Keys MA: Valproate in the treatment of behavioral agitation in elderly patients with dementia. J Neuropsychiatry Clin Neurosci 7:314–319, 1995

McElroy SL, Keck PE Jr, Pope HG, et al: Clinical and research implications of the diagnosis of dysphoric or mixed mania or hypomania. Am J Psychiatry 149:1633–1644, 1992

McFarland BH, Miller MR, Straumfjord AA: Valproate use in the older manic patient. J Clin Psychiatry 51:479–481, 1990

Meunier H, Carraz G, Meunier V, et al: Proprietes pharmacodynamiques de l'acide n-propylacetique. Therapie 18:435–438, 1975

Mitchell P: Valproate for rapid-cycling unipolar affective disorder. J Nerv Ment Dis 179:503–504, 1991

Murray N, Hopwood S, Balfour DJK, et al: The influence of age on lithium efficacy and side effects in out-patients. Psychol Med 13:53–60, 1983

Papatheodorou G, Kutcher SP, Katic M, et al: The efficacy and safety of divalproex sodium in the treatment of acute mania in adolescents and young adults. J Clin Psychopharmacol 15:110–116, 1995

Petty F, Rush AJ, Davis JM, et al: Plasma GABA predicts response to divalproex in mania. Biol Psychiatry 37:593–683, 1995

Pope HG Jr, McElroy SL, Keck PE Jr, et al: Valproate in the treatment of acute mania: a placebo-controlled study. Arch Gen Psychiatry 48:62–68, 1991

Prien RF, Himmelhoch JM, Kupfer DJ: Treatment of mixed mania. J Affect Disord 15:9–15, 1988

Puzynski S, Klosiewicz L: Valproic acid amide as a prophylactic agent in affective and schizoaffective disorders. Psychopharmacol Bull 20:151–159, 1984

Sovner R: The use of valproate in the treatment of mentally retarded persons with typical and atypical bipolar disorders. J Clin Psychiatry 50:40–43, 1989

Swann AC, Secunda SK, Koslow SH, et al: Mania: sympathoadrenal function and clinical state. Psychiatry Res 37:195–205, 1991

Swann AC, Stokes PE, Casper R, et al: Hypothalamic pituitary-adrenocortical function in mixed and pure mania. Acta Psychiatr Scand 85:270–274, 1992

Swearer JM, Drachman DA, O'Donnell BF, et al: Troublesome and disruptive behaviors in dementia: relationship to diagnosis and disease severity. J Am Geriatr Soc 36:784–790, 1988

CHAPTER 17

EFFICACY OF LAMOTRIGINE IN BIPOLAR DISORDER

Preliminary Data

Joseph R. Calabrese, M.D.

Lithium, valproate, and carbamazepine possess moderate to marked antimanic properties but only poor to moderate antidepressant effects (Calabrese et al. 1994). Increased morbidity is associated with the depressed and mixed phases of bipolar disorder, as well as the rapid-cycling pattern of presentation (Calabrese et al. 1993). The use of antidepressants puts bipolar patients at increased risk for drug-induced hypomania or mania and rapid cycling. There is a need to develop a mood stabilizer that has moderate to marked antidepressant efficacy with little or no increased risk for drug-induced mania and rapid cycling.

Two case reports have indicated that a recently released anticonvulsant, lamotrigine, may have efficacy in the treatment of bipolar disorder, particularly in the management of the depressed phase of the illness (Calabrese et al. 1996; Weisler et al. 1994). Lamotrigine was approved by the U.S. Food and Drug Administration (FDA) in December 1994 for use as adjunctive therapy in the treatment of partial seizures in adults with epilepsy. This drug has been studied in clinical trials in more than 3,000 patients with epilepsy and is marketed in more than 70 countries as an antiepileptic (Gilman 1995). Approximately 200,000 patients with epilepsy have been exposed to lamotrigine in clinical practice. It is believed to act by inhibiting the stimulated presynaptic release of glutamate and may have antidepressant and mood-stabilizing properties.

PHARMACOLOGY

Lamotrigine is structurally related to the antimalarial pyrimethamine but, in contrast to it, has potent anticonvulsant properties, weaker antifolate properties, and no hematological potential (see Figure 17–1). This drug appears structurally and pharmacologically unique. Its mechanism of action is fundamentally different from that of other anticonvulsant drugs. Lamotrigine inhibits sodium currents by selectively binding to the inactivated state of the sodium channel (Xie 1995). Lamotrigine subsequently suppresses the release of the excitatory amino acid glutamate. In addition, lamotrigine has been observed to inhibit cortical and amygdala kindling (Gilman 1995).

When compared with the currently available agents used in the management of bipolar disorder, lamotrigine appears to have unique pharmacokinetic features. It is absorbed rapidly (peak concentration, 2.5 hours) and has a comparatively long half-life (29 hours). It has no significant effect on the hepatic oxidase system and is almost entirely bioavailable (98%). It is moderately protein bound (55%) and has no effect on birth control pills. The available evidence suggests that it lacks teratogenicity, and routine monitoring chemistries, complete blood counts, and blood pressure, heart rate and electrocardiogram, and body weight measurements do not appear necessary. In the management of epilepsy, no correlation between blood level and efficacy is apparent. Special dosing considerations are required with the administration of lamotrigine because hepatic inducers, such as carbamazepine, accelerate the

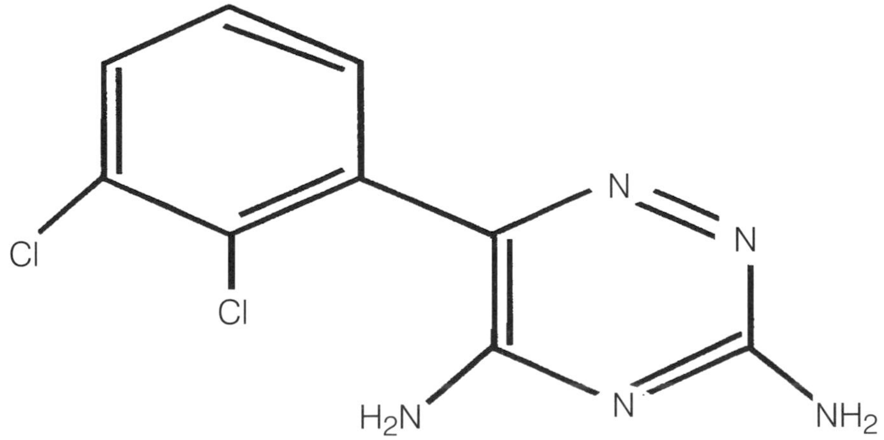

Figure 17–1. Chemical structure of lamotrigine: 6-(2,3-dichlorophenyl)-1,2,4-triazine-3,5-diamine.

metabolism of the drug, and hepatic inhibitors, such as valproate, inhibit its metabolism. Adverse events are usually mild and resolve without drug discontinuation. In order of decreasing frequency, the side effects associated with lamotrigine include dizziness, headaches, diplopia, ataxia, nausea and vomiting, somnolence and asthenia, and rash. Although the rash is usually mild to moderate and resolves without drug discontinuation, it can be serious and does lead to drug discontinuation. Drug discontinuations are most likely caused by rash and are usually associated with valproate use during the first 6 weeks of treatment. These more serious rashes are primarily erythematous, morbilliform, and generalized. Weight gain and tremors are not common. This observation suggests that lamotrigine may have properties that complement lithium and the other anticonvulsants in the treatment of bipolar disorder.

Two case reports involving three patients have led to the development of an ongoing study designed to evaluate the "spectrum of efficacy" of lamotrigine when used as add-on or monotherapy treatment of bipolar disorder in patients nonresponsive to or intolerant of pharmacotherapy (Calabrese et al. 1996; Weisler et al. 1994).

Initially, Weisler et al. (1994) reported on two cases of treatment-refractory bipolar disorder that responded to lamotrigine. The first involved a 77-year-old woman with recurrent major depression dating back to the 1930s. Since her first documented manic episode in 1985, she had failed many medication trials, including lithium, carbamazepine, divalproex, thiothixene, and many antidepressants. Although she experienced marked acute antidepressant efficacy from electroconvulsive therapy, she had to be given treatments no more than 2–3 weeks apart to maintain a response, thereby making this an impractical solution. She was admitted to the hospital in the depressed phase of the illness with catatonic symptoms; she was unable to speak, eat, or ambulate independently. Treatment with lamotrigine was initiated at 50 mg twice daily and then increased to 100 mg twice daily 1 week later. The patient began to show steady clinical improvement over the next few weeks and eventually experienced a complete remission of both depression and manic episodes. At the time of publication, her response was ongoing and had lasted longer than 9 months, the longest period of stability she had experienced in the past 4–5 years as documented by the patient and her family.

The second patient, a 43-year-old man, presented in the depressed phase of bipolar II disorder accompanied by rapid cycling (eight tandem cycles per year). After his condition did not respond to treatment with lithium, carbamazepine, divalproex, and many antidepressants, an augmentation trial of lamotrigine was begun. Lamotrigine was started at 25 mg every morning and 50 mg at bedtime, and this was added to lithium, 300 mg twice daily; bupropion, 75 mg/day; and levothyroxine, 0.05 mg/day. Within 7 days, the patient reported improvement in mood with increased energy. Over 3 months, the lamotrigine dose was gradually increased to 400 mg/day in divided doses, and the bupropion was discontinued. After 7 months of treatment, the patient experienced a relapse when he ran out of his lamotrigine supply; he relapsed into severe depression, as reflected by a total score of 34 on the 31-item Hamilton Rating Scale for Depression (Ham-D). After resuming his prior dose of lamotrigine for 1 week, his Ham-D score decreased to 2.

The starting dose and rate of escalation of lamotrigine were well tolerated in both patients described in the preceding paragraphs. However, the recommended rate of dose escalation is much slower and described further in the package insert.

More recently, Calabrese et al. (1996) systematically demonstrated marked acute and prophylactic bimodal mood-stabilizing properties in another bipolar patient with rapid cycling. This 49-year-old male disabled general contractor presented medication-free and in the depressed phase of bipolar I rapid-cycling disorder. He reported episodes of classic mania followed by a severe depression. During periods of classic mania, he reported foolish business ventures that left him hundreds of thousands of dollars in debt. The depression was accompanied by crying spells, decreased physical and sexual energy, irritability, and suicidal thoughts. Previously, he had failed a 3-year trial of lithium, a 4-year trial of fluoxetine monotherapy (which caused him to cycle into a high), and a 3-week trial of carbamazepine. The carbamazepine trial was complicated by intolerable nausea.

His rapid cycling started at age 14 years, and during the last 35 years, he noted that his depressions had become more frequent, longer, and more severe. His "highs" had become less frequent and severe but longer. His longest past depression continued for 180 days, and mania persisted for 60 days. Before his depressions assumed a circular pattern of cycling, they normally followed his highs. In the year prior to study entry, he experienced eight episodes without symptom-free euthymic intervals, four "highs," and four depressions.

Baseline ratings included scores on the 31-item Ham-D, Global Assessment Scale (GAS), and Schedule for Affective Disorders and Schizophrenia—Change Version (SADS-C) Mania Rating Scale (MRS), which were 46, 32, and 12, respectively; ratings were repeated at 1, 2, 4, 6, 8, 12, 16, and 20 weeks. Treatment was begun with lamotrigine monotherapy at 25 mg/day for 2 weeks, 50 mg/day for 2 weeks, 100 mg for 1 week, 150 mg for 1 week, and then 200 mg/day thereafter. During the first 20 weeks of treatment, the patient's Ham-D scores decreased as follows: 46, 36, 22, 30, 26, 22, 13, 16, 9. At the same time, his GAS score increased from 32 to 69. Side effects included fatigue and swelling of his lower extremities, which required treatment with furosemide. Over 12 months of follow-up, this patient continued taking lamotrigine. He remains euthymic without rapid cycling. This case also presents evidence of a potential acute and prophylactic antidepressant effect of lamotrigine in the absence of any mania-inducing properties in a rapid cycler who was nonresponsive to lithium monotherapy and predisposed to antidepressant-induced mania.

These two clinical reports provide preliminary data of lamotrigine's mood-stabilizing properties, particularly antidepressant effects. The following are preliminary data from a study that was designed to evaluate the "spectrum of efficacy" and safety of lamotrigine when used as add-on or monotherapy treatment of bipolar disorder nonresponsive to or intolerant of pharmacotherapy.

DRUG TRIAL DATA

Sixty-seven patients (mean age, 43.6 years; 61% female, 39% male) with treatment-refractory bipolar disorder (bipolar I disorder, 72%; bipolar II disorder, 25%; bipolar disorder not otherwise specified, 3%) underwent an open, prospective 12-month trial at five United States and European sites (Calabrese et al. 1999a). Fifty patients, most of whom were in the depressed phase of their illness, received lamotrigine as an add-on to other psychotropics, and 17 received lamotrigine monotherapy. The mean number of psychotropic medications to which lamotrigine was added was 2.2 (range, 1–5). Lamotrigine was used to augment lithium in 18 patients, carbamazepine in 6, valproate in 18, antidepressant medications in 18, and antipsychotic agents in 22. Concomitant psychotropic medications were not added and doses were not increased during lamotrigine titration; adjunctive chloral hydrate and lorazepam were permitted. The mean last dose of lamotrigine coadministered with anything but carbamazepine and divalproex was 142 mg/day, with carbamazepine was 169 mg/day, and with divalproex was 83 mg/day.

The 31-item Ham-D, SADS-C MRS, GAS, and Clinical Global Impression (CGI) Scale were completed every 2–4 weeks. Fifty patients have been exposed to lamotrigine for an average of 88.4 days and continue in the trial. Six have dropped out because of lack of efficacy and 8 because of adverse events (6 because of rashes). In the 39 patients (58%) who presented in the depressed phase of their disorder, the mean baseline total Ham-D score was 31.5 ± 9.2 and decreased to 18.0 ± 15.2 (Mann-Whitney test, $P < 0.0001$) on their most recent evaluation (see Figure 17–2). Nine of the 39 patients (23%) showed moderate improvement (25%–49% decrease in Ham-D scores), and 18 (46%)

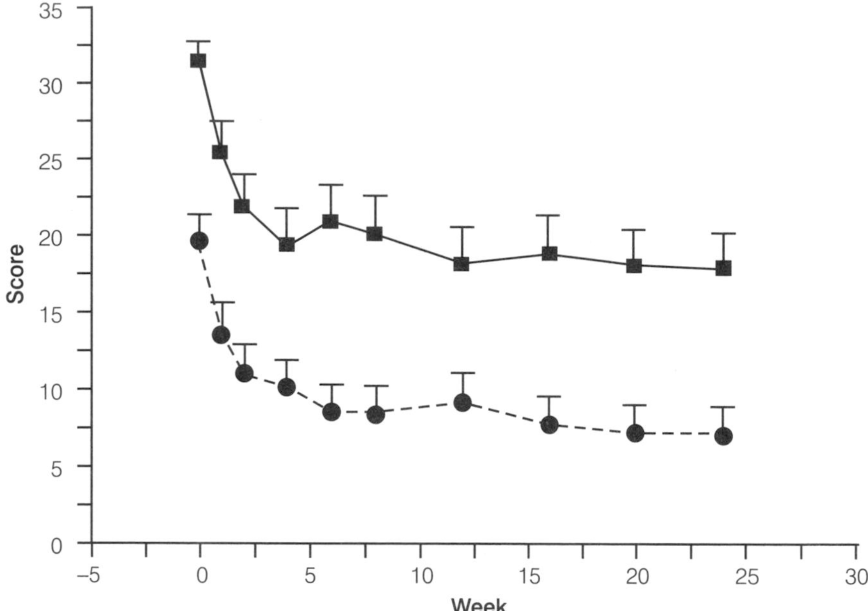

Figure 17–2. Spectrum of efficacy of lamotrigine in patients with treatment-refractory bipolar disorder. Top line in graph (filled squares), scores on the item Hamilton Rating Scale for Depression of patients who had presented in the depressed phase of the disorder (n = 39). Bottom line in graph (filled circles), scores on the Schedule for Affective Disorders and Schizophrenia—Change Version Mania Rating Scale of patients who had presented in the hypomanic (n = 7), manic (n = 9), or mixed (n = 9) phase of the disorder (total n of second group = 25). Three patients were excluded because they presented in unspecified phases of the illness.

showed marked improvement (≥50% decrease in Ham-D scores); 28 continue taking lamotrigine. The baseline GAS score was 49.4 and improved to 57.4 ($P < 0.01$), and the CGI—Severity Scale (CGI-S) score was 4.7 and decreased to 3.6 (Mann-Whitney test, $P < 0.002$). Mean CGI—Improvement Scale (CGI-I) score was 2.9, with 9.4% very much improved, 25% much improved, 43.8% minimally improved, 12.5% no change, 6.3% minimally worse, and 3% much worse. Of the 10 depressed patients who received lamotrigine monotherapy, none were moderate responders and 5 were marked responders.

In the 25 patients who presented in hypomanic (7), manic (9), or mixed (9) states, the baseline SADS-C MRS scores decreased from 21.1 ± 8.0 to 8.0 ± 9.9 (Mann-Whitney test, $P < 0.0001$). Four patients (16%) showed moderate improvement and 15 (60%) showed marked improvement on the SADS-C MRS. The baseline GAS score was 50 ± 8.6 and improved to 61.6 ± 14.9 ($P < 0.01$), and the CGI-S score decreased from 4.6 to 3.3 ($P < 0.002$). The mean CGI-I score was 2.5, with 18.2% very much improved, 36.4% much improved, 22.7% minimally improved, 13.6% no change, 4.5% minimally worse, 4.5% much worse, and 0% very much worse. In order of decreasing frequency, adverse events occurring in at least 10% of patients included headache, sedation, rash, nausea, dizziness, and tremors.

Although the design of this ongoing study was not double-blind, the data from this trial were consistent with two prior clinical case reports and suggested that lamotrigine had a broad spectrum of efficacy in bipolar disorder, including hypomania, mania, mixed states, and depression. Moderate to marked antidepressant responses were seen in 69% of the patients. Moderate to marked antimanic responses were seen in 76% of the patients. Efficacy appeared to be similar in rapid cyclers. Adverse events were usually mild and resolved without drug discontinuation. Serious adverse events were uncommon, and drug discontinuations resulted from rash. In an attempt to replicate these preliminary open, prospective findings, a multicenter, double-blind, placebo-controlled evaluation of the acute efficacy of lamotrigine in the depressed phase of bipolar I disorder has been designed and is ongoing.

The following is a summary of the first study in this series, which was conducted to evaluate the efficacy and safety of two doses of lamotrigine compared with placebo in the treatment of a major depressive episode in 195 patients with bipolar I disorder (Calabrese et al. 1999b). Outpatients received lamotrigine (50 or 200 mg/day) or placebo as monotherapy for 7 weeks. Psychiatric evaluations, including the Ham-D, Montgomery-Asberg Depression Rating Scale (MADRS), MRS, CGI-S, and Clinical Global Impression-I (CGI-I), were completed at 4 days and then weekly. Lamotrigine, 200 mg/day, showed significant antidepressant efficacy on the 17-item Ham-D, Ham-D Item 1, MADRS, CGI-S, and CGI-I compared with placebo. Improvements were seen as early as week 3. Lamotrigine, 50 mg/day, also showed efficacy compared with placebo on several measures. The MADRS appeared to separate efficacy differences between placebo and lamotrigine more robustly than the 17-item Ham-D. The proportion of patients who showed a marked response on CGI-I was 51%, 41%, and 26% for lamotrigine 200 mg/day, lamotrigine 50 mg/day, and placebo groups, respectively. Adverse events (including switch rates) and other safety results were similar across treatment groups, except for the higher incidence of headaches in the lamotrigine groups. The conclusion was that lamotrigine monotherapy was an efficacious and well-tolerated treatment of bipolar depression. These new data suggest that lamotrigine has the potential to complement the spectrum of activity of lithium and valproate (Calabrese et al. 1999b).

REFERENCES

Calabrese JR, Woyshville MJ, Kimmel SE, et al: Mixed states and bipolar rapid cycling and their treatment with valproate. Psychiatric Annals 23:70–78, 1993

Calabrese JR, Bowden CL, Woyshville MJ: Lithium and anticonvulsants in bipolar disorder, in Psychopharmacology: The Fourth Generation of Progress. Edited by Bloom FE, Kupfer DJ. New York, Raven, 1994, pp 1099–1111

Calabrese JR, Fatemi SH, Woyshville MJ: Antidepressant effects of lamotrigine in bipolar rapid cycling (letter). Am J Psychiatry 153:1236, 1996

Calabrese JR, Bowden CL, McElroy SL, et al: Spectrum of activity of lamotrigine in treatment refractory bipolar disorder. Am J Psychiatry 156:1019–1023, 1999a

Calabrese JR, Bowden CL, Sachs GS, et al: A double-blind placebo-controlled study of lamotrigine monotherapy in outpatients with bipolar I depression. J Clin Psychiatry 60:79–88, 1999b

Gilman JT: Lamotrigine: an antiepileptic agent for the treatment of partial seizures. Ann Pharmacother 29:144–151, 1995

Weisler R, Risner ME, Ascher J, et al: Use of lamotrigine in the treatment of bipolar disorder. Paper presented at the annual meeting of the American Psychiatric Association, Philadelphia, PA, May 21–26, 1994

Xie X: Interaction of the antiepileptic drug lamotrigine with recombinant rat brain type IIA Na+ channels and with native Na+ channels in rat hippocampal neurones. Archives of the European Journal of Physiology 430:437–446, 1995

CHAPTER 18

ATYPICAL ANTIPSYCHOTIC AGENTS IN MANIA

Clinical Studies

Mauricio Tohen, M.D., Dr.P.H., and
Gary D. Tollefson, M.D., Ph.D.

Since antipsychotic drugs first became available, they have been used in the treatment of bipolar disorder. Even after mood-stabilizing drugs, such as lithium and anticonvulsants, entered the therapeutic arena, antipsychotic use in bipolar disorder continued. Antipsychotic agents generally have been used in the treatment of severe behavioral disruptions or psychotic symptoms during acute manic episodes. It has been estimated that at least 30% of bipolar patients are nonresponsive to mood-stabilizing agents (Tohen et al. 1990). In general, antipsychotics are currently used for patients who do not respond to or do not tolerate lithium or anticonvulsant (carbamazepine, valproate) treatment. A recent meta-analysis reported that 84.7% of all bipolar patients appear to receive treatment with antipsychotic drugs. The rate for inpatient treatment was 90.7% (Tohen et al. 1998). In this chapter, we review the use of antipsychotic agents, with a special focus on the atypical drugs, in the treatment of bipolar disorder.

The introduction of chlorpromazine almost half a century ago focused on the treatment of acute agitated states (Delay et al. 1952). The early experience of antipsychotic agents in bipolar disorder remains, to some extent, unclear because of the diagnostic overlap that existed between manic-depressive illness and schizophrenia (Hegarty et al. 1994).

TYPICAL ANTIPSYCHOTIC AGENTS IN THE TREATMENT OF ACUTE MANIA

Several open and controlled studies have compared typical antipsychotics (neuroleptics) with lithium in the treatment of acute mania. Janicak and colleagues (1992) conducted a meta-analysis of randomized, double-blind studies comparing neuroleptics with lithium in the treatment of acute mania. A statistically significant superiority of lithium was reported, with 89% of patients responding to lithium compared with only 35% responding to neuroleptics ($P = 0.0003$) (Janicak et al. 1992; Johnson et al. 1968, 1971; Shopsin et al. 1975; Spring et al. 1970; Takahashi et al. 1975). In contrast, numerous studies have reported that neuroleptics have a documented advantage of a faster onset of action compared with lithium (Garfinkel et al. 1980; Johnson et al. 1968, 1971; Prien et al. 1972; Shopsin et al. 1975).

A recent study by McElroy et al. (1996) compared valproate with haloperidol in a randomized open design. This study found no difference in terms of efficacy but a higher degree of extrapyramidal adverse effects in patients who received haloperidol.

Other studies have explored the efficacy and safety of the concurrent use of neuroleptics and lithium (Biederman et al. 1979; Carman et al. 1981; Small et al. 1975). Biederman and collaborators (1979) found that the combination was superior to lithium plus placebo in a double-blind study of patients with schizoaffective disorder. Other studies reported a possible neurotoxic effect when lithium was combined with neuroleptics (Addonizio 1985; Cohen and Cohen 1974).

The use of neuroleptics in the treatment of mania remains common practice even in patients with their first episode of mania. In the McLean/Harvard First-Episode Mania Project, 50% of all patients received a neuroleptic agent. In 87% of the cases, the neuroleptic was of intermediate potency, such as perphenazine (Tohen et al. 1996b).

Neuroleptics and Dosing

Rifkin et al. (1990) conducted a fixed-dose study of three dosages of haloperidol—10, 30, and 80 mg/day—for up to 6 weeks in the treatment of mania. They found no advantage of using haloperidol at doses higher than 10 mg/day. Dosage also appears to vary according to illness stage. Doses of 500–600 mg of chlorpromazine equivalents have been reported in patients with multiple episodes (Gerner and Stanton 1992; Sernyak et al. 1994), whereas the average dose of neuroleptics for acute treatment was 175 mg in a sample of patients with a first episode (Tohen and Zarate 1998).

NEUROLEPTICS AND MAINTENANCE TREATMENT

Although the use of neuroleptics as maintenance treatment of bipolar disorder is common practice, no systematic study has focused on this important issue. Outcome studies have shown high use of neuroleptics not only during acute treatment but also during maintenance treatment. A recent meta-analytic review found that in patients with a median of minimum exposure to neuroleptics of 2.5 months, the use of neuroleptics was 96% (Tohen et al. 1998).

Other studies (Gelenberg 1994; Schou 1989) have found similar high use rates of neuroleptics as maintenance treatment despite the known risks associated with long-term use, such as tardive dyskinesia, which is reported to occur more often in patients with affective disorders (Addonizio 1985; Kane 1988; Keck et al. 1989). In the McLean/Harvard study, 55% of the patients were receiving neuroleptics at discharge, and 4 years later, 46% were still taking neuroleptics (Tohen et al. 1990). Other studies have reported higher rates of neuroleptic use. Mukherjee et al. (1986) reported that 124 of 131 bipolar patients (95%) received neuroleptics at some point during their illness. Similarly, Dinan and Kohen (1989) found that all of the patients in an outpatient group had been exposed to neuroleptics for at least 2 months. A recent review by Tohen and Zarate (1998) pooled data from many studies (Dinan and Kohen 1989; Hunt and Silverstone 1991; Licht et al. 1994; Sachs 1990; Sernyak and Woods 1993; Waddington and Youssef 1988; Waddington et al. 1989; Yassa et al. 1983), and in the full sample of 869 patients, on average, 592 (68%) had received neuroleptics at some time during their illness (range, 31%–100%). Because the sample was taken from different studies, and different diagnostic criteria and treatment settings were used, the findings should be cautiously interpreted. Also, because many of the patients were selected from inpatient settings, the sampling could have been biased toward the population with a high degree of behavioral impulsivity who would thus be prone to initial treatment with neuroleptics because of lithium's slow onset of action.

Several studies have reported high use rates of neuroleptics in hospitalized bipolar patients, but a report by Sernyak and colleagues (1994) found that the majority (95%) of patients discharged on neuroleptics continue to take them 6 months after discharge. In a similar study conducted by Keck et al. (1996), 68% of bipolar patients were taking neuroleptics at discharge and at the 6-month follow-up. In the McLean/Harvard First-Episode Mania Project (Tohen et al. 1996b), 84% of all bipolar patients (46 of 55) were discharged on neuroleptics. Interestingly, only 31% of them were still taking neuroleptics at the 6-month follow-up. The differences between the multiple-episode and first-episode samples suggest that the use of neuroleptics for maintenance treatment is more common in multiple-episode than in recent-onset patients. Analyzing the data from these three studies suggests an association between longer duration of bipolar disorder and use of neuroleptic drugs. Patients with a mean duration of illness of 13 years had a 95% use of neuroleptics compared with 68% in those with a 10-year duration and 31% in those with less than a 1-year duration. Because the percentages are from different studies, the only conclusion that can be drawn is that an association exists between duration of illness and rate of exposure to neuroleptics.

DEPOT NEUROLEPTICS

The efficacy of depot neuroleptics in the maintenance treatment of schizophrenia is well established (Janicak et al. 1993). For bipolar disorder, several open studies evaluated the use of depot neuroleptics as adjunctive treatment to lithium or carbamazepine (Lowe and Batchelor 1986; Naylor and Scott 1980; White et al. 1993). These open studies indicated that depot neuroleptics appear to be effective when added to mood stabilizers.

Also, several studies have compared depot neuroleptics with lithium carbonate (Ahlfors et al. 1981; Esparon et al. 1986; Kielholz et al. 1979). Kielholz and colleagues (1979) compared lithium carbonate with flupentixol in a 2-year follow-up of 30 patients. The authors found that both treatments were equally effective in preventing relapse to mania or depression. Ahlfors and colleagues (1981) conducted a similar study of 3 years' duration and found that neuroleptics appeared to significantly decrease the frequency and duration of manic episodes but simultaneously increase the frequency and duration of depressive episodes. Esparon and colleagues (1986) found no benefits in the addition of flupentixol to lithium carbonate in a double-blind crossover 2-year study of 15 patients with bipolar disorder.

NEUROLEPTICS AND ADVERSE EFFECTS

Some reports have suggested that typical antipsychotic agents may exacerbate symptoms of depression in bipolar patients (Ahlfors et al. 1981; Kukopulos et al. 1980; Levine 1986; Morgan 1972; White et al. 1993). A reported depressogenic quality of neuroleptics in bipolar disorder limits their use, especially in maintenance treatment.

In a study of flupentixol decanoate, Ahlfors et al. (1981) found an increased risk of relapse to depression compared with that of lithium carbonate. White et al. (1993) also found a higher risk of length of illness caused by depression when depot neuroleptics were compared with lithium or carbamazepine. In another large study that included almost 500 patients, Kukopulos et al. (1980) reported a higher risk of depression and, to some extent, a tendency toward multiple cycles in some bipolar patients. McElroy et al. (1996) suggested that neuroleptics have a unidirectional effect in bipolar disorder, with antimanic effects but no antidepressant or mood-stabilizing properties.

Furthermore, patients with affective disorders may have a higher risk of extrapyramidal adverse effects and tardive dyskinesia than do patients with schizophrenia (Chacko et al. 1993); some authors suggest a risk twice as high in patients with bipolar disorder (Kimmel et al. 1993). Nasarallah et al. (1988) found a 26% risk in a sample of 46 patients with bipolar disorder and 5.9% in a similar sample of 135 patients with schizophrenia. Investigators have also suggested that the concomitant use of typical antipsychotic drugs and lithium may increase the risk of extrapyramidal adverse effects and of neuroleptic malignant syndrome (Addonizio 1985; Cohen and Cohen 1974), the latter having possible lethal consequences.

Lenox et al. (1992) found no difference between haloperidol and a benzodiazepine when both were used as adjunctive treatment to lithium carbonate. Only one study (McElroy et al. 1996) has compared a neuroleptic (haloperidol at 0.2 mg/kg/day) with divalproex (20 mg/kg/day). The study found that both agents were equally effective, but divalproex had superior tolerability.

SUMMARY OF THE EFFECTS OF TYPICAL NEUROLEPTICS IN BIPOLAR DISORDER

In summary, the use of typical neuroleptics in bipolar disorder is not ideal. Although good data support their efficacy in the treatment of manic symptoms, their use may in fact worsen the course of the illness by increasing the risk of depressive symptoms and possibly increasing cyclicity. In addition, inherent adverse effects common to neuroleptics, such as extrapyramidal adverse effects and tardive dyskinesia, may be increased in patients with affective disorders. Nonetheless, typical antipsychotic agents have until now played an important

schizoaffective disorder (n = 81), psychotic depression (n = 114), and schizophrenia (n = 40) (Banov et al. 1994). Results showed that patients with bipolar disorder, manic episodes, and schizoaffective bipolar disorder had significantly better outcomes than did patients with schizoaffective depressed disorder and psychotic depression. In addition, bipolar and schizoaffective disorder patients had significantly greater improvement in social functioning than did schizophrenic patients who had similar basic measures of social functioning. This study suggested that clozapine appears to have a superior response in patients with affective psychosis compared with that in patients with schizophrenia.

A recent review (Tohen and Zarate 1998) posting data from different studies found a 70% response rate in patients with bipolar disorder who received clozapine. This review found that clozapine is more effective in treating bipolar and schizoaffective disorder (85%) than in treating schizophrenia (46%). These studies, however, must be approached with caution because they were small open-label studies. Despite what appears to be very promising antimanic and mood-stabilizing effects of clozapine, it is unlikely that this drug will become a first-line treatment of bipolar disorder because life-threatening adverse effects, such as agranulocytosis, limit its use.

Risperidone

Risperidone (serotoninergic 5-HT_2/dopaminergic D_2 receptor antagonist) has also been reported to be effective in the treatment of bipolar and schizoaffective disorder (Keck et al. 1995; Tohen et al. 1996a). In 1992, Hillert and colleagues reported a reduction in depressive and psychotic symptoms in patients with schizoaffective disorder, depressed type, treated with risperidone. Recent publications by Dwight et al. (1994) and Koek and Kessler (1996) suggested a possible induction of mania in patients with bipolar or schizoaffective bipolar disorder. However, a recent review by Stoll (1996) examined five open-label studies (total of 122 bipolar and schizoaffective bipolar-type patients) that showed good to excellent antimanic and antipsychotic efficacy and no clear evidence of induced mania or hypomania. Jacobsen (1995) found a favorable response in 16 bipolar I and II patients who received a mean dosage of 3.3 ± 1.9 mg/day of risperidone for approximately 9 weeks. Ghaemi et al. (1997) found an equally good response in 14 bipolar I patients who received concomitant risperidone (mean dose of 2.8 ± 1.8 mg/day) and mood stabilizers. Tohen et al. (1996a) reported a favorable response in 15 patients with psychotic mania. Of the 13 patients who completed 2 weeks of treatment, all 13 had at least 25% improvement and 8 had 50% improvement in their BPRS scores. Also, of the 8 patients who completed 6 weeks of treatment, 7 had a 50% improvement and all 8 had a 25% improvement in their BPRS scores. Risperidone was well tolerated, and no exacerbations to hypomania or mania occurred.

More recently, Segal et al. (1998) conducted a randomized, double-blind study of 45 patients to compare risperidone with lithium and haloperidol in the treatment of mania. A similar pattern of improvement was seen after 28 days, and no significant difference in extrapyramidal side effects was found between risperidone and haloperidol. The authors concluded that risperidone has efficacy equivalent to that of lithium and haloperidol in the management of acute mania. However, to adequately demonstrate no difference between treatments, a larger sample size is needed powered for noninferiority (i.e., a sample size large enough to have the statistical power to detect that one agent is not inferior to another).

Olanzapine

Olanzapine is a thienobenzodiazepine atypical antipsychotic agent with affinity to dopaminergic D_1, D_2, D_3, D_4; serotoninergic 5-HT_2, 5-HT_3, 5-HT_6; α_1; muscarinic M_1; and histaminergic H_1 receptors. Studies suggest that olanzapine is effective in the treatment of affective symptoms. Tollefson et al. (1997) found that olanzapine was statistically significantly superior to haloperidol, as measured by baseline-to-endpoint changes in the Montgomery-Asberg Depression Rating Scale (MADRS) score in patients with schizophrenia. Olanzapine also has been used in the treatment of schizoaffective bipolar disorder. Tran et al. (1996) and Tohen et al. (1997) reported that patients with schizoaffective bipolar disorder who received olanzapine showed a statistically significant greater improvement from baseline to endpoint on the MADRS than did those who received haloperidol. In addition, these studies showed that olanzapine was superior to haloperidol in schizoaffective bipolar patients by using the BPRS. Furthermore, in a recent study to assess the efficacy of olanzapine in the treatment of an acute episode of bipolar disorder, olanzapine was statistically significantly superior to placebo in mean reductions of YMRS total, Positive and Negative Syndrome Scale for Schizophrenia (PANSS) total, and PANSS positive scores from baseline to endpoint (Tohen et al. 1999). In addition, the number of responders (those patients showing a 50% or greater decrease in the YMRS score from baseline to last measurement in acute treatment) was statistically greater with olanzapine than with placebo (48.6% vs. 24.2%, $P = 0.004$). Thus, olanzapine appears to have mood-stabilizing properties.

CONCLUSION

The efficacy of antipsychotic agents in the treatment of psychotic mania is well established with the use of neuroleptics. Open studies have also suggested efficacy with the atypical agents. Efficacy of atypical agents in maintenance treatment requires further study because the use of neuroleptics for maintenance treatment has several drawbacks, including the lack of mood-stabilizing effects, possible exacerbation of depressive symptoms, and increased risk of extrapyramidal side effects and tardive dyskinesia. Thus, some recent reports have expressed caution in the use of neuroleptics for maintenance treatment (Gelenberg and Hopkins 1996; McElroy et al. 1996). Atypical antipsychotic agents have an advantage over neuroleptics, especially for maintenance therapy, considering that many patients do not receive adequate protection with mood stabilizers. Atypical antipsychotics also have a superior adverse-event profile. Other areas that need to be further explored regarding the use of atypical agents include the treatment of nonpsychotic mania, bipolar depression, mixed states, and bipolar II disorder.

REFERENCES

Addonizio G: Rapid induction of extrapyramidal side effects with combined use of lithium and neuroleptics. J Clin Psychopharmacol 5:296–298, 1985

Ahlfors UG, Baastrup C, Dencker SJ, et al: Flupenthixol decanoate in recurrent manic-depressive illness. Acta Psychiatr Scand 64:226–237, 1981

Banov MD, Zarate CA Jr, Tohen M, et al: Clozapine therapy in refractory affective disorders: polarity predicts response in long-term follow-up. J Clin Psychiatry 55:295–300, 1994

Biederman J, Lerner Y, Belmaker RH: Combination of lithium carbonate and haloperidol in schizoaffective disorder: a controlled study. Arch Gen Psychiatry 36:327–333, 1979

Calabrese JR, Kimmel SE, Woyshville MJ, et al: Clozapine for treatment-refractory mania. Am J Psychiatry 153:759–764, 1996

Carman JS, Bigelow LB, Wyatt RJ: Lithium combined with neuroleptics in chronic schizophrenic and schizoaffective patients. J Clin Psychiatry 42:124–128, 1981

Chacko RC, Hurley RA, Jankovic J: Clozapine use in diffuse Lewy body disease. J Neuropsychiatry Clin Neurosci 5:206–208, 1993

Cohen WJ, Cohen NH: Lithium carbonate, haloperidol and irreversible brain damage. JAMA 230:1283–1287, 1974

Delay J, Deniker P, Harl J: Utilization therapeutique psychiatrique d'une phenothiazine d'action cetrale elective (4560RP). Annales Medico-Psychologiques 110: 112–117, 1952

Dinan TG, Kohen D: Tardive dyskinesia in bipolar affective disorder: relationship to lithium therapy. Br J Psychiatry 155:55–57, 1989

Dwight MM, Keck PE Jr, Stanton SP, et al: Antidepressant activity and mania associated with risperidone treatment of schizoaffective disorder. Lancet 344:1029–1030, 1994

Esparon J, Kolloori J, Naylor GJ, et al: Comparison of the prophylactic action of flupenthixol with placebo in lithium treated manic-depressive patients. Br J Psychiatry 148:723–725, 1986

Garfinkel PE, Stancer HG, Persad E: A comparison of haloperidol, lithium carbonate and their combination in the treatment of mania. J Affect Disord 2:279–288, 1980

Gelenberg AJ: Neuroleptics for bipolar maintenance. Biological Therapeutics in Psychiatry 17:46–47, 1994

Gelenberg AJ, Hopkins HS: Antipsychotics in bipolar disorder. J Clin Psychiatry 57 (suppl 9):49–52, 1996

Gerner RH, Stanton A: Algorithm for patient management of acute manic states: lithium, valproate, or carbamazepine? J Clin Psychopharmacol 12:57–63, 1992

Ghaemi SN, Sachs GS, Baldassano CF, et al: Acute treatment of bipolar disorder with adjunctive risperidone in outpatients. Can J Psychiatry 42:196–199, 1997

Hegarty JD, Baldessarini RJ, Tohen et al: One hundred years of schizophrenia: a meta-analysis of the outcome literature. Am J Psychiatry 151:1409–1416, 1994

Hillert A, Maier W, Wetzel H, et al: Risperidone in the treatment of disorders with a combined psychotic and depressive syndrome: a functional approach. Pharmacopsychiatry 25:213–217, 1992

Hunt N, Silverstone T: Tardive dyskinesia in bipolar affective disorder: a catchment area study. Int Clin Psychopharmacol 6:45–50, 1991

Jacobsen FM: Risperidone in the treatment of affective illness and obsessive-compulsive disorder. J Clin Psychiatry 56:423–429, 1995

Janicak PG, Newman RH, Davis JM: Advances in the treatment of manic and related disorders: a reappraisal. Psychiatric Annals 22:92–103, 1992

Janicak PG, Davis JM, Preskorn SH, et al: Treatment With Antipsychotics: Principles and Practice of Psychopharmacotherapy. Baltimore, MD, Williams & Wilkins, 1993, pp 93–184

Johnson G, Gershon S, Hekiman LJ: Controlled evaluation of lithium and chlorpromazine in the treatment of manic states: an interim report. Compr Psychiatry 9:563–573, 1968

Johnson G, Gershon S, Burdock EI, et al: Comparative effects of lithium and chlorpromazine in the treatment of acute manic states. Br J Psychiatry 119:267–276, 1971

Kando JC, Tohen M, Castillo J, et al: Concurrent use of clozapine and valproate in affective and psychotic disorders. J Clin Psychiatry 55:255–257, 1994

Kane JM: The role of neuroleptics in manic-depressive illness. J Clin Psychiatry 49 (suppl l):12–14, 1988

Keck PE Jr, Pope HG Jr, Cohen BM, et al: Risk factors for neuroleptic malignant syndrome: a case-control study. Arch Gen Psychiatry 46:914–918, 1989

Keck PE Jr, Wilson DR, Strakowski SM, et al: Clinical predictors of acute risperidone response in schizophrenia, schizoaffective disorder, and psychotic mood disorders. J Clin Psychiatry 56:466–470, 1995

Keck PE Jr, McElroy SL, Strakowski SM, et al: Factors associated with maintenance antipsychotic treatment of patients with bipolar disorder. J Clin Psychiatry 57: 147–151, 1996

Kielholz P, Terzani S, Poldinger W: The long-term treatment of periodical and cyclic depressions with flupenthixol decanoate. International Pharmacopsychiatry 14:305–309, 1979

Kimmel SE, Calabrese JR, Meltzer HY: Clozapine in treatment refractory mania (Abstract 21:80), in 1993 CME Syllabus and Proceedings Summary, American Psychiatric Association Annual Meeting, San Francisco, CA, May 22–27, 1993. Washington, DC, American Psychiatric Association, 1993

Koek RJ, Kessler CC: Probable induction of mania by risperidone (letter). J Clin Psychiatry 57:174–175, 1996

Kukopulos A, Reginaldi D, Laddomada P, et al: Course of the manic-depressive cycle and changes caused by treatments. Pharmakopsychiatrie Neuropsychopharmakologie 13:156–167, 1980

Lenox RH, Newhouse PA, Creelman WL, et al: Adjunctive treatment of manic agitation with lorazepam versus haloperidol: a double-blind study. J Clin Psychiatry 53:47–52, 1992

Levine S: The management of resistant depression. Acta Psychiatrica Belgica 86:141–151, 1986

Licht RW, Gouliaev G, Vestergaard P, et al: Treatment of manic episodes in Scandinavia: the use of neuroleptic drugs in clinical routine setting. J Affect Disord 32:179–185, 1994

Lowe MR, Batchelor DH: Depot neuroleptics and manic-depressive psychosis. Int Clin Psychopharmacol 1 (suppl 1):53–62, 1986

McElroy SL, Keck PE Jr, Strakowski SM: Mania, psychosis and antipsychotics. J Clin Psychiatry 57 (suppl 3):14–26, 1996

Morgan HG: The incidence of depressive symptoms during recovery from hypomania. Br J Psychiatry 120:537–539, 1972

Mukherjee S, Rosen AM, Caracci G, et al: Persistent tardive dyskinesia in bipolar patients. Arch Gen Psychiatry 43:342–346, 1986

Nasarallah HA, Churchill CM, Hamdan-Allan GA: Higher frequency of neuroleptic-induced dystonia in mania than in schizophrenia. Am J Psychiatry 145:1455–1456, 1988

Naylor GJ, Scott CR: Depot injections for affective disorders. Br J Psychiatry 136:105–108, 1980

Prien RF, Point P, Caffey E, et al: Comparison of lithium carbonate and chlorpromazine in the treatment of mania. Arch Gen Psychiatry 26:146–153, 1972

Rifkin A, Karajgi B, Doddi S, et al: Dose and blood levels of haloperidol in treatment of mania. Psychopharmacol Bull 26:144–146, 1990

Sachs GS: Use of clonazepam for bipolar affective disorder. J Clin Psychiatry 51 (suppl 5):31–34, 1990

Schou M: Lithium prophylaxis: myths and realities. Am J Psychiatry 146:573–576, 1989

Segal J, Berk M, Brook S: Risperidone compared with both lithium and haloperidol in mania: a double-blind randomized controlled trial. Clin Neuropharmacol 21:176–180, 1998

Sernyak MJ, Woods SW: Chronic neuroleptic use in manic-depressive illness. Psychopharmacol Bull 29:375–379, 1993

Sernyak MJ, Griffin RA, Johnson RM, et al: Neuroleptic exposure following inpatient treatment of acute mania with lithium and neuroleptic. Am J Psychiatry 151:133–135, 1994

Shopsin B, Gershon S, Thompson H, et al: A controlled comparison of lithium carbonate, chlorpromazine, and haloperidol. Arch Gen Psychiatry 32:34–42, 1975

Small JG, Kellams JJ, Milstein V, et al: A placebo-controlled study of lithium combined with neuroleptics in chronic schizophrenic patients. Am J Psychiatry 132:1315–1317, 1975

Spring G, Schweid D, Gray C, et al: A double-blind comparison of lithium carbonate and chlorpromazine in the treatment of manic states. Am J Psychiatry 126:1306–1310, 1970

Stoll AL: Risperidone induction of mania: fact or fallacy? International Drug Therapy Newsletter 31:5–6, 1996

Takahashi R, Sakuma A, Itoh K, et al: Comparison of efficacy of lithium carbonate and chlorpromazine in mania. Arch Gen Psychiatry 32:34–42, 1975

Tohen M, Zarate CA Jr: Antipsychotic agents and bipolar disorder. J Clin Psychiatry 59 (suppl 1):38–48, 1998

Tohen M, Waternaux CM, Tsuang MT: Outcome in mania: a 4-year prospective follow-up of patients utilizing survival analysis. Arch Gen Psychiatry 47:1106–1111, 1990

Tohen M, Zarate CA Jr, Centorrino F, et al: Risperidone in the treatment of mania. J Clin Psychiatry 57:249–253, 1996a

Tohen M, Zarate CA Jr, Zarate SB, et al: The McLean/Harvard First-Episode Mania Project: pharmacological treatment and outcome. Psychiatric Annals 26:5444–5448, 1996b

Tohen M, Sanger TM, McElroy S, et al: Olanzapine versus haloperidol in the treatment of schizoaffective bipolar patients (NR206), in 1997 New Research Program and Abstracts, American Psychiatric Association 150th Annual Meeting, San Diego, CA, May 17–22, 1997

Tohen M, Zhang F, Taylor CC, et al: Neuroleptic use in bipolar disorder: a pharmacoepidemiologic review. Paper presented at the 151st annual meeting of the American Psychiatric Association, Toronto, ON, May 30–June 4, 1998

Tohen M, Sanger TM, McElroy SL, et al: Olanzapine versus placebo in the treatment of acute mania. Am J Psychiatry 156:702–709, 1999

Tollefson GD, Beasley CM Jr, Tran PV, et al: Olanzapine versus haloperidol in the treatment of schizophrenia and schizoaffective and schizophreniform disorders: results of an international collaborative trial. Am J Psychiatry 154:457–465, 1997

Tran PV, Sanger T, Beasley C, : Olanzapine in the treatment of schizoaffective disorder. Paper presented at the 36th annual meeting of New Clinical Drug Unit, Boca Raton, FL, May 28–31, 1996

Waddington JL, Youssef HA: Tardive dyskinesia in bipolar affective disorder: aging, cognitive dysfunction, course of illness, and exposure to neuroleptic and lithium. Am J Psychiatry 145:613–616, 1988

Waddington JL, Brown K, O'Neill JO, et al: Cognitive impairment, clinical course and treatment history in outpatients with bipolar affective disorder: relationship to tardive dyskinesia. Psychol Med 19:897–902, 1989

White E, Cheung P, Silverstone T: Depot antipsychotics in bipolar affective disorder. Int Clin Psychopharmacol 8:119–122, 1993

Yassa R, Ghadirian AM, Schwartz G: Prevalence of tardive dyskinesia in affective disorder patients. J Clin Psychiatry 44:410–412, 1983

Zarate CA Jr, Tohen M, Baldessarini RJ: Clozapine in severe mood disorders. J Clin Psychiatry 56:411–417, 1995a

Zarate CA Jr, Tohen M, Banov MD, et al: Is clozapine monotherapy a mood stabilizer? J Clin Psychiatry 56:109–113, 1995b

CHAPTER 19

CALCIUM CHANNEL BLOCKERS

Paul J. Goodnick, M.D., and Amparo Benitez, D.O.

Lithium has been the treatment of choice for mania since its usefulness was first reported by Cade. Lithium has been shown to have varied effects on multiple biological systems, including electrolyte flux and neurochemistry. It has been reported to have calcium channel blocking properties, as do the phenothiazines that have been used to treat mania (Dubovsky 1986; Dubovsky and Franks 1983; Himmelhoch and Garfinkel 1986; Johnson et al. 1993; Wood 1985). Thus, elevated plasma calcium levels subsequent to therapy with lithium have been reported (Carman and Wyatt 1979; Gerner et al. 1977; Linder et al. 1993).

This effect of lithium on calcium levels is important, because a series of calcium-related abnormalities have been reported in mood disorders. Hypercalcemia has been associated with depression, stupor, and coma; hypocalcemia, with irritability, anxiety, and mania. Cerebrospinal fluid (CSF) studies have reported elevations in depressed patients and reductions in patients with mania (Carman and Wyatt 1979; Dubovsky and Franks 1983). Recovery from depression led to reductions in CSF calcium. There have been a series of studies of intracellular calcium, reviewed by Dubovsky et al. (1992). In two studies reviewed, Dubovsky et al. found both baseline and agonist-stimulated levels (nM) highest in untreated manic patients, followed by untreated bipolar depressed patients, untreated unipolar depressed patients, and then control subjects. For example, the sequence found in the initial study by Dubovsky et al. for baseline intracellular calcium was 157 ±65.1, 136 ±44.8, 124 ±24.9, and 98 ±15 (Dubovsky et al. 1992).

Calcium channel blockers (CCBs) inactivate the voltage-sensitive calcium channel, thus blocking calcium influx (Dubovsky 1986; Dubovsky and Franks 1983; Hoschl 1991; Physicians' Desk Reference 1994; Pollack et al.

1987). This leads to inhibition of smooth muscle contraction, neurotransmitter synthesis and release, and neural signal transmission. As a consequence, it is not surprising that in 1982, Dubovsky reported the first case of acute mania successfully treated by verapamil (Dubovsky et al. 1982).

PHARMACOLOGY

The CCBs as a group are chemically heterogeneous. Currently, there are four varieties available in the United States: verapamil, diltiazem, nifedipine, and nimodipine. These can be broken down into two chemical classes: 1) non-dihydropyridine—verapamil and diltiazem—and 2) dihydropyridine—nifedipine and nimodipine. These two chemical classes bind to different parts of the calcium channel. In terms of kinetics, following oral administration, there is extensive metabolism by the liver in a first-pass effect, and the drug accumulates with repeated dosing. Thus, the elimination half-life will also increase—for example, that of verapamil from an initial range of 2–8 hours to one of 5–12 hours after the first few days of administration.

The pharmacological profiles of the individual CCBs are as follows:

- Verapamil has been established in the United States for therapy of both tachyarrhythmias and angina with a dosage of 240–480 mg/day (Physicians' Desk Reference 1994). Dilation of the main coronary arteries and prevention of coronary vasospasm are the major cardiovascular benefits. Further, the rate of cardiac conduction is reduced through the atrioventricular (AV) node (Pollack et al. 1987). It is highly lipophilic and readily crosses the blood-brain barrier (Doran et al. 1985; Hoschl 1991). Following oral or parenteral use, cerebrospinal concentration is 7% of serum levels (Doran et al. 1985). Verapamil is more than 90% absorbed from orally administered dosages, with a bioavailability of 20%–35%. Peak plasma concentrations occur 1–2 hours after oral administration. Mean elimination half-life in single-dose studies is 2.8–7.4 hours and, after repeated dosing, 4.5–12 hours. Elimination half-life is prolonged in the elderly. It is extensively metabolized in the liver, with 70% excreted as metabolites in the urine. Verapamil is 90% bound to plasma proteins. In case of liver compromise, half-life may increase to 14–16 hours. Regarding serotonin, verapamil has been shown to inhibit 5-HT_3 receptor function (Hargreaves et al. 1997). Verapamil has also been shown to alleviate haloperidol-induced catalepsy; higher doses attenuate and lower doses potentiate haloperidol (Kozlovskii et al. 1996) as is the case with diltiazem and nimodipine. It also produces partial inhibition (similar to nifedipine and diltiazem) of contractions produced by noradrenaline, phenylethylamine, and dopamine (Bhugra and Gulati 1996).

- Diltiazem, a benzothiazepine class antagonist, is also approved for treatment of angina at a dosage of 120–240 mg/day (Physicians' Desk Reference 1994). Similarly, it reduces AV node conduction. Diltiazem is well absorbed; it has a bioavailability rate of 40, with 96% of drug excreted as metabolites in the urine. Its elimination half-life is 3.0–4.5 hours; in patients with liver compromise, the half-life is significantly increased. Renal function problems do not affect pharmacokinetics. Diltiazem is 70%–80% bound to plasma proteins. The interaction of diltiazem with serotonin, haloperidol, and NA is similar to that of verapamil (see above) (Bhugra and Gulati 1996; Hargreaves et al. 1997; Kozlovskii et al. 1996).
- Nifedipine has a similar profile for treatment of angina, with a dosage range of 30–120 mg/day and a maximum of 180 mg/day. It is more likely than verapamil to produce both hypotension and reflex tachycardia. Peak blood levels occur after 30 minutes; elimination half-life is 2 hours. Eighty percent of the parent drug and metabolites are eliminated via the kidneys. As with verapamil and diltiazem, the presence of liver disease increases the half-life of nifedipine. Plasma protein binding is 92%–98%. Results on nifedipine's serotonin and catecholamine effects are similar to those of verapamil (see above) (Bhugra and Gulati 1996; Hargreaves et al. 1997; Kozlovskii et al. 1996). In addition, similar to nimodipine, nifedipine has been shown to have little effect on serotonin parameters (Viveros et al. 1996) but also to inhibit a serotonin-activated inward channel of potassium but not prevent serotonin-induced constriction of blood vessels (Jalonen et al. 1997; Semkina et al. 1996). Nifedipine has been shown to cause increases in striatal dopamine and dihydroxyphenylacetic acid (DOPAC) (Viveros et al. 1996).
- Flunarizine is well absorbed, with peak plasma concentrations within 2–4 hours. It is 90% bound to plasma proteins, with a very long elimination half-life of 18 days (Reynolds 1993). This medication has been shown to block reuptake of serotonin in a dose-dependent fashion (Jensen et al. 1994). Flunarizine has been shown to counteract depletion of serotonin induced by *d*-fenfluramine (Mennini et al. 1996). (Flunarizine is not available in the United States at the time of writing.)
- Nimodipine is the most lipophilic of the CCBs and crosses the blood-brain barrier the most easily to prevent cerebral vasospasm following

subarachnoid hemorrhage (Langley and Sorkin 1989; Pazzaglia et al. 1993). It also has anticonvulsant properties and decreases cocaine-induced hyperactivity (DeFalco et al. 1992; Pazzaglia et al. 1993). Dosage ranges are usually 180–360 mg/day, with a maximum of 720 mg/day. Nimodipine, however, has relatively little effect on the myocardium (Brunet et al. 1990). Nimodipine is rapidly absorbed, with peak concentrations within 1 hour after administration. The elimination half-life has two phases: 1) early: 1–2 hours and 2) terminal: 8–9 hours. It is more than 95% bound to plasma proteins; more than 99% is recovered from urine in metabolite form. Bioavailability is only 13%; with liver disease, both elimination half-lives and bioavailability are increased. As with the results summarized above for other CCBs, nimodipine inhibits 5-HT_3 receptor function as well as serotonin-activated inward potassium channels but does not prevent serotonin-mediated vessel constriction or have any effect on striatal levels of serotonin or 5-hydroxyindoleacetic acid (5-HIAA) (Hargreaves et al. 1997; Jalonen et al. 1997; Semkina et al. 1996; Viveros et al. 1996). Regarding catecholamine effects, nimodipine produces partial inhibition of NA and DA-induced contractions while alleviating haloperidol-induced catalepsy (Bhugra and Gulati 1996; Kozlovskii et al. 1996). Finally, it causes increases in striatal DA and DOPAC (Viveros et al. 1996).

STUDIES IN MOOD DISORDERS

The following review of the current state of knowledge concerning the use of CCBs in mood disorders progresses from that more highly researched (e.g., mania) to that with less available results (e.g., prophylaxis). The review also proceeds from case reports to open studies to double-blind results.

Mania

All four CCBs have been studied in treatment of mania: it is logical to apply the CCBs because the blocking of calcium channels prevents the release of the norepinephrine that can induce development of the manic state (see summary, Table 19–1). The earliest report was that of Dubovsky et al. (1982), who in a double-blind on-off-on (ABA) design found that 160 mg/day of verapamil was effective in reducing manic symptoms in a 21-day protocol. A reduction in the Manic-State Rating Scale from 35 to 13 was reported, followed by relapse within 9 days of being back on placebo.

Table 19–1. Summary of calcium channel blockers in treatment of mania

Medication		Study type			Dose (mg/day)	% success
		CR	OS	DB		
Verapamil	Reports	10/11	5/7	6/7	160–480	84
	Patients	14/17	28/37 (5 studies)	16/20 (3 studies)		78
Diltiazem	Reports	0/0	1/1	0/0	120–360	100
	Patients	0/0	5/7	0/0		72
Nimodipine	Reports	2/2	2/2	1/1	90–720	100
	Patients	3/3	15/18	5/9		71

Note. Numbers divided by slashes mean number improved/total number included. CR = case report; OS = open study; DB = double-blind.

This result was then repeated in 1983 at dosages of 160–480 mg/day (Dubovsky and Franks 1983). Since then, there have been 9 other case reports; with the exception of Kennedy et al. (1986), all others have reported some degree of response to verapamil in mania (Gitlin and Weiss 1984; Goodnick 1993; Helmuth et al. 1989; Jacobsen et al. 1987; Mathis et al. 1988; Patterson 1987; Solomon and Williamson 1986; Wehr et al. 1988). For example, Patterson (1987) said that a patient with combined mania and psychosis responded to 320 mg/day in a 10-day period with clearing of both conditions. Sleep stabilized within 24 hours, and delusions cleared in 4 days. Another case report (Goodnick 1993) then indicated the safe and effective use of verapamil in mania during pregnancy. Deicken (1990) presented a case report of successful use of verapamil in bipolar depression. There have been seven open and single-blind studies of the use of verapamil in mania: Barton and Gitlin (1987), Brotman et al. (1986), Dinan et al. (1988), Goodnick (1995), Hoschl et al. (1986), Lenzi et al. (1995), and Walton et al. (1996). Rates of response have been reported respectively as 5/5, 6/6, 0/8, 5/6, 12/12, and most of 15 (no report on individual patients in Walton et al. 1996). The Barton and Gitlin study stands out in contrast to the others in using dosages of 160–240 mg/day; five of the others used dosages of 120–480 mg/day (no dosage data were provided for the Lenzi et al. study). The response was not related to duration of treatment: Barton and Gitlin (21 days), Brotman et al. (10 days), Dinan et al. (21 days), Goodnick (14 days), and Hoschl et al. (30 days). A unique factor in the Goodnick study is the significant correlation of reduction in the Young Mania Rating Scale (YMRS) to the increase of plasma calcium ($r = .61$, $P = .034$).

There have been eight double-blind, controlled studies of the use of verapamil in mania; however, the controls have varied from placebo (Dose et al. 1986; Dubovsky et al. 1986; Janicak et al. 1998) to lithium-controlled (Garza-Trevino et al. 1992; Giannini et al. 1984) to neuroleptic- or clonidine-controlled (Giannini et al. 1986; Hoschl and Kozeny 1989; Walton et al. 1996). Without exception, the dosage of verapamil has been allowed to be increased up to 320–480 mg/day. Periods of dosing have varied from 7 to 35 days. Comparison doses of active placebo have been as follows: lithium to produce a serum level of 0.8–1.5 mEq/L; clonidine of 17 µg/kg; and neuroleptic of 375 mg chlorpromazine equivalent. Most studies have used the Brief Psychiatric Rating Scale (BPRS) to monitor response. Reported overall percentage improvements were as follows: verapamil 4%–68%, lithium 27%–73%, neuroleptic 39%, and placebo 4%–22%. Overall, patients placed on verapamil at doses of 360 mg or greater showed a 50% decrease in mania ratings that was, in general, equivalent to active control subjects and better than those placed on placebo. (See detail in Table 19–2.)

For other CCBs, reports are scarce. Diltiazem was reported as successful in the treatment of mania in five of seven patients (Caillard 1985). It was administered for 14 days at dosages of 120–360 mg/day in an open design. The two patients who were not helped by diltiazem had a secondary mania by Feighner criteria (i.e., organic mood disorder). The few side effects reported included headache, transient edema of the extremities, and vertigo. D-600 was administered in a double-blind, placebo-controlled 15-day protocol; five of nine had substantial clinical improvement, including three ultrarapid cyclers (Aldenhoff et al. 1986). Side effects included peripheral flushing, mild orthostasis, and stomach upset. Furthermore, diltiazem has been shown to reduce the effects of dextroamphetamine in healthy volunteers (Fabian 1997). In a placebo-controlled study that used measures of subjective and sleep changes determined by visual analogue scales, diltiazem attenuated the cardiovascular changes more than the subjective changes induced by amphetamine. Consistent with potential effects of flunarizine to reduce symptoms of mania is a case report of a patient who became depressed upon its administration (Patten and Thompson 1995). Probably because of flunarizine's long elimination half-life, the depressive symptoms persisted for 8 weeks after discontinuation.

Nimodipine was initially tested in a 7-day open trial (Brunet et al. 1990). At a dosage of 360 mg/day, all six patients were reportedly significantly improved. Mood and "speech activity" were seen as most improved, with least change in sleep patterns. Two patients required prn droperidol. There were no adverse side effects, no sedative effects, and no changes in vital signs, electrocardiograms, or electroencephalograms. All patients had resultant elevated plasma calcium levels, which remained in the normal range; this result complements the one regarding response to verapamil reported above (Goodnick 1995). The earliest study of rapid cyclers showed that in 9 of 12 patients receiving a dose of 90 mg/day, those receiving a combination of nimodipine and lithium did better than those taking either drug alone (Manna 1991) in terms of both number of episodes and total number of days with symptoms ($P < 0.05$). For combined therapy, lithium alone, and nimodipine alone, the results for number of episodes were 1.7, 2.3, and 2.5, and those for number of days with symptoms were 15, 28, and 30 days, respectively. Pazzaglia et al. (1993) reported a double-blind, placebo-controlled study of nimodipine in acute and prophylactic treatment of patients with lithium- and carbamazepine-refractory mania and in one patient with depression. Eleven patients diagnosed with bipolar disorder underwent an ABA design with placebo phases of approximately 7.6 weeks and active drug periods of approximately 11.6 weeks. Five of nine patients who completed the trial showed significant improvement, including all three with ultrarapid-cycling bipolar disorder (i.e., with cycle durations of less than 24 hours). On the rating scale used (Mood Analogue Scale), the respective improvements from placebo to drug in these three

Table 19–2. Verapamil (V) treatment of mood disorders

Study (*N*)	Dosage, mg/day (duration, days)	Diagnoses/ Design	Outcome
Mania			
Case reports			
Dubovsky et al. 1982 (1)	160 (21)	BP (DSM-III) ABA (3 weeks)	MSRS (35 to 13) P (9-day relapse)
Dubovsky and Franks 1983 (2)	160–480 (21)	BP (DSM-III); ABA (3 weeks)	Dramatic improvement
Gitlin and Weiss 1984 (1)	80 (14) 240 (1 year)	Added to Li	Marked reduction in symptoms Controlled hypomania
Kennedy 1986 (1)	320 (30)	BP	No response
Solomon and Williamson 1986 (2)	320 (4 months)	RC/hypomania	Euthymia, then depression Response to antidepressant Without hypomania
Jacobsen et al. 1987 (1)	160 (6 months)	BP/RC	Remission of RC
Patterson 1987 (1)	320 (10)	BP psychosis	Discharged in remission
Mathis et al. 1988 (4)	320 (?)	BP	2/4 improved
Wehr et al. 1988 (2)	?	BP/RC	Remission in nonresponders
Helmuth et al. 1989 (1)	360 (7)	Mania	Euthymia but choreoathetosis; V withdrawal led to relapse
Deicken 1990 (1)	320 (24 months)	BP	Euthymia; relapse on V withdrawal
Goodnick 1993 (1)	240 (14)	BP	Controlled manic symptoms in pregnancy
Open studies			
Brotman et al. 1986 (6)	240–320 (21)	Li nonresponders Mania: BP/SAD	Improved in 10 days 3/6 discharged in 21 days

Hoschl et al. 1986 (5)	120–480 (30)	Mania	Remission
Barton and Gitlin 1987 (8)	160–240 (21)	Mania (RDC)	0/8 responded; 4 became dysphoric
Dinan et al. 1988 (6)	320–400 (21)	BP: mania (DSM-III Petersen)	5/6 improved in 2 weeks
Goodnick 1996 (12)	360 (14)	Mania (DSM-III-R; YMS)	12/12 responded: –60.5%
Double-blind controlled studies			
Giannini et al. 1984 (12)	320 (30)	BP: mania (DSM-III) BPRS: Li control crossover	V: –68%; Li: –73%
Dose et al. 1986 (8)	320–480 (7)	BP; IMPS; P controlled	7/8 responded in 3–7 days; 5 relapsed on P
Dubovsky et al. 1986 (7)	480 (24)	BP: mania (DSM-III); BPRS: P controlled	V: –53%; P: –22%; 6/7 remission
Giannini et al. 1986 (20)	320 (20)	BP: mania (DSM-III); BPRS: clonidine control crossover	V ≥ clonidine
Hoschl and Kozeny 1989 (46)	240–480 (35)	BP (DSM-III); NL and Li controlled	V: –45%; Li + NL: –27%; Li: –39%: BPRS
Garza-Trevino et al. 1992 (20)	320 (28)	BP: mania (DSM-III-R); Li controlled	V: –44%; Li: –39%: Petersen
Janicak et al. 1998 (32)	480 (21)	BP: mania (DSM-III-R); P controlled	V: 3/17; P:1/15
Prophylaxis			
Case reports			

(continued)

Table 19–2. Verapamil treatment of mood disorders *(continued)*

Study (*N*)	Dose, mg/day (duration, days)	Diagnoses/ Design	Outcome
Gitlin and Weiss 1984 (1)	320	BP: AD-induced	Remission 1.3 years
Dubovsky et al. 1985 (1)	400	BP: AD-induced	Remission 2 years
Deicken 1990 (1)	320	BP	Remission 1 year twice; relapse on brief stoppage
Goodnick 1993 (2)	240	BP	Remission in pregnancy
Controlled studies			
Barton and Gitlin 1987 (4)	240–320	BP (RDC)	2/4 remission for 18 months
Giannini et al. 1987 (20)	320	BP (DSM-III); crossover	V > Li in 6-month study

Note. In the Outcome column, the minus-quantity percentages indicate the mean percentage reduction in rating scale scores of baseline pathology. ABA = on-off-on; AD = antidepressant; BP = bipolar disorder; SAD = schizoaffective disorder; BPRS = Brief Psychiatric Rating Scale; IMPS = Inpatient Multidimensional Psychiatric Scale; Li = lithium; MSRS = Manic-State Rating Scale; NL = neuroleptic; P = placebo; Petersen = Petersen Mania Scale; RC = rapid cycling; RDC = Research Diagnostic Criteria; V = verapamil; YMS = Young Mania Scale.

patients were 1.09 to 0.12, 2.55 to 1.74, and 2.34 to 1.63. Side effects noted included peripheral flushing, mild orthostasis, and gastrointestinal upset. Goodnick (1995) recently published reports on two patients with rapid-cycling bipolar disorder who had not been helped in treatment attempts with lithium, carbamazepine, valproate, verapamil, elevated thyroid, either singly or in combination, who responded to nimodipine as it was increased from a first-week dosage of 30 mg tid to a second-week dosage of 60 mg tid. In each case, at the end of 10–14 days, patients had achieved mood stability with resolution of abnormalities in energy, sleep, and so on. In 1996, another case report showed the benefit of combining administration of nimodipine with lithium in a patient with DSM-IV (American Psychiatric Association 1994) mania who previously had not responded to lithium or to lithium plus antipsychotics (Grunze et al. 1996). As nimodipine was increased in stages from 90 to 270 mg/day after 10 days, mania rating scores improved within 15 days from 16 to 3 (Bech-Rafaelson Mania Scale) and 49 to 20 (BPRS). This has most recently been followed by a further elaboration of a previous study (Pazzaglia et al. 1998). That report showed that 10 of 30 patients had a clinically substantial response with a Clinical Global Impression (CGI) Scale score of moderate or marked improvement. Substitution of verapamil for nimodipine in two bipolar patients produced recurrence of symptoms; reintroduction of nimodipine reestablished response.

Prophylaxis

Because of cost and labor requirements, there are many fewer reports concerning the use of CCBs for prophylaxis of bipolar disorder. There have been four case reports on the use of verapamil: Gitlin and Weiss (1984; 1), Dubovsky et al. (1985; 1), and Goodnick (1993; 2). Gitlin and Weiss published a case of a 32-year-old woman with a history of multiple antidepressant-induced manias despite lithium prophylaxis at 1.2 mEq/L. At a dosage of 80 mg tid, verapamil successfully treated hypomania and maintained mood stability for at least 1 year. Dubovsky et al. successfully treated phenelzine-induced hypomania with verapamil at 400 mg/day. After 2 weeks of verapamil, the reintroduction of phenelzine did not induce mood changes; when the patient was recrossed to placebo instead of verapamil, hypomania reemerged. It again resolved when verapamil was begun again; the patient stayed in remission thereafter on a combination of verapamil and phenelzine. Goodnick reported that the use of 240 mg controlled-release verapamil once a day prevented the reoccurrence of mania in two pregnant patients who had previously had mania in all pregnancies.

Deicken (1990) reported on the successful prophylaxis of bipolar depression with verapamil. In open trials, Barton and Gitlin (1987) reported that two of four patients taking 240–320 mg/day for 18 months showed mild prophylactic efficacy. In the same year, in 20 bipolar patients, Giannini et al. (1987) reported results of a dosage of 320 mg/day versus lithium at a serum level of 0.8–1.0 mEq/L in a 6-month crossover design. These researchers found that verapamil was superior to lithium in long-term prophylaxis and that after crossover, patients previously on lithium showed further stability on verapamil.

Again, there are even fewer reports with other CCBs. Flunarizine has been reported as effective prophylactically by Lindelius and Nilsson (1992). Their patient had a 20-year history of illness, with annual recurrences, and had intolerance to lithium-associated side effects. A dosage of 10 mg/day of flunarizine stopped repeat episodes for at least 3 years and produced no adverse side effects. One episode of depression after 3 years was successfully treated with electroconvulsive therapy with no complications. Regarding nimodipine, Manna (1991) found in a randomization study of prophylaxis of nimodipine alone, lithium alone, or nimodipine plus lithium that the combination was the most effective in reducing the number and duration of relapses into either mania or depression. Furthermore, Pazzaglia et al. (1993), as stated above, found that nimodipine at dosages of up to 720 mg/day was particularly effective in the treatment and prophylaxis of rapid- and ultrarapid-cycling bipolar disorder.

OTHER PSYCHIATRIC APPLICATIONS

Other neuropsychiatric application attempts have included substance intoxication, dementia, panic disorder, and schizophrenia. Case reports have shown possible efficacy in agitation with phencyclidine (PCP) intoxication and geriatric dementia (Dubovsky 1986; Hoschl 1991). In panic disorder, verapamil at 240 mg/day or diltiazem at 60 mg/day has been associated with a positive response in four of seven "treatment resistant" patients (Goldstein 1985; Pollack et al. 1987). In contrast, several double-blind studies have clearly concluded that verapamil is not effective in chronic schizophrenia (Grebb et al. 1986; Pickar et al. 1987).

PRACTICAL POINTS

Regarding possible side effects and drug interactions, several points need to be remembered. The most commonly reported side effects of verapamil include nausea, vertigo, headache, dry mouth, and constipation (Hoschl 1991). Nifedipine, as contrasted to verapamil, has an increased likelihood of producing hypotension and reflex tachycardia. Nimodipine is generally well tolerated; there are only a few reports of nimodipine-induced low blood pressure (Brunet et al. 1990). One case report has related toxic blood levels of verapamil to side effects of weakness, bradycardia, hypotension, and abdominal pain (Kaufman 1996).

Regarding drug interactions, verapamil administration has reportedly led to both lithium toxicity and decreased lithium levels (Hoschl 1991; Prien and Gelenberg 1989). Significant bradycardia has been reported with concomitant use of verapamil and lithium (Dubovsky et al. 1987). Neurotoxicity has been reported with the combined use of carbamazepine and verapamil, as well as of carbamazepine and diltiazem (Chou 1991). Diltiazem has been reported to increase serum digoxin levels (Pollack et al. 1987).

CONCLUSION

Despite the need for further investigation of alternatives to lithium in the treatment and prophylaxis of bipolar disorder, research has progressed slowly because of the relative lack of federal and private research support. Currently, it appears that the CCBs may act effectively by blocking release of neurotransmitter from neurons. In practical applications, reports appear to indicate that verapamil at dosages of 240–480 mg/day may be successful in the treatment of mania with few side effects and no need for blood level monitoring. Nimodipine may become of particular value in the treatment of rapid-cycling and ultrarapid-cycling bipolar disorder. Reports concerning other CCBs as well as reports on the prophylactic use of CCBs in mood disorders are too few to draw any conclusions, except that further investigation is warranted.

More research on these agents is indicated, with larger sample sizes to establish efficacy, particularly in double-blind studies. Unfortunately, funding for such studies has been slow in coming, whether from public or private sources (Dubovsky 1994). They may be particularly of value in patients who cannot tolerate side effects or will not comply with the blood level monitoring required in the other standard treatments: lithium, carbamazepine, and valproate. Furthermore, the CCBs may become the treatment of choice for bipolar disorder occurring or at risk of occurring during pregnancy, with reduced teratogenic risk. At this point, given the limited knowledge of CCBs, it is reasonable to reserve them for use in patients who are lithium- or anticonvulsant-refractory or -intolerant.

REFERENCES

Aldenhoff JB, Schlegel S, Hauser I, et al: Antimanic effects of the calcium-antagonist D-600: a double-blind placebo controlled study. Clin Neuropharmacol 9:553–555, 1986

American Psychiatric Association: Diagnostic and Statistical Manual of Mental Disorders, 3rd Edition. Washington, DC, American Psychiatric Association, 1980

American Psychiatric Association: Diagnostic and Statistical Manual of Mental Disorders, 3rd Edition, Revised. Washington, DC, American Psychiatric Association, 1987

American Psychiatric Association: Diagnostic and Statistical Manual of Mental Disorders, 4th Edition. Washington, DC, American Psychiatric Association, 1994

Barton BM, Gitlin MJ: Verapamil in treatment mania: an open trial. J Clin Psychopharmacol 7:101–103, 1987

Bhugra P, Gulati OD: Interaction of calcium channel blockers with different agonists in aorta from normal and diseased rats. Indian J Physiol Pharmacol 40:109–119, 1996

Brotman AW, Farhadi AM, Gelenberg AJ: Verapamil treatment of acute mania. J Clin Psychiatry 47:136–138, 1986

Brunet G, Cerlich B, Robert P, et al: Open trial of a calcium antagonist, nimodipine, in acute mania. Clin Neuropharmacol 13(3):224–228, 1990

Caillard V: Treatment of mania using a calcium antagonist: preliminary trial. Neuropsychology 14:23–26, 1985

Carman JS, Wyatt RJ: Calcium: bivalent cation in the bivalent psychoses. Biol Psychiatry 14:295–336, 1979

Chou JC: Recent advances in treatment of acute mania. J Clin Psychopharmacol 11(1):3–21, 1991

DeFalco FA, Bartiromo U, Majello L, et al: Calcium antagonist nimodipine in intractable epilepsy. Epilepsia 33:343–345, 1992

Deicken RF: Verapamil treatment of bipolar depression. J Clin Psychopharmacol 10:148–149, 1990

Dinan TG, Silverstone T, Cookson JC: Cortisol, prolactin, and growth hormone levels with clinical ratings in manic patients treated with verapamil. Int Clin Psychopharmacol 3:151–156, 1988

Doran AR, Norang PK, Meigs CY, et al: Verapamil concentrations in the cerebrospinal fluid after oral administration. N Engl J Med 312:1261–1262, 1985

Dose M, Emrich HM, Cording-Tommel C, et al: Use of calcium antagonists in mania. Psychoneuroendocrinology (Oxford) 11:241–243, 1986

Dubovsky SL: Calcium antagonists: a new class of psychiatric drugs? Psychiatric Annals 16:724–728, 1986

Dubovsky SL: Why don't we hear more about the calcium antagonists? Biol Psychiatry 35:149–150, 1994

Dubovsky SL, Franks RD: Intracellular calcium ions in affective disorders: a review and an hypothesis. Biol Psychiatry 18:781–797, 1983

Dubovsky SL, Franks RD, Lifschitz M, et al: Effectiveness of verapamil in the treatment of a manic patient. Am J Psychiatry 139:502–504, 1982

Dubovsky SL, Franks RD, Schrier D: Phenelzine-induced hypomania: effects of verapamil. Biol Psychiatry 20:1009–1014, 1985

Dubovsky SL, Franks RD, Allen S, et al: Calcium antagonists in mania: a double blind study of verapamil. Psychiatry Res 18:309–320, 1986

Dubovsky SL, Franks RD, Allen S: Verapamil: a new antimanic drug with potential interactions with lithium. J Clin Psychiatry 48:371–372, 1987

Dubovsky SL, Murphy DL, Christiano J, et al: The calcium second messenger in bipolar disorders: data supporting new research directions. J Neuropsychiatry 4:3–14, 1992

Fabian J: Diltiazem, a calcium antagonist, partly attenuates the effects of dextroamphetamine in healthy volunteers. Int Clin Psychopharmacol 12:113–120, 1997

Garza-Trevino ES, Overall JE, Hollister LE. Verapamil versus lithium in acute mania. Am J Psychiatry 149:121–122, 1992

Gerner RH, Post RM, Spiegel AM, et al: Effects of parathormone and lithium treatment on calcium and mood in depressed patients. Biol Psychiatry 12:145–151, 1977

Giannini AJ, Houser WL, Loiselle RH, et al: Antimanic effects of verapamil. Am J Psychiatry 141:1602–1603, 1984

Giannini AJ, Loiselle RH, Price WA, et al: Comparison of antimanic efficacy of clonidine and verapamil. J Clin Pharmacol 25:307–308, 1986

Giannini AJ, Tarasz R, Loiselle RH, et al: Verapamil and lithium in the maintenance therapy of manic patients. J Clin Pharmacol 27:980–982, 1987

Gitlin MJ, Weiss J: Verapamil as maintenance treatment in bipolar illness: a case report. J Clin Psychopharmacol 4:341–343, 1984

Goldstein JA: Calcium channel blockers in the treatment of panic disorder (letter). J Clin Psychiatry 46:546, 1985

Goodnick PJ: Verapamil prophylaxis in pregnant women with bipolar disorder (letter). Am J Psychiatry 150:1560, 1993

Goodnick PJ: Nimodipine treatment of rapid-cycling bipolar disorder. J Clin Psychiatry 56:330, 1995

Goodnick PJ: Verapamil response in mania and changes in plasma calcium and magnesium. South Med J 89:225–226, 1996

Grebb JA, Shellon RC, Tayer ER, et al: A negative, double-blind, placebo-controlled clinical trial of verapamil in chronic schizophrenia. Biol Psychiatry 21:691–694, 1986

Grunze H, Walden J, Wolf R, et al: Combined treatment with lithium and nimodipine in a bipolar I manic syndrome. Prog Neuropsychopharmacol Biol Psychiatry 20:419–426, 1996

Hargreaves AC, Gunthorpe MJ, Taylor CW, et al: Direct inhibition of 5-hydroxytryptamine 3 receptors by antagonists of l-type Ca +2 channels. Mol Pharmacol 50:1284–1294, 1997

Helmuth D, Ljaljevic Z, Ramirez L, et al: Choreoathetosis induced by verapamil and lithium treatment. J Clin Psychopharmacol 9:454–455, 1989

Himmelhoch JM, Garfinkel ME: Sources of lithium resistance in mixed mania. Psychopharmacol Bull 22:613–620, 1986

Hoschl C: Do calcium antagonists have a place in the treatment of mood disorders? Drugs 42:721–729, 1991

Hoschl C, Kozeny J: Verapamil in affective disorders: a controlled, double-blind study. Biol Psychiatry 25:128–140, 1989

Hoschl C, Blahos J, Kabes J: The use of calcium channel blockers in psychiatry, in Biological Psychiatry 1985. Edited by Shagass CE, Josiassen RC, Bridger WH, et al. New York, Elsevier, 1986, pp 330–332

Jalonen TO, Margraf RR, Wielt DB, et al: Serotonin induces inward potassium and calcium currents in rat cortical astrocytes. Brain Res 758:69–82, 1997

Janicak PG, Sharma RP, Pandey G, et al: Verapamil for the treatment of acute mania: a double-blind, placebo-controlled trial. Am J Psychiatry 155:972–973, 1998

Jacobsen FM, Sack DA, James SP: Delirium-induced hypomania: effect of verapamil. Biol Psychiatry 20:1009–1014, 1987

Jensen PN, Smith DF, Poulsen JH, et al: Effect of flunarizine and calcium on serotonin uptake in human and rat blood platelets and rat synaptosomes. Biol Psychiatry 36:118–123, 1994

Johnson FN, Birch NJ, Carstens M, et al: Mechanisms of lithium action. Reviews of Contemporary Pharmacotherapy 4:287–318, 1993

Kaufman K: Irish Journal of Psychological Medicine 13:100–101, 1996

Kennedy S, Ozersky S, Robillard M: Refractory bipolar illness may not respond to verapamil. J Clin Psychopharmacol 6:316–317, 1986

Kozlovskii VL, Prakhe IV, Kenunen OG: The influence of calcium channel blockers on effects of haloperidol and phenamine in mice and rats. Eksp Klin Farmakol 59:12–15, 1996

Langley MS, Sorkin EM: Nimodipine: a review of its pharmacodynamic and pharmacokinetic properties, and therapeutic potential in cerebrovascular disease. Drugs 37:669–699, 1989

Lenzi A, Marazziti D, Raffaelli S, et al: Effectiveness of the combination verapamil and chlorpromazine in the treatment of severe manic or mixed patients. Prog Neuropsychopharmacol Biol Psychiatry 19:519–528, 1995

Lindelius R, Nilsson CG: Flunarizine as maintenance treatment of a patient with bipolar disorder (letter). Am J Psychiatry 149:139, 1992

Linder J, Levin K, Saaf J, et al: Influence of lithium treatment on calcium and magnesium in plasma and erythrocytes. Lithium 4:115–123, 1993

Manna V: Disturbi affettivi bipolari e ruolo del calcio interneuronale: effetti terapeutici del trattamento con sali di litio e/o calcio antagonista in pazienti con rapida inversione di polarita [Bipolar affective disorders and role of intraneuronal calcium: therapeutic effects of the treatment with lithium salts and/or calcium antagonist in patients with rapid polar inversion]. Minerva Med 82:757–763, 1991

Mathis P, Schmitt L, Moron P: Efficacite du verapamil dans les acces maniaques. Encephale 14:127–132, 1988

Mennini T, Govvi M, Crespi D, et al: In vivo and in vitro interaction of flunarizine with d-fenfluramine serotonergic effects. Pharmacol Biochem Behav 53:155–161, 1996

Patten S, Thompson J: Organic depression associated with flunarizine. Can J Psychiatry 40:111–112, 1995

Patterson JF: Treatment of acute mania with verapamil. J Clin Psychopharmacol 7:206–207, 1987

Pazzaglia PJ, Post RM, Ketter TA, et al: Preliminary controlled trial of nimodipine in ultra-rapid cycling affective dysregulation. Psychiatry Res 49:257–272, 1993

Pazzaglia PJ, Post RM, Ketter TA, et al: Nimodipine monotherapy and carbamazepine augmentation in patients with refractory recurrent affective illness. J Clin Psychopharmacol 18:404–413, 1998

Physicians' Desk Reference, 48th edition. Montvale, NJ: Medical Economics, 1994

Pickar D, Wolfkowitz OM, Doran AR, et al: Clinical and biochemical effects of verapamil administration in schizophrenic patients. Arch Gen Psychiatry 44:113–118, 1987

Pollack MH, Rosenbaum JF, Hyman SE: Calcium channel blockers in psychiatry. Psychosomatics 28(7):356–369, 1987

Prien RF, Gelenberg AJ: Alternatives to lithium for preventative treatment of bipolar disorder. Am J Psychiatry 46:840–848, 1989

Reynolds JEF (ed): Martindale: The Extra Pharmacopoeia. London, Pharmaceutical Press, 1993

Solomon L, Williamson P: Verapamil in bipolar illness. Can J Psychiatry 31:442–444, 1986

Semkina GA, Masievskii DD, Mirzoian RS: Nimodipine, nifedipine, and cerebrovascular effects of serotonin. Eksp Klin Farmakol 59:13–16, 1996

Viveros MP, Martin S, Ormazabal MJ, et al: Effects of nimodipine and nifedipine upon behavior and regional brain monoamines in the rat. Psychopharmacology (Berl) 127:123–132, 1996

Walton SA, Berk M, Brook S: Superiority of lithium over verapamil in mania: a randomized, controlled, single-blind trial. J Clin Psychiatry 57:543–546, 1996

Wehr TA, Sack BA, Rosenthal NE, et al: Rapid cycling affective disorder: contributing factors and treatment responses in 51 patients. Am J Psychiatry 145:179–184, 1988

Wood K: The neurochemistry of mania: the effect of lithium on catecholamines, indoleamines, and calcium mobilization. J Affect Disord 8:215–223, 1985

INDEX

*Page numbers printed in **boldface** type refer to tables or figures.*

A

B

C

D

G

H

T

U

V